>> THIRD EDITION >>>>>>>

Developing Occupation-Centered Programs With the Community

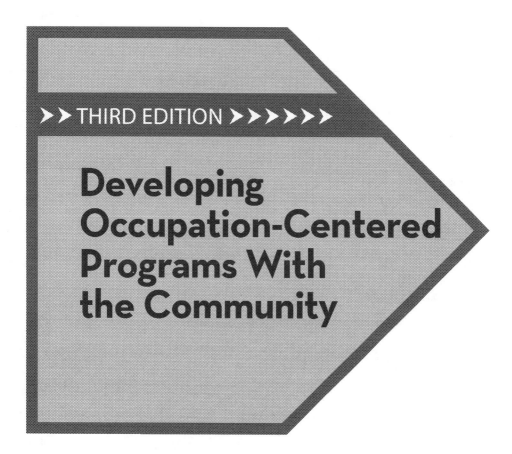

>> THIRD EDITION >>>>>>

Developing Occupation-Centered Programs With the Community

Linda S. Fazio, PhD, OTR/L, LPC, FAOTA

Professor of Clinical Occupational Therapy
Associate Chair of Academic and Community Program Support and Development
Mrs. T.H. Chan Division of Occupational Science and Occupational Therapy
University of Southern California
Los Angeles, California

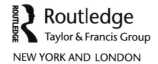

Routledge
Taylor & Francis Group

NEW YORK AND LONDON

Developing Occupation-Centered Programs With the Community, Third Edition includes ancillary materials specifically available for faculty use. Included are PowerPoint Slides. Please visit www.routledge.com/9781630912598 to obtain access.

First published 2017 by SLACK Incorporated

Published 2024 by Routledge
605 Third Avenue, New York, NY 10158

and by Routledge
4 Park Square, Milton Park, Abingdon, Oxon OX14 4RN

Routledge is an imprint of the Taylor & Francis Group, an informa business

Library of Congress Cataloging-in-Publication Data

Names: Fazio, Linda S., author.
Title: Developing occupation-centered programs with the community / Linda S.
  Fazio.
Other titles: Developing occupation-centered programs for the community
Description: Third edition. | Thorofare, NJ : Slack Incorporated, [2017] |
  Preceded by Developing occupation-centered programs for the community /
  Linda S. Fazio. 2nd ed. c2008. | Includes bibliographical references and
  index.
Identifiers: LCCN 2017001851 (print) | ISBN
  9781630912598 (paperback : alk. paper)
Subjects: | MESH: Occupational Therapy--organization & administration |
  Community Health Services--organization & administration | Program
  Development--methods | Community Health Planning
Classification: LCC RC487 (print) | NLM WB 555 | DDC
  362.2/2--dc23
LC record available at https://lccn.loc.gov/2017001851

ISBN: 9781630912598 (pbk)
ISBN: 9781003523802 (ebk)

DOI: 10.4324/9781003523802

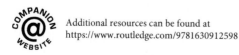

Additional resources can be found at
https://www.routledge.com/9781630912598

Dedication

To my daughters, April and Holly, who are always at the center of my community, sharing in many of my occupations, and untiring in their contributions to the meaning in my life.

CONTENTS

Developing Occupation-Centered Programs With the Community, Third Edition includes ancillary materials specifically available for faculty use. Included are PowerPoint Slides. Please visit www.routledge.com/9781630912598 to obtain access.

ACKNOWLEDGMENTS

I have been privileged to enjoy the company of students for most of my professional life, more than 40 years. This ever-changing community of students has challenged me to expand my knowledge and creativity, and to find solutions to problems I didn't know existed. As many have said, *to be a teacher is to be a student.*

Students have taught me not only to think "outside of the box," but to create so many "new boxes" that we've built veritable villages of ideas when it comes to the creation of community programs. Students are explorers and often "just do" and, in the process, they create amazing things.

Thank you all for letting me tag along on the journeys!

About the Author

Linda S. Fazio, PhD, OTR/L, LPC, FAOTA was born and lived her early life on a wheat and dairy farm in Southeast Kansas, where she attended a one-room school as the only student in her grade for 8 years. From there, she went to a small rural high school, and then received a scholarship to Ottawa University, Ottawa, Kansas, to study poetry and art, then to the University of Kansas in Lawrence, Kansas as an art and craft major. Her path then led to occupational therapy.

She received her Bachelor's Degree in Occupational Therapy, Psychology and Sociology in 1964 from Texas Woman's University in Denton, Texas. Her first employment was with the Veteran's Administration Medical Center in Northampton, Massachusetts, as a psychiatric staff occupational therapist. It was here that she started her first community-based program with a pottery production workshop for outpatient veterans. Following her marriage to then–psychology doctoral student Anthony Fazio, her work moved to the Boston, Jamaica Plain, Veterans Administration Medical Center.

When her husband accepted a faculty position at the University of Wisconsin-Milwaukee, Dr. Fazio began employment at Curative Workshops in Milwaukee as a home rehabilitation therapist. At this time, she began graduate studies toward an MFA in fiber arts and began teaching weaving and fiber art for the Shorewood Opportunity School in Milwaukee. About this time, she realized that her interests were swinging toward historical textile production and she entered graduate studies in anthropology, where she received her MS degree in Anthropology with a specialty in Museology/Textile Conservation in 1977. Her work as an occupational therapist moved to St. Michael's Hospital, Milwaukee, as a psychiatric therapist, and Coordinator of Volunteers which gave her more flexibility as she raised her two daughters and attended graduate studies.

In 1977, she moved back to Texas Woman's University as an Instructor in Occupational Therapy and began doctoral studies in Counseling, Higher Education/Medical Education, and Administration. She received her Licensed Professional Counselor (LPC) license and began a part-time practice in counseling and occupational therapy with a group of Psychology Associates. She received her PhD from the University of North Texas in Denton in 1985. The following year, she completed Post-Doctoral study in Sexuality and Disability at the Texas Institute of Rehabilitation and Research in Houston; at this time, she was an Associate Professor of Occupational Therapy at Texas Woman's University and Assistant Dean.

In 1987, she came to the University of Southern California in Los Angeles and began to teach and develop a course in community program development that has continued to the present. Her roles at USC have been full-time teaching and administration. She has held the administrative roles of Academic Fieldwork Coordinator, Coordinator of the Professional and Undergraduate Programs, Assistant Chair, Director of Post-Professional and International Students, and, most recently, Associate Chair of Academic and Community Program Support and Development.

Dr. Fazio has previously published the first and second editions of *Developing Occupation-Centered Programs for the Community* and has co-edited two editions of *Play in Occupational Therapy With Children* with Dr. Diane Parham. She has also authored numerous chapters and articles. She has consulted widely in occupational therapy and occupational therapy assistant program design and curriculum development and has initiated many new academic programs over the course of her career. She has been a continuous member of the American Occupational Therapy Association volunteer sector since 1978, serving as an Accreditation Evaluator, Chair of the Commission on Education, and member of various appointed and elected committees. She has received 43 service awards from the American Occupational Therapy Association.

PREFACE

Since the *Second Edition* of *Developing Occupation-Centered Programs for the Community* was published in 2008, there have been some important changes in the direction of community programming and in the roles and responsibilities of programmers. In 2008, we were beginning to talk about sustainability, but the word was not mentioned in the text. We were saying a little about the strengths of our participants, but we were not recognizing our formal roles as incorporating asset finding and building capacity in our populations. We were still primarily interested in identifying and "fixing" needs. Today, we are still interested in recognizing needs and in helping to solve them, but more and more, these responsibilities are met by the community, with our expertise and assistance. Thus, there is a small but significant title change in this edition from *Developing Occupation-Centered Programs for the Community* to *Developing Occupation-Centered Programs With the Community*.

This book has always been written to support and assist those who "care," and those who care enough to do something. Over the course of the past several years, likely decades, people of the world have become more disengaged, helpless, and despondent. Our planet is under attack by complacency. Generations are losing hope that anyone cares about a greater good, let alone work to bring it about. Yet, when we hear that someone has done this, we are encouraged; we may even shed tears in our recognition that someone has cared enough to promote a change toward the better.

It is my intention to offer you a set of tools to recognize the need for help, and to do something about it—not the tools just to "fix" people's problems, but to help them acknowledge their problems and create their own solutions. In the words of Peter Block (2009), these tools can help us "to shift our conversations from the problems of community to the possibility of community" (p. 177).

When I was a graduate student in anthropology at the University of Wisconsin-Milwaukee, I was fortunate to hear anthropologist Margaret Mead speak these words:

> *Never doubt that a small group of thoughtful committed citizens can change the world.*
> *Indeed, it's the only thing that ever has.*
> —Lecture, University of Wisconsin-Milwaukee (1973)

I was so intrigued by her words that I have kept them with me since that day, and I am reminded of them often. I published them in the preface of the *First Edition*, and again in the *Second*, and they are here for you to read today…still very true, and still relevant. As I continued to practice as an occupational therapist while reading and studying in various disciplines, I became more and more convinced that an orientation to occupation was a way to bring about change in a community, and to "right" the "wrongs." Occupational engagement provided a language that everyone could understand. I have shared this belief with students for some time and have, with their help, devised ways to bridge their admission into community practice utilizing occupation.

Today, we have new research, and new language to better help us as we translate our programs into helping models that will encourage our communities to recognize and build their own resources and assets toward sustainable communities who are optimistic and hopeful.

The glue that holds the world together is community—in place, in spirit, and in meaning—working (with) our populations for a better future that we will all share.

Reference

Block, P. (2009). *The art of community: Building the new age of participation.* San Francisco ,CA: Berrett-Koehler.

Linda S. Fazio, PhD, OTR/L, LPC, FAOTA

INTRODUCTION

As in the first two editions, this *Third Edition* will provide a basic "workbook" guide to the design and development of community programming that celebrates engagement in meaningful occupation by the participants. There are assumptions made in the content offerings that students are enrolled in, or have completed, entry-level occupational therapy education. This education will have included the study of occupation, occupational therapy history, and foundations of occupational therapy practice in disability/illness and in health and wellness, and it will have had some introduction to health services administration.

Occupational therapy education has evolved since the first and second editions of this text, and this *Third Edition*, as those previously, is written to appeal to various levels of practice entry. It can be used in a structured classroom setting that may include lecture, discussion, and completion of exercises that are included in the chapters, along with PowerPoint slides that are available to instructors. Following the organization of the text and completing the exercises along the way will lead the student or student group to the completion of a proposal for the further development of a program. This proposal can be presented in the form of a "poster" for others to view, such as is done in regional and national professional meetings. This offers the student or student group an opportunity to make a professional presentation and often to explain to non-occupational therapy students what they are proposing to do. The text can also be utilized as a handbook should the experiential portion of the work be carried out in an off-site service learning, fieldwork, or internship model with visits from a preceptor or perhaps returning to campus for seminars. Academic programs are structured differently, so instructors will know how best to offer these opportunities to students.

During the writing of this edition, the author has consulted with several developing occupational therapy doctoral programs (OTD) and has been influenced to broaden and adapt the text for the design of OTD residencies for programs who wish their graduates to have expertise in program design and development.

In response to therapists who have practiced in what may be considered more conventional/traditional ways and now wish to expand their venues and challenge themselves in service to perhaps a larger, and more varied community, the book content and references may be used to stimulate their thinking and to teach the steps to follow toward the realization of their plans and dreams.

Part I of the text is designed to prepare the reader to appreciate the many meanings of community and what it means to practice occupation in the community. Following completion of Part I, the reader will have a better sense of his or her preparedness for community programming work and will have a beginning grasp of what he or she wishes to do.

Part II traces the process of designing and planning a community program, and it does so in small increments, one chapter at a time. It is in Part II that the profiles are researched and developed; needs, assets, and capacity are investigated toward the realization of programming that is sustainable. The phase of planning that includes selection of organizing theories, and the identification of goals, objectives, impact, and outcome is completed.

Part III deals with important practical decisions from determining your staff, space, equipment, and supplies and what they will cost to funding your program. The final chapter in Part III provides direction toward successful ways to market your programming.

Part IV describes the layers of evaluation that are critical in helping you build and sustain your program.

Part V is a compilation of "stories" highlighting the needs and assets of different populations; each chapter emphasizes one or more aspects of the program design and development process. Chapters in this section of the text are referred to in earlier chapters to illustrate particular points and concepts.

Part VI has been developed to provide you with some programming ideas for, in some cases, populations in need that are emerging; in other cases, populations and programming may have been represented in our interests, and work of previous eras but for various reasons appear to have been forgotten, such as programming utilizing the arts. Several of these communities of need are well-suited to occupation-centered practice and there is some programming being done, but very little by occupation-centered practitioners. It is hoped that you will add to these chapters through your selection of innovative and thoughtful programming. These "stories in the making" are invitations to you.

Linda S. Fazio, PhD, OTR/L, LPC, FAOTA

I

Building a Foundation

1

Understanding Community

LEARNING OBJECTIVES

1. To appreciate the many definitions and meanings associated with the concept of *community*

2. To understand the distinction between *community* and *the community*

3. To understand *community* as an organizing theme in our development of occupation-centered programs

4. To appreciate the potential role of occupation-centered practitioners as community change agents and builders of capacity and consensus

KEY TERMS

1. Locale
2. Community
3. Social capital
4. Reciprocity
5. Cultural shifting
6. Change agent
7. Builders of consensus, capacity, and assets
8. Gatekeepers/key informants
9. Chaos theory/change curve

Fazio, L. S. *Developing Occupation-Centered Programs With the Community, Third Edition* (pp 3-19).
© 2017 Taylor & Francis Group.

What Is Community?

Hacker (2013) suggests that one of our first challenges is likely to lie in defining community and our "community of interest." What are they? Do they have boundaries? If they do, are these boundaries geographic (a city, a neighborhood, or something broader than these), or is there no geographical boundary but rather a common culture, ethnicity, grouping, or condition (e.g., parents of children on the autism spectrum) or perhaps a shared concern (access to public transportation)? The truth of it is that people have been trying to define *community* and to carve out roles within it for a very long time.

EARLY FOUNDATIONAL WORK

Community, with its accompanying definitions and scope of investigation, has long been a central theme in the study of sociology. In fact, most of the earlier theoretical work was done by sociologists. When we review the sociological literature, we find that this discipline has established a number of definitions for the term *community*: Lyon (1987) noted some 94 in the sociological literature of 1955 (p. 5). Although he noted many definitions in his review of the literature at the time, he was able to establish three common characteristics: locale, or geographic area; common ties; and social interactions. Other sociological researchers, including Park (1936) and Bernard (1973), concurred with these common characteristics. In general, though, the use of **locale,** or reference to place, as a central definition and descriptor for community has been widely accepted across disciplines.

Anthropology, sociology, public health, and psychology have all looked at communities slightly differently. Cultural anthropology tends to take an ethnographic perspective of community, examining the structure, norms, and social beliefs that bring people together (Mckeown, Rubinstein, & Kelly, 1987).

Sociology builds on concepts of social capital (Lee & Newby, 1983). Public health identifies the social and political responsibility of community and sees the community as a population. Psychology introduces shared emotional connections and the feeling of a "sense of community" (McMillan & Chavis, 1986; Sarason, 1974).

Anthropologists have long shared an interest in community, particularly as defined by locale. Although Hillery (1955) supported the view that locale is a central characteristic of community, he proposed that groups of people differing in terms of place and time may also differ in their interpretations of meaning surrounding locale. He distinguished between community and *the* community. His distinction separated the idea of common ties and social interactions from locale. In his view, community is the most powerful of the two concepts, emphasizing moral commitment, social cohesion, and continuity in time, or what might be described by the German term *Gemeinschaft*. In his examples, which are based on modes of subsistence, agricultural peoples attach a fixed settlement to their meaning of locale, whereas hunters/gatherers who subsist by traveling over large geographic areas define *locale* as a less identifiable place. It is likely that even hunters/gatherers along with nomadic groups who also travel over wide areas designate locales and attach significance to them (i.e., sources of water, ceremonial/burial sites, and so on). These locales may be designated sites where nomadic bands or groups join together to form communities, albeit with a looser definition of community than that of an agricultural group that stays in one place. Those who have studied the transitions from hunter/gatherer to agriculturist have noted that when groups begin to first tend plants and then grow them, they become locked to a site or locale (Childe, 1953; Heiser, 1973). Perhaps these groups then become locked to a broader concept of community as well.

Also discussing community from an anthropological perspective, Moore (1996) reminded us that in biology, *community* refers to a breeding population. His discussions centered around bands as the elemental human communities of hunters and gatherers (p. 105). As biological creatures, humans also have breeding population communities, but community means a good deal more to humans than a group with which one may breed. According to Moore, community is "the unit that orchestrates individual movements in space over time," and in our cultural world, "community is the setting in which, from one generation to the next, human beings learn how to be fully human" (p. 96). In fact, this community unit is also where cultural creativity and innovation take place.

McKnight (1988) emphasized a common goal as the motivating reason people come together. For him, community was a collective association driven toward a common theme or goal. Green and Kreuter (1991) focused on common values and mutual concern for "their" group (pp. 504-505). Additionally, Nisbet (1972) emphasized that community thrives on self-help and equal consent. He suggested that people come together to do something that cannot be done in isolation. These are all important points for those of us who wish to encourage change in the individual, the group, and the larger community as well.

In 1995, Ray used community as a metaphor for what he described as a worldwide paradigm shift. In his analysis, the world is in crisis, offering both danger and opportunity. He saw community building as the only viable way to maintain society as the world is transformed (p. 18). Jarman and Land (1995) suggest that most would describe the best of all possible worlds, thus "to live among people without fear, where trust is given and received freely, a place of belonging, where a sense of connectedness and unity provides the foundation for life-sustaining and enhancing interactions" (p. 22). The underlying ideal is that everyone in the community is accepted and treated as a valuable, integral member. An ideal, yes, but to be achieved in its entirety is not too likely; however, can we aspire to create such microcosms in our programming? I would suggest that we can. In the preface to this text, Margaret Mead is quoted as having said, "Never doubt that a small group of thoughtful committed citizens can change the world. Indeed, it's the only thing that ever has" (Mead, 1973). To sum it up nicely, MacQueen and colleagues (2001) conducted a series of interviews in an attempt to determine what *community* meant and proposed a combined, common definition: "A group of people with diverse characteristics who are linked by social ties, share common perspectives, and engage in joint action in geographical locations or settings" (pp. 1932-1934).

Exercise 1-1

We have introduced several terms and ideas to advance our understanding of how and why people come together to form communities. Locale, common ties, and social interaction are three. Make some notes and discuss with others how these terms may be translated into your own motivation for joining a particular community. Maintaining contact with your family, organizations you joined as a child or adolescent, and your college "community" may be starting points.

_____

_____

_____

_____

_____

WHAT DOES COMMUNITY MEAN TODAY?

Contemporary Definitions and Concepts

Many people are writing about and referring to "community" these days. It is a word that continues to be used widely in the professional and research literature as well as in newspapers and magazine articles, brochures, and flyers (Martin, 2015). People are continuing to define and redefine the word. Bacon (2009), writing about what he describes as "the art" of community, proposes the following definition: "A community is a collection of people who interact together in the same environment" (p. 4). His interest in collective groupings is not necessarily new, but he proposes that it offers the stimulus for an emphasis on the interactions that occur within groupings. These interactions offer opportunities for new definitions of participation and a renewed faith in a sense of belonging that can be mobilized to "build communities," and others agree (Bacon, 2009; Block, 2009; Green & Haines, 2016).

Block (2009) emphasizes the experience of belonging (to a community). For him, it means to be part of something—a membership—and with that membership comes accountability; it is because of this accountability that transformation and change can occur. For Block, it is about community building, and this is to increase the amount of belonging or relatedness that exists in the world (2009, p. xii). Block is interested in promoting "healthy" communities where people are interdependent. Members are investors, owners, and creators (Block, 2009, p. 3). Belonging to a community would then prompt conversations regarding such matters as our relatedness and willingness to provide hospitality and generosity—two elements to be nurtured as we create, strengthen, and restore communities.

Green and Haines (2016) are also interested in developing and building community. They suggest that a fundamental tenet of community development is to help people belonging to communities learn to help themselves (p. 8). This is referred to as *capacity building*. The agenda is to help people become change agents rather than simply the objects of changes that may be orchestrated around them. Capacity building involves these key components: (1) a sense of community, (2) a level of commitment, (3) the ability to solve problems, and (4) access to resources (Green & Haines, 2016 pp. 8-9). We see in these components of capacity building many potential routes for occupation-centered practitioners; perhaps most obvious to us is the assistance we can offer in identifying and analyzing problems and in facilitating the skills and knowledge to solve them.

Hacker (2013), in her discussions of community-based participatory research, cautions us that the lack of an accepted definition of community can lead different collaborators to form contradictory or incompatible assumptions about community and, in so doing, preventing the achievement of their objectives. In Hacker's work, these comprise public health agendas (p. 23). Hacker recommends that our first challenge should be to define the community of interest. We would ask ourselves, "What is this population of interest? What are the boundaries of this community? Is the community geographically bounded (e.g., a city, a neighborhood, a county) or is it defined by a common culture (e.g., race/ethnicity, etc.) or condition (e.g., older adults who are without access to public transit and do not drive), or another concern?" It is "condition" that is often the first community of interest for occupation-centered practitioners. We will return to these concerns and focus specifically on these questions as well as your own definition of "your" community in Chapters 7 and 8.

All of these definitions and discussions shed light on our understanding of the present-day metropolitan and urban communities in which we want to encourage programs. Many people today often relocate in the course of their lives; most reside far from their communities (locales) of origin. It is likely that more transient attachments may be formed for those who move from one locale to another in pursuit of career and economic opportunity, and a sense of community with accompanying commitments and responsibilities may be more tenuous. Of course, any privileges or rights attached to community might also be forfeited—at least those that are offered following a period of investment or tenure. This view of community would appear to place more responsibility for the attributes and privileges of community, as described by Moore (1996), on the family and/or the individual.

Exercise 1-2

We might ask ourselves, "Do these individuals and families have the information and skills to establish communities for themselves? Is this an area we might wish to consider as we develop programming?" Consider some of the earlier discussion highlighting historical elements associated with community. Can you think of individuals or groups that appear to be without connection to a community or who are in danger of losing that connection? Note and discuss the information and skills you might offer those who appear to be isolated from your understanding of community:

_____

_____

_____

_____

_____

Metropolitan communities, where many cultures come together, may also redefine our interpretation of community. Consider these questions in your discussion with others. Will these communities provide stress and disengagement, or will they offer us new definitions of cultural creativity and innovation?

_____

_____

_____

_____

_____

Will we evolve new ways of learning to be "human"? If so, will occupation-centered practitioners have a role in facilitating this new learning? What might be some examples?

_____

_____

_____

_____

_____

How will we identify what kinds of services a community might need, want, and value? It is likely that desired services may vary considerably from one locale to another and from one constituency to another. Cognizant of this potential dilemma, Warren (1987) proposed that we must understand and appreciate that community, particularly the urban community, which represents a "local web of relationships around the locality-relevant functions" (p. ii). In his interpretation, various formal and informal networks within a community are connected to others outside of the locality. When one seeks to establish a program within a community, it will be necessary to appreciate and understand what likely will be an intricate and complex series of relationships "between" communities. Even if we are planning a program that appears fairly isolated in locale or in conceptualization, we must consider extended and overlapping communities and systems, particularly in the present era of heightened communication and access to information. Most members of established and forming communities in the United States have at least one or more computers in their households. What may have been once potentially isolated individuals and families now have access to the virtual community, its resources, and its potential liabilities. Parsons (1951) reminded us that, even within a community, substantial complexity may be displayed by the interplay between cultures and the varied levels of society. In fact, by introducing a program within a community, we are introducing yet another layer of complexity that may cause temporary shifts in balance. However, these potential shifts can be tempered by establishing the program in developmental increments, as we describe in this text.

The foregoing information is important for us to know as we are helping our service populations to design relevant and meaningful programs. As you begin to develop your community profile in Chapter 7, you will want to consider the following questions:

1. What can we learn about the community itself?

2. Is the community one that appears well established or is it one that is in process?

3. What is the nature of common ties, and what are the patterns of social interaction?

4. What is the configuration of "families"? Are children present? Older adults?

Do we know how the presence of children and older adults affects our understanding of community? Are the interactions, communications, and expectations influenced by their presence? These are provocative questions to be investigated, and they may influence and affect our understanding of so-called specialized communities: those serving older adults; young, childless adults; and institutions serving specific populations representing various needs.

Locale, Unity, Technology, and the Future

As we have seen, a community may be represented by no fixed locale at all, yet Nisbet (1967) suggests that such communities may offer a strong sense of unity. This may be a significant point of understanding in what we have described as the transient world of today. Nisbet's interpretation of community may help us to understand such questions as how and why retirees who move from their long-established homes to high-rise senior residences can either feel that they are part of a community or that they are not, as well as why many elders prefer to "age in place"—to remain in the homes and communities to which they have become accustomed and that they "belong to." Nisbet's interpretation can further help us as care providers to encourage the building of community for those who feel excluded.

Shifting paradigms responsive to the fluidity of attachment to locale by present-day populations heavily invested in technology may, in fact, define a new, more global sense of community. There are very few persons in the world today who are not aware of the virtual community created by the Internet; many avail themselves of the information and connections it provides as a component of their daily round of occupational engagement. In 1993, Rheingold provided an account of living in a virtual community in *Virtual Community: Homesteading on the Electronic Frontier*. Today, virtual communites have become commonplace (Bacon, 2009). With the ever-present Internet and social networking, communities cross geographic boundaries as well as the bounds of age, gender, and race/ethnicity. Often we communicate but are invisible to one another. As all of these tools become available to more people, we will have to continuously rethink our definitions of *community*. In 1990, Wellman and Wortley argued that community locus/physical geography is less important than personal networks. In fact, in our evolving world today, this seems to be the case.

Although the advantages of a global community may be appreciated by many, others see it as a threat to the very essence of communities. Bacon (2009) sees online communities as offering a wide range of opportunities from access in the form of supporting a cause to marketing products and services. Certainly these communities appear to offer vast opportunities for community building, but do they offer a sense of belonging that may be without substance or responsibility? Block expresses the concern that the effects of globalization (connection, availability of diverse information) does not include belonging (2009, p. 1). As he describes it, this "belonging" is measured by an emotional, spiritual, and/or psychological sense of "membership."

Present and future community practices will certainly correspond with and within virtual worlds. However, as we have seen from our discussions, we might question this reliance on technology. Is it one that encourages a perceived and real sense of community, or does it contribute to isolation and despair? Does the information highway take us home? Does it establish the boundaries of community in a way that we find comforting and satisfying? Does this global thinking and loss of attachment to locale prompt individuals today, more than ever before, to lust more for the real and assumed benefits of community? Nisbet (1953, 1967) suggested this to be the case decades ago. Perhaps we are simply redefining and reframing locale to be without boundaries (and restraints), and perhaps we are placing our emphasis on other aspects of community that we deem to be more significant; but is the world becoming a better place because of it?

Exercise 1-3

Consider the preceding questions. Note your thoughts and discuss the potential impact on community (both positive and negative) resulting from the reliance on technology and expansion of virtual worlds. Begin by considering how technology and virtual communities have affected you and your network of social connections:

_____

_____

_____

_____

_____

Our Professional Responsibilities to Communities

Community may also be conceptualized in a way that negates both locale and emotional investment; this refers to those communities defined by common interests, intellectual bonds, and/ or professional bonds (Goode, 1957; Nisbet, 1953). The community of occupational therapists, the medical community, and the community of women/men are all examples. We may now also include the evolving "community" of community practitioners representing many disciplines, interests, and areas of expertise.

Etzioni (1995) describes strengthening connections within and between communities with what he describes as attention to "communitarian design, architecture, and planning" (p. 113). In a very practical sense, we can make our physical environments (both private and public spaces), as well as all of the contexts of practice more community-friendly. The author goes on to suggest that people should be provided with shared space within which to mingle, and that development should be planned in ways that enhance rather than hinder the sociological mix that sustains a community (p. 314). Many American and European communities being developed today offer the opportunity of community building through meticulous design, as Etzioni has suggested. Block also talks about designing physical spaces that support community (2009, pp. 151-162). In his description, spaces that are formally planned as meeting places are most often designed for control, negotiation, and persuasion rather than communal intimacy. This causes us to question our agendas when we prepare to meet with members of our communities and design/arrange spaces to help rather than hinder community building. The simple addition of round tables for participants with no obvious "leader" may be all that is needed. Occupational therapy practitioners have long been interested in ensuring accessibility and space for everyone; we can now incorporate these interests of encouraging and sustaining community in our plans as well.

Campbell (1995) offers one of the most engaging discussions of contemporary community and sustainability. She describes attributes that, to her, demonstrate a "sense of the whole," or community. Most notably, she envisions a sense of community ownership, engagement in meaningful work, ecological sustainability, and respect for differences (p. 189). In her observations, these principles or attributes promote a shared experience of belonging and contributing to something larger than oneself. This is the essence of community, and we can find further evidence in our programming examples. We may need the author's definition of "ecological sustainability" to see just how this concept may fit in with what we do. For Campbell, the tenets of ecological sustainability suggest that a "sustainable way of life recognizes that Earth's resources (food, water, air, etc.) are finite and the growth of all living systems is limited" (pp. 193-194). Campbell suggests that, when our lifestyles are aligned with principles of sustainability, we feel more secure and self-respecting. When they are not, we often feel vaguely uneasy. I commend students who design programs with an interest in ecological sustainability, and we are seeing more of these, many providing service learning opportunities to high school and college students. There are several programs in this text designed to sustain the human system through meaningful engagement in occupation and activity. It is perhaps the health and well-being of the human occupants of this planet that may be the most vulnerable to extinction, and it has always been a core value of occupational therapy to preserve and protect the person and his or her engagement in a life of choice. Today, sustainability has taken on even greater importance and has evolved and branched into new meanings. These are discussed further in Chapter 9.

COMMUNITY-CENTERED PRACTITIONERS: WANTING TO HELP

In 1892, Addams delivered a lecture at the summer session of the School of Applied Ethics in Plymouth, Massachusetts. The lecture was later printed in the form of two essays: *The Subjective Necessity for Social Settlements* (Addams, n.d.b) and *The Objective Value of a Social Settlement* (Addams, n.d.a). At this time, Hull House had been operating for nearly three years. Hull House in Chicago and other social settlements in America (the College Settlement Association in New York and Andover House in Boston) were gathering places for individuals dedicated to developing new solutions to the social problems of the day. According to Addams, Hull House was opened in part on the theory that the dependence of classes on each other is reciprocal. In the *Subjective Necessity*, Addams descries the benefits to humanity in the transition of emotion into motive and action. The *Objective Value* discusses Hull House itself and the activities described as social, educational, humanitarian, and civic. The two essays form a philosophical and practical discussion of the beginnings of social settlements in America—a discussion that would continue to address the needs of communities for more than 100 years to come. I would recommend these essays as required reading for anyone who proposes to help communities make positive changes.

The work of Hull House and other settlement houses prompted massive philanthropic efforts as well as vast changes in the health and well-being of men, women, and children; it gave a glimmering of birth to several professions, namely social work and occupational therapy. There were also changes and advances in existing nursing care and medicine as well as public works and policy.

Nurses

A discussion of community-centered services cannot be complete without mention of the community legacy of the nursing profession. Arguably, the first practitioner to consider community as a point of service as well as investigation has been the nurse. Early on, home- and community-based practices of conventional nursing were recognized as among the most efficient and effective ways to deliver service to individuals and families (Clark, 2003). Initially, as with occupational therapists, the community was recognized as a site where a person might live, work, and play;

it was within this natural environment that services were delivered, but beyond individual care, the concerns of nursing have always actively included public health issues. From the late 1800s onward, the nursing profession has concerned itself with altering unsafe physical environments, addressing health-threatening hygienic conditions of individuals and populations, and promoting the immunization of children (Stevens & Hall, 1992). These authors also note that, more recently, the nursing profession has been devising theoretical structures to address additional community-centered issues such as oppressive social arrangements, poverty, and political disenfranchisement. All of these are recognized as threats to the safety and well-being of aggregate communities. The practices advocated by the nursing profession are referred to as *emancipatory*, designed to free individuals and groups from oppressive situations through education, practice, and action. Clark (2003) discusses the concern of community-centered nursing with the recognition and prevention of societal violence. Her discussions include not only the physical and sexual abuse of children and adults, but also concerns of critical incident stress, elder abuse, intimate partner violence, and neglect (pp. 757-771). Certainly, nursing care today is addressing the multiple needs of whole communities as well as of target groups within communities. Occupational therapists and occupational therapy assistants are entering this broader perspective of community practice a bit later than nurses but are quickly adapting to the extension of services and concerns to address the health care, prevention, and wellness needs of complex communities as well as general societal concerns.

Psychologists and Social Workers

Psychologists also include community in their practice perspectives. Orford (1993) refers to theories of person-in-context social support as well as power and control as concerns of community psychology. Recognizing that communities must be empowered to understand and change organizations and the conventional ways of accessing self-help and nonprofessional help, psychologists in the community are seen as changemakers as well as providers of professional care. Social workers, of course, have seated the core of their practices in communities through aggregates of individuals as well as individuals and families within the larger community. Drawing from sociological theories, these practitioners have developed their own theoretical constructs to address the needs of individuals within communities and the structures of organizations that, at times, may assist or impede a successful individual and family interface with the larger community (Hardcastle, Wenocur, & Powers, 2004).

The Meaning of Community for Occupational Therapists

An appreciation of the early discussions of the meaning of community and the various definitions that have evolved over time establishes a foundation for our work as community-based practitioners, particularly as we first learn to develop programming in the community. As practitioners in the community, we will address not only the needs of the person, but also societal and environmental factors that affect the health and well-being of individuals and populations. We may say that, in its simplest form, a **community** is a person's natural environment, but we know that community is more than location or locale, as described earlier; it also comprises relationships and the strong sense of "belonging" or membership. To fully appreciate the concept of community, however, it is necessary to keep in mind that it is based not only on relationships, but also partnerships and coalitions. According to Brownson (1998), the inclusion of relationships in the definition of community has implications for occupational therapy practice that go beyond the locations of practice. Consideration of relationships expands our thinking across and beyond the boundaries that the term *community* may initially suggest. Context, or actual space, may also be important because it influences these relationships. As we have learned, being present in a delimited space is not enough to constitute community, and neither are communities bound by familiar geography. Consider the global nature of the programs described by Kronenberg, Algado, and Pollard in their text *Occupational Therapy Without Borders: Learning from the Spirit of Survivors* (2005).

Warren (1987) studied the functions of community and identified several factors or functions of particular interest to occupation-centered program designers. Community can serve (1) as a "sociability arena" where members are able to develop friendships through regular interaction; (2) as an "organizational base" where the members feel a kindred notion of commonality, leading to an organization or unique banding together; and (3) as a "reference group" suggesting an identification. Condeluci (2002) reminds us that the term *community* is the blending of the prefix *com*, which means "with," and the root word *unity*, which means "togetherness and connectedness." He goes on to suggest that when people come together in unity for the sake of a unified theme, a community is formed (p. 11). All of these elements—a dimension for social enactment, the creation of organizations to form a point of reference/identification ("I belong to...")—result in potential unity and are central to much of our occupation-centered programming.

Exercise 1-4

Think of the organizations of which you have been a member. How did they provide an opportunity for enacting social connections and bonds, for establishing identity, and for developing unity? Make some notes and discuss your thoughts:

_____

_____

_____

_____

Can you further think of community programs with which you may have volunteered, or perhaps one that you are thinking of developing—particularly programs intended to empower adults, adolescents, and/or children? Discuss how you think such programs help to build a sense of community for the particular population you have in mind:

_____

_____

_____

_____

_____

Elements of Community Reflected in Occupation-Centered Programming

Condeluci (2002) describes elements of community that would include (1) a common theme: all communities share a common theme and, for many of our community programs, this "shared theme" is expressed in our mission and goals. Sometimes, a shared theme is also the reason for meeting, as in the structure of clubs (discussed in a later chapter); and (2) the element of membership, or gathering around a theme/purpose that provides a structure for membership. Sometimes, membership is formal, as in the structure of the *Roots and Shoots Club* program described in Part V, Chapter 19. Other times, it is informal, as in the gathering of mothers in the waiting area of a pediatric clinic. Whether formal or informal, both examples offer potential for effective community programming (Condeluci, 2002, pp. 15-21). Elements of (3) ritual are also important to community building (Condeluci, 2002, pp. 20-23). Again, rituals may be formal or informal. Saying a pledge, establishing the "behavioral" rules of the day, and putting on your club T-shirt may be formal indicators that you are meeting for an agreed purpose. Although more of an informal ritual, gathering for a cup of coffee and conversation before initiating work in a community garden is no less meaningful. Also important as elements of community are patterns, jargon, and memory (Condeluci, 2002, pp. 23-27). Patterns are the movements and territories of the members; jargon is the shared language a group may use to discuss the common theme; and memory is built up over time as the group, the community, creates a shared history. Patterns, jargon, and memory are central to the functions and character of many ongoing programs.

> An excellent example of programming utilizing components of patterns and memory is the Tule Indian Tribal History Project of Gelya Frank and occupational therapy students at the University of Southern California. This project involved students and faculty as well as younger members of the tribe as they helped tribal elders to document their heritage. Pictures and stories were recorded and archived to trace lineages and events; in the process, all members of the tribe experience a renewed sense of community (Gelya Frank, personal communication, May 2005; Frank & Goldberg, 2010).

Exercise 1-5

We often enter established communities in an effort to bring about elements of change. Sometimes, these communities appear closed to us because they are largely translated through established patterns, rituals, jargon, and shared memory. These characteristics may be utilized to support programming, as the Tule Indian project suggests, but at other times, they may appear to be intimidating and inhibiting. Working with street gangs in the community or with inmates in the prison system can be examples of potentially intimidating layers of established patterns, rituals, jargon, and shared memory. Can you think of any such experiences that you may have encountered? Note how your example or examples demonstrate these characteristics and discuss your answers:

_____

_____

_____

_____

_____

Social Capital and Reciprocity

Social relationships and networks serve as a form of capital because they require investments of time and energy, with the anticipation that individuals will be able to tap into these resources when necessary. The more individuals invest in these resources (social capital), the more likely they are to receive benefits in the future. The most frequently used indicators of social capital are voter turnout, newspaper readership, participation in voluntary organizations, and attendance at local organizational meetings. For community development practitioners, social capital is important. Lin (2001) argues that social capital can operate and provide benefits in several ways: (1) social networks are an important channel or source for information; (2) social ties and networks can be a source of influence; (3) they can be a form of social credentials (finding jobs, for example); and (4) social capital helps reinforce identity. Interaction with one's network is the primary source of social identity and self-concept. Changing social constructions in today's society, particularly around family, have caused many individuals to feel isolated. Putnam (2000) refers to this phenomenon as a decline in **social capital** or the connectedness between people (the relationships) in their communities (p. 19). Putnam's (2000) *Bowling Alone* provided statistical evidence of the decline in citizen participation over the past 50 years and its negative implications for what he described as *democratic life* (pp. 18-19). Putnam talks about bonding and bridging—two types of social capital.

Bonding social capital involves dense social networks among small groups of people that bring them closer together. It accumulates in the daily lives of families and people living in communities through the course of informal interactions. Bridging social capital is composed of loosely connected networks of large numbers of individuals typically linked through indirect ties. It is outward-looking, connecting communities and people to others. Temkin and Rohe (1998) found that both bonding and bridging social capital is needed to create positive community change. In general, social capital depends on the ability of people to trust each other, to reciprocate actions for the benefit of each other, and, through this, to experience a sense of cohesion and participation (Putnam, 2000; Roberts & Chada, 2006). It is in response to the decline in social capital that many of our community programming goals are established.

> It was the re-establishment of social capital that prompted the Lunalilo Home program for institutionalized elders on the island of Oahu, Hawaii. This program was constructed on concepts of empowerment, self-determination, engagement, and social connectedness—all contributing factors to the building of social capital. Since its initiation in 2009, this program has evolved into a working farm that grows flowers for the production of Hawaiian leis as well as plants for other purposes (Kealli Lum, personal communication, 2014). The lei is, of course, a visual example of reciprocity and social capital in action. See Chapter 22 for a further description of this program and the farm.

Another characteristic implicit in social capital and of importance to programming is that of **reciprocity**. In its simplest form, *reciprocity* means to look out for one another, or give and take. I give to you, and you (in turn) give to me. Our most effective programs will build social capital not only between those we help, but also with the broader community. For many who are differently abled, the relationships that constitute their social capital are with other people who are differently abled; successful programming will encourage reciprocity between and with the many layers of community. Jarman and Land suggest that "most communities are very good at identifying and welcoming those who are like them but fall woefully short in embracing diversity" (1995, p. 22). In further discussions of the concept of social capital, Condeluci (2002) would caution us to carefully consider our programming for individuals with disabilities. By separating them from the greater community, as many of our programs do, we may believe that we are creating reserves of social capital or connectedness, building reservoirs as it were. However, we may be further contributing to their isolation by not offering programming that enables the building of relationships, active "reciprocal" relationships, with others who are not disabled.

Cultural Shifting: Bringing Communities Together

Cultural shifting is a phrase Condeluci (2002) uses to describe the bridging of two or more communities to foster the inclusion of people with disabilities within the mainstream. Finding a "fit" for our clients/patients/members in existing communities and not establishing pockets of isolated communities is our imperative. Bear in mind, though, that not all programs targeting only your population are isolative; many populations must first be empowered (provided with information and skill building) and encouraged to advocate for themselves before inclusion can occur. Empowering our clients also means that *they* choose the community they wish to occupy, and inclusion may not be their choice.

> Programs that are intended to blend or bridge cultures require careful design and, in many ways, may seem more complex because each program goal is bridging two or perhaps more existing communities. Take, for example, the *Ice Cream Cart* program described in
>
> *(continued)*

Chapter 19. Middle school students who were differently abled learned to operate a small business alongside students who were not identified as differently abled. Selling ice cream during lunch was the venture. When this core of students moved to junior high school, they mentored other students to take up their business, and they "all" were mentors, not just the able students.

Condeluci (2002) suggests that all of us have moved people into the community; in fact, most of our programs are right in the middle of the larger community, but these programs have not led to inclusion for the vast majority. To establish a program to change the person (with the identified "problem"), Condeluci describes this as "chasing the wrong butterfly" (2002, p. 36). We need to remedy what may be the larger problem as well—that of the attitudes, knowledge, and behavior of the larger culture/community. Attempting to respond to this charge is exactly what many programs are doing today: raising awareness and offering solutions to the larger community while meeting the needs of their selected populations. The abled and differently abled middle school students in our previous *Ice Cream Cart* example, the *Painted Brain* program described in Chapter 26, and the developing program for trafficked young women discussed in Chapter 24 are all examples. The collaborations and partnerships we build are examples of reciprocity in process. By extending notions of reciprocity beyond our immediate population of interest, we are ensuring greater individual connectedness and future successes. We might suggest that true community establishes bonds based on the reciprocal sharing of differences. Jarman and Land (1995) suggest that this can happen only if individuals and ideas are made to connect in new ways (p. 30). To be most effective, all of our program designs must factor in goals for creating relationships beyond the immediate boundaries of our population-driven objectives to build coalitions and relationships with many disimilar communities.

OCCUPATIONAL THERAPY PRACTITIONERS AS ORGANIZERS, DEVELOPERS, AGENTS OF CHANGE, AND CAPACITY BUILDERS

In some programming efforts, you may wish to consider yourself, the occupation-centered practitioner, as the **change agent**. In this capacity, you design and plan a community program that will bring about change. It is important not to lose sight of the fact that the role of the programmer, including his or her role as change agent, may be changing as well. Ohmer and DeMasi (2009), Green and Haines (2016), and Hacker (2013) describe **consensus building**, asset building, and participation as the new or renewed interests of community programming and development; therefore, the change agent may remain in this role, but in a very different capacity than what we might have expected in the recent past. A fundamental tenet of community programming today is the ultimate goal of helping them (communities) learn to help themselves, regardless of how large or small they may be. This is often referred to as **capacity building**, or becoming active agents of change rather than the objects of change (Green & Haines, 2016, p. 8). There are likely several key components to capacity building: (1) a sense of community, (2) a level of commitment, (3) the ability to solve problems, and (4) access to resources. Occupation-centered practitioners can work to build community capacity in any of these ways, but perhaps offering knowledge, skills, and access to resources for problem solving may be the most natural to the way we have learned to practice.

Another venue for programmers is to help a community **build assets**. Community building and development is a participatory effort to mobilize community assets that increases the capacity of residents to improve the quality of their lives. Kretzmann and McKnight (1993) defined assets as the "gifts, skills, and capacities of individuals, associations, and institutions" within a community (p. 25). Focusing our efforts on building assets rather than on needs represents a significant shift in how community development practitioners and programmers have approached their work over the past few decades. Kretzmann and McKnight (1993) and Green and Haines (2016) encourage us to look to community assets as a way of identifying strengths and resources that can contribute to a strategic planning process. They suggest that a focus on needs assessment may be both an advantage and a disadvantage to communities. Focusing on need identifies problems and mobilizes communities to address local issues; however, it may prompt residents to look to others outside the community (professionals) for help. Communities can focus too much on outside resources and become more dependent than they were previously. We see this happening all over the world. A balance between identifying problems/needs and strengths/assets is the way to build sustainable programs.

If your goal is to bring about change that will blend communities, before you attend to the needs and the assets of your population, first identify the larger community (this is part of your profile but may require a more in-depth observation than first considered). The first step is to find the point of connection. The second step is what Condeluci (2002) describes as finding the venue or play point (p. 37). For us, this is the actual program and the context within which it will take place—where the two communities come together. Also, remember that for us, as occupational therapy practitioners, context has a wider meaning than physical space. It also encompasses culture; social dimensions; and personal, spiritual, and temporal elements. The complexity of this analysis gives us an opportunity to make a "just-right fit."

There is one more critical element needed for the bridging of communities—that of **gatekeeper:** the person who will introduce and endorse your programming. This gatekeeper may be an indigenous member of the community who has either formal or informal influence. Those of you who may have considered programming with a Native American population or a street gang know the importance of a gatekeeper. For the Tule River project, the tribal elders were strongly identified as the gatekeepers who would introduce the team of researchers and practitioners and also endorse their project. It was also the endorsement of this group, the gatekeepers, that would release the funds to permit this project to happen. Gatekeepers occupy many positions and may not even be physical members of the local community; funders and legislators are examples. In many of our programming efforts, the gatekeeper is an organization that has already successfully bridged a relationship with the population/community of interest. Sometimes known by other descriptors, this is nevertheless the person or persons you must partner with, often to gain access to the community and, more importantly, to ensure the success of your program.

Clark (2003) refers to **key informants** as those who, because of their position in the community, possess information and insights about the community (p. 322). Key informants may be both formal and informal community leaders. Examples may include public officials, school and health care personnel, prominent businesspeople, police, and local clergy. For the *Ice Cream Cart* program, the gatekeepers were simply the members of the student council and members of the athletic teams; however, gatekeepers are not always those who are in leadership roles (formal leaders), and it may take some investigation to find the right person or persons.

Impetus for Large-Scale Change That Will Affect Communities

In their book, *Surfing the Edge of Chaos*, Pascale, Millemann, and Gioja (2000) present us with another perspective as we continue to investigate the nature of change in communities. They suggest that innovations of any nature rarely emerge from systems with high degrees of order and stability. Systems in equilibrium lose diversity. What they describe as the condition of being "on the edge of chaos" is the precondition for transformation to take place (p. 66). In this era of overwhelming societal problems (real and potential), we can consider any change agent to certainly be operating in this unstable zone. If we, as occupation-centered practitioners who understand what we do about the nature of occupation as it is embedded in individuals within their complex communities, can manage to stay afloat (on the surfboard as it were), we stand a good chance of encouraging positive changes. The world is ripe for them; it has seldom been closer to the "edge of chaos."

In their book, *Seven Life Lessons of Chaos*, Briggs and Peat (1999) remind us that humans have had to deal with change since the beginning, but only recently has science recognized change as a fundamental force in the universe. **Chaos theory** was, early on, developed to understand the movements that caused thunderstorms, hurricanes, and other similar phenomena. In today's language, it is being applied to almost every body of information, including the nature of social dynamics, particularly how organizations form and change. *Leadership Acumen* (MacNamara, 2003), a publication focusing on executive leadership and senior management, devoted an issue to "change, chaos, and globalization" or, in their words, "other windmills." The point of referring to Don Quixote's windmills is to say that common belief that business leaders, or anyone, can manage change is a fallacy (2003, p. 2). What we may do, including those of us who wish to engage in developing community programs, is to understand the "change curve." The idea of a **change curve** was originally identified by Kubler-Ross (1975) in her book dealing with death and dying. The change curve process is a recognition that change is not cyclical but rather an ongoing process that never returns to status quo. Our community programs, to grow and flourish, must have a built-in understanding that adaptation and reinvention in response to inevitable change will be a necessary working mechanism.

Briggs and Peat (1999) suggest that "chaos" is evolving into a cultural metaphor (p. 32). When considered as a metaphor, we can ask a wide range of questions relevant to our interest in communities: why they change, how to program when change is most likely, and perhaps how to predict the consequences of change. Chaos theory suggests that, instead of resisting life's uncertainties, we should embrace the possibilities they offer.

Young (1994) focuses specifically on change in social systems. He refers to chaos theory as an elegant mathematical grounding for a postmodern social science that affirms variety and change as natural attributes or characteristics of social systems. Of particular interest are his explanations of chaos theory, the new and evolving science of complexity, which offers support and direction for postmodern understandings that honor change, variety, and disorder (Young, 1994, p. 5). His description of attractors, as those agents compelling change, is complementary to the work of Pascale et al. (2000, pp. 69-75). Attractors are of interest to those wishing to understand change; they are defined as analogous to a compass, "orienting a living system in one particular direction," and "they provide organisms with the impetus to migrate out of their comfort zone" (Pascale et al., 2000, p. 69). These authors provide complex and relevant explanations for how attractors draw a complex system in a particular direction. They speak of strange attractors as those who lure systems to the very edge of chaos. There is an interplay between the survival instinct and a hostile environment. We might consider occupational therapy and the changes that have occurred in practice respondent to the complex demands of managed health care as an example. Certainly, those working in the community to bring about change—and isn't that what we always desire?—are in a position to utilize attractors to shake up the comfort zones of our communities and to make change the desirable outcome for all those involved.

COMMUNITY AND OCCUPATION-CENTERED PRACTICE: A SUMMARY

This chapter has introduced a number of ways in which to describe and define *community*. As our descriptions have evolved, so have our potential roles and responsibilities as program designers and developers. We have identified the growing complexity of not only our interpretations of community, but in our real and potential responsibilities to make sure that communities are empowered to believe in themselves and in their capacities to take charge of their futures.

Our descriptions and interpretations may lead us to think that communities are always large, unwieldy, and scary. How could we hope to work within such a system and be effective? However, we need to be reminded that there are all kinds of communities, large and small. When we think about our programming process as described in this text, we begin by identifying a population. Usually we think of this population as having needs that we can remediate and strengths and assets that we can identify and help to build. As our work evolves, we are building and strengthening a community, or maybe several such.

With the words *community- and occupation-centered practice*, we bring together the elements of a theme that will organize our work in the community. Certainly occupational therapy practitioners have been in the community before (perhaps always), but now occupation will be at the center of our practice. Centering our practice in occupation frees us to utilize our knowledge and skills in many new, creative, and marketable venues. By locating our programs in the community as defined by locale or spirit, we are accepting the challenge of responding to that community's need with what must be new and innovative "ways of being." We have identified some of the strategies to bring about change and to provide a map for what we have termed new and innovative ways of being. Yearly vast populations are excluded from access to health care; therefore, it is imperative that we do more than ever before to help prevent illness and trauma and that we provide information, access, skills, and caring to "even out the odds" and empower those who are at risk for becoming new members of the disenfranchised.

Spurred by a desire to extend democracy beyond what she described as its political expression and sensitive to a strong need to extend humanitarian values and concerns, Jane Addams (1893–1990) was dedicated to the community represented by the evolving Chicago location of Hull House. Her commitment and resulting work, which was followed by Julia Lathrop and Eleanor Clark Slagle (Slagle, 1922; Slagle & Robeson, 1933), established our legacy by placing meaningful engagement/occupation strongly at the center of community. Their combined philosophies and commitment to the community they served provide the cognitive and emotional map that will guide us as we establish our presence in service to our communities.

REFERENCES

Addams, J. (n.d.a). The objective value of a social settlement. Retrieved from http://www.swarthmore.edu/library/peace/DG001-025/DG001JAddams/objvalue.pdf

Addams, J. (n.d.b). The subjective necessity for social settlements. Retrieved from http://teachingamericanhistory.org/library/document/the-subjective-necessity-of-social-settlements/

Bacon, J. (2009). *The art of community: Building the new age of participation.* Sebastopol, CA: O'Reilly Media.

Bernard, J. (1973). *The sociology of community.* Glenview, IL: Scott Foresman.

Block, P. (2009). Community: The structure of belonging. San Francisco, CA: Berrett-Koehler.

Briggs, J., & Peat, D. D. (1999). *Seven life lessons of chaos.* New York, NY: Harper and Row.

Brownson, C. (1998). Funding community practice: Stage 1. *American Journal of Occupational Therapy, 52*(1), 60-64.

Campbell, S. (1995). A sense of the whole: The essence of community. In K. Gozdz (Ed.), *Community building* (pp. 189-197). San Franciso, CA: Sterling and Stone.

Childe, V. G. (1953). *New light on the most ancient East.* New York, NY: W. W. Norton.

Clark, M. J. (2003). *Community health nursing: Caring for populations.* Upper Saddle River, NJ: Prentice Hall.

Condeluci, A. (2002). *Cultural shifting: Community leadership and change.* St. Augustine, FL: Training Resources Network.

Etzioni, A. (1995). Back to we: The communication nexus. In K. Gozdz (Ed.), *Community building* (pp. 305-317). San Francisco, CA: Sterling and Stone.

Frank, G., & Goldberg, C. (2010). *Defying the odds: The Tule River tribe's struggle for sovereignty in three centuries.* Lamar series in western history. New Haven, CT: Yale University Press.

Goode, W. J. (1957, April). Community within a community: The professions. *American Sociological Review, 22,* 194-200.

Green, G., & Haines, A. (2016). *Asset building and community development.* Thousand Oaks, CA: Sage.

Green, L. W., & Kreuter, M. W. (1991). *Health promotion planning: An educational and environmental approach* (2nd ed.). Mountainview, CA: Mayfield Press.

Hacker, K. (2013). *Community-based participatory research.* Thousand Oaks, CA: Sage.

Hardcastle, D., Wenocur, S., & Powers, P. (2004). *Community practice: Theories and skills for social workers.* New York, NY: Oxford University Press.

Heiser, C. (1973). *Seed to civilization.* San Francisco: W. H. Freeman.

Hillery, G. (1955). Definitions of community: Areas of agreement. *Rural Sociology, 20,* 194-204.

Jarman, B., & Land, G. (1995). Beyond breakpoint: Possibilities for new community. In K. Gozdz (Ed.), *Community building* (pp. 21-33). San Francisco, CA: Sterling and Stone.

Kretzmann, J., & McKnight, J. (1993). *Building communities from the inside out: A path toward finding and mobilizing a community's assets.* Evanston, IL: Center for Urban Affairs and Policy Research, Northwestern University.

Kronenberg, F., Algado, S., & Pollard, N. (Eds.). (2005). *Occupational therapy without borders: Learning from the spirit of survivors.* London: Elsevier.

Kubler-Ross, E. (1975). *Death: The final stage of growth.* Englewood Cliffs, NJ: Prentice Hall.

Lee, D., & Newby, H. (1983). *The problem of sociology: Introduction to the discipline.* London, Unwin Heyman.

Lin, N. (2001.) *Social capital: A theory of social structure and action.* New York, NY. Cambridge University Press.

Lyon, L. (1987). *The community in urban society.* Chicago, IL: Dorsey Press.

MacNamara, D. (2003, October 13). Leadership acumen. *Banff Executive Leadership, Inc.* Retrieved from http://www. banffexeclead.com/Newsletter04/newsletter.html

MacQueen, K. M., McLellan, E., Metzger, D. S., Kegeles, S., Strauss, R. P., Scotti, R., … Trotter, R. T. (2001). What is community? An evidence-based definition for participatory public health. *American Journal of Public Health, 91*(12), 1929-1938.

Martin, T. (2015). Philadelphia orchard project. *Country Gardens, 24*(4), 27-29.

Mckeown, T. C., Rubenstein, R. A., & Kelly, J. G. (1987). Anthropology, the meaning of community and prevention. In L. A. Jason, R. E. Hess, R. D. Felner, & J. N. Moritsugu (Eds.), *Prevention: Toward a multidisciplinary approach* (pp. 35-64). New York, NY: Haworth Press.

McKnight, J. (1988). *Beyond community services.* Evanston, IL: Center of Urban Affairs and Policy Research.

McMillan, D. W., & Chavis, D. M. (1986). Sense of community: A definition and theory. *American Journal of Community Psychology, 14*(1), 6-23.

Mead, M. (1973). Lecture. Personal Collection of M. Mead, University of Wisconsin, Milwaukee, WI.

Moore, A. (1996). The band community: Synchronizing human activity cycles for group cooperation. In R. Zemke & F. Clark (Eds.), *Occupational science: The evolving discipline* (pp. 95–106). Philadelphia, PA: F. A. Davis.

Nisbet, R. (1953). *The quest for community.* New York, NY: Oxford University Press.

Nisbet, R. (1967). *The sociological tradition.* New York, NY: Basic Books.

Nisbet, R. (1972). *Quest for community.* New York, NY: Oxford University Press.

Ohmer, M., & DeMasi, K. (2009). *Consensus organizing.* Los Angeles, CA: Sage.

Orford, J. (1993). *Community psychology: Theory and practice.* Hoboken, NJ: John Wiley and Sons.

Park, R. (1936). Human ecology. *American Journal of Sociology, 17*(1), 1–15.

Parsons, T. (1951). *The social system.* Glencoe, IL: Free Press.

Pascale, R., Millemann, M., & Gioja, L. (2000). *Surfing the edge of chaos.* New York, NY: Crown.

Putnam, R. (2000). *Bowling alone: The collapse and revival of American community.* New York, NY: Simon and Schuster.

Ray, M. (1995). A metaphor for a worldwide paradigm shift. In K. Gozda (Ed.), *Community building* (pp. 9-19). San Francisco, CA: Sterling and Stone.

Rheingold, H. (1993). *Virtual community: Homesteading on the electronic frontier.* New York, NY: Harper.

Roberts, J., & Chada, R. (2006). What's the big deal about social capital? In H. Khan & R. Muir (Eds.), *Sticking together: Social capital and local government* (pp. 25-30). London, UK: Institute for Public Policy Research.

Sarason, S. D. (1974). *A psychological sense of community: Prospects for a community psychology.* San Francisco, CA: Jossey Bass.

Slagle, E. C. (1922). Training aides for mental patients. *Papers on occupational therapy.* Utica, NY: State Hospital Press.

Slagle, E. C., & Robeson, H. A. (1933). Syllabus for training of nurses in occupational therapy. Utica, NY: State Hospital Press.

Stevens, P., & Hall, J. (1992). Applying critical theories to nursing in communities. *Public Health Nursing, 1*(9), 2-9.

Temkin, K., & Rohe, W. (1998). Social capital and neighborhood stability: An empirical investigation. *Housing Policy Debate, 9*(1), 61-88.

Warren, R. (1987). Foreword. In L. Lyon, *The community in urban society.* Chicago, IL: The Dorsey Press.

Wellman, B., & Wortley, S. (1990). Different strokes from different folks: Community ties and social support. *American Journal of Sociology, 96*(3), 558-588.

Young, T. R. (1994). Chaos theory and social dynamics: Foundations of postmodern social science. In: A. Robertson & A. Combs (Eds.), *Proceedings of the 2nd Annual Conference on Chaos Theory.* Philadelphia, PA: World Scientific Pub Co.

2

Practicing Occupation in the Community

LEARNING OBJECTIVES

1. To identify elements of occupation appropriate for guiding community practice
2. To understand the complexity of the practice environment of community as a system
3. To appreciate the diversity of occupation-centered practice available in the context of community
4. To understand the relationship between community health interventions and occupation-centered community practice
5. To identify the history and future of occupational therapy practice in prevention of illness and injury and in the promotion and maintenance of health and well-being
6. To distinguish between primary, secondary, and tertiary prevention
7. To understand the nature of occupational dysfunction and how it may affect communities

KEY TERMS

1. Occupation
2. Systems model
3. Community-based and community-level interventions
4. Community health interventions
5. Client-centered rehabilitation model
6. Community-based rehabilitation model
7. Independent living model
8. Prevention and promotion
9. Primary, secondary, or tertiary (prevention)

(continued)

Fazio, L. S. *Developing Occupation-Centered Programs With the Community, Third Edition* (pp 21-40).
© 2017 Taylor & Francis Group.

> **10.** Lifestyle redesign
>
> **11.** Occupational dysfunction: imbalance, deprivation, and alienation
>
> **12.** Spirit of Survivors Occupational Therapists Without Borders (SOS–OtwB)
>
> **13.** Occupational justice/occupational injustice
>
> **14.** Occupational apartheid

The second key concept, **occupation**, accompanies community in helping us to define the theme for this text. There is no need for an in-depth discussion of occupation since these core ideas, supporting our professional practices, provide the content for several of your occupational therapy courses. Historically, many central ideas were expressed by the early founders of occupational therapy; among them are moral treatment, balance in occupations, and purposeful activity. These central ideas, and the addition of emphasis on participation and engagement, continue to guide the work of practitioners today.

Exercise 2-1

Briefly review your knowledge base regarding our early history as a developing profession and your thoughts regarding each of the basic tenets, already mentioned, underlying the development of the profession. Make some notes and discuss with others the origins of these ideas and how you think they influence practices that you have observed, and, particularly, how do these ideas influence practices in the community?

_____

_____

_____

_____

_____

Of course, we must remember that no profession exists in a vacuum, either in its establishment or in its continued existence. Professions are established to meet the needs of society; however, these needs may be translated. The need for engagement in a meaningful occupation and its connection to well-being was recognized early in the development of our profession as a core theme that would, in fact, remain timeless.

Through the 1900s, occupational therapists continued to define and refine occupation as an organizing concept for the profession. As researchers investigated occupation as a unifying concept for organizing knowledge in occupational therapy and as they published their ideas, all occupational therapists were able to again explore the potential of occupation for providing the most effective change for their patients and for unifying our profession. The beliefs of the founders were not lost; they were only sleeping and waiting for the time when they could be further developed and matched to other areas of expanding knowledge in the disciplines of philosophy, sociology, biology, and anthropology. Mary Reilly (1962) united the past with the present when, in her 1961 Eleanor Clarke Slagle lecture, she proposed that the original hypothesis of occupational therapy can be stated as follows: "that man, through the use of his hands, as they are energized by mind and will, can influence the state of his own health" (pp. 1-9). This lecture and the writings to follow elaborated an occupational behavior paradigm of practice that renewed our beliefs in the philosophical principles established by the founders. Following Reilly, others continued to develop the tenets of occupation. Yerxa began to explore the development of a basic science of occupation. Her work and the work of her colleagues built on the foundations of many disciplines and, through that work, she has reminded us that humans attach meaning to their occupations through their cultures (Clark, Wood, & Larson, 1998; Yerxa et al., 1990). Others remind us that humans are resourceful in mobilizing occupation to act on their world and to manipulate and transform their world (Engelhardt, 1977; Reilly, 1962; Rogers, 1983). Additionally, Hall (1969) establishes for us that in utilizing our occupations, we are responsive to time. In our continued investigations of occupation, we have also developed our knowledge of play, daily living tasks, and work (Kielhofner, 1985, 1995; Reilly, 1974; Shannon, 1970). Kielhofner (1995) has brought all of these ideas together in the definition of human occupation as "doing culturally meaningful work, play or daily living tasks in the stream of time and in the contexts of one's physical and social world" (p. 3).

Over time, others have contributed definitions, and these are useful in helping us to establish the parameters of what we call *occupation*. Nelson (1977, 1988) defines *occupation* as based on occupational form and occupational performance, and Gray (1998) defines it in response to occupation as ends and as means. Some of the most recent work in elaborating this concept is that of occupational science; the definition of *occupation* particular to this science is "the daily activities that can be named in the lexicon of the culture and that fill the stream of time" (Clark et al., 1998; Yerxa et al., 1990). In July 2007, the World Federation of Occupational Therapists executive group approved this definition of *occupation*: "In occupational therapy, occupation refers to the everyday activities that people do as individuals, in families and with communities to occupy time and bring meaning and purpose to life. Occupations include things people need to, want to and are expected to do." This one dovetails nicely with what we are describing as occupation-centered programming for communities and can be used to frame most of the work described in this text. Undoubtedly, there will be other definitions forthcoming as we continue to explore and elaborate occupation as the central unifying concept around which we will develop present and future practice. Regardless of definition, there seems to be little doubt that the belief in occupation as well as the dedication to meaningful activity remains strong. Occupation-centered intervention unites us as practitioners.

Kielhofner (1992) wrote these words: "occupational therapy first emerged and continues to exist because it has an implicit social contract to address the problems of those members of society who have limited capacity to perform in their everyday occupations" (p. 3). The years of epidemic illness (tuberculosis and polio) and the injuries resulting from two world wars served to further establish that skillfully orchestrated therapy through the utilization of occupation could, in fact, influence an individual's ability to again function in and contribute to his or her community. This belief in occupation continues into the present and is being utilized by practitioners to not only help individuals regain and maintain function, but also to act on their worlds in ways that they find most meaningful and satisfying. It may be that what Kielhofner (1992) referred to as "our implicit social contract" has maintained our active interest in social justice over time. We will return to the ideas of social justice as we examine the needs of present-day society a bit later in this chapter.

Exercise 2-2

We know that there are many societal issues to confront today. Child and adult obesity and resulting illnesses, childhood and adolescent crime, and problems of the military and returning veterans are but a few. Can you name others?

_____

_____

_____

_____

_____

What did Kielhofner mean by "our implicit social contract"? Do your ideas for community programming address societal issues/social justice? How and in what way will you address these concerns?

_____

_____

_____

_____

_____

The previous exercise explored the connection between society and the individual through the identification of issues of concern to all of us. Individuals act in and on the society and community of which they are members. None of us are exempt.

UNDERSTANDING SYSTEMS AS A WAY OF THINKING ABOUT COMMUNITY PRACTICE

Belief in occupation unites us, and concern for community and the society in general motivates us. How do we act on these beliefs to help individuals make the changes they desire for themselves, for their families, and for their communities? We first need a way to think about the issues at hand; we need a map. In understanding the community as our context for intervention, we will use a **systems model** to initiate our thinking; this is the beginning of our "map." *General systems theory* is the term used to describe the scientific efforts to identify the structural, behavioral, and developmental features of living organisms and how they influence each other (Boulding, 1956; von Bertalanffy, 1968). The use of systems thinking is a way to help us understand things that interact. Gray, Kennedy, and Zemke (1997) suggest to us ways in which dynamic systems theory may be applied to occupation, thus blending key components of occupation-centered practice—the components of occupation and the multiplicity of systems that make up community. For our usage in community intervention, we are interested in how the human (an open system) receives and is influenced by information (input), the processing of this information, and the behavioral change that occurs as a result (output). Whether our role is prevention, promotion, or remediation, we are interested in the dynamics of this process within the larger system of environment/community.

If we wish to develop a new way to think about the practice of occupation in the community, then it would likely be from this dynamic systems perspective as a foundation of understanding. We might then adopt or perhaps develop a theory, frame of reference, or paradigm from which to view our practice in the community—that is, a way of thinking about the community and the relationship of individuals to each other and to the many layers that constitute the community. We are not suggesting that this is a simple process. The community is a complex open system with many interrelated levels of function. For our purposes, we would believe that these multiple systems must interrelate in such a way to produce meaningful occupation. As facilitators of this process, we are active participants and add to the complexity of this open system.

Once we have gained an appreciation of the complexity of the system within which we are practicing, we will want to further develop our map to best reach our destination. McColl, Gerein, and Valentine (1997) suggest that the occupational therapy practitioner who is able to assess the situation and choose between a number of models is perhaps best able to meet the challenges of practice. These authors are speaking from a "response to disability" perspective, and we might assume that it is even more true in the complex open system presented to us by the community. In the environment of community, we must respond not only to the needs of our clients with disability, but also to the needs of those who may require prevention or wellness services as well as social, political, and economic attention. To be eclectic in our choices means that we must have a thorough understanding of all of those perspectives from which we may choose to ensure the appropriate and effective delivery of programming.

COMMUNITY HEALTH INTERVENTIONS FOR OCCUPATION-CENTERED PRACTICE

Scaffa and Brownson (2005) distinguish between **community-based intervention** and **community-level intervention**. Community-based practices place the practitioner in the community. This practice venue is familiar to occupational therapy practitioners and many other professionals. In 2014, Scaffa wrote that "community-based practice described a broad range of health-related services that included prevention and health promotion, acute and chronic medical care, habilitation and rehabilitation; and direct and indirect service provision" (p. 5). Community-level interventions are those that attempt to modify the sociocultural, political, economic, and environmental context of the community to achieve health goals. These interventions are population-based approaches to health and do not focus on individual health behavior change (Scaffa, 2014; Scaffa & Brownson, 2005). Community health may be viewed as a continuum from community-based to community-level to community-centered interventions (Scaffa & Brownson, 2005). Community-centered interventions come from the community itself. These initiatives are often generated by leaders/members of the community who are interested in developing and utilizing community resources. Community-centered interventions are gaining in importance as we can see from recent literature describing asset building and consensus organizing in community development (Green & Haines, 2016; Ohmer & DeMasi, 2009). Clearly partnerships and coalitions become ever more important as intervention follows this trajectory. Clark (2003) refers to the building of these alliances or coalitions as a responsibility of the health care practitioner—of finding those individuals who may unite to address a common interest and helping them to mobilize their interests. Ohmer and DeMasi (2009) refer to this as *consensus organizing*.

A community-centered intervention occurs when community members come together through partnerships and coalitions to identify common concerns and solve community problems.

The Rural Community Empowerment Program may be described in this way. It represents a series of partnerships between the rural communities of the United States and federal and state agencies, local and tribal governments, private businesses, foundations, and nonprofits that engage the resources and commitments of these organizations to carry out portions of the community's strategic plan (http://www.ezec.gov/welcome/index.html). Agendas for the various communities that may be of interest to occupational therapy practitioners, particularly those working in rural areas, include youth health and employment-creating jobs.

The Dudley Street Neighborhood Initiative (DSNI) is likely one of the best known success stories in community developing in recent years. The philosophy behind this project was to build on local assets rather than to focus on the needs of residents. The community came together to establlish the DSNI with a 31-member board of directors, the majority consisting of local residents. There were many community-chosen projects including removal of illegal dumping and even provision of affordable housing. A number of abandoned parcels of land were converted to parks, gardens, and public spaces (Lipman & Mahan, 1996; Medoff & Sklar, 1994).

According to Scaffa and Brownson, **community health interventions** are "intended to address the physical, mental, social and spiritual health of communities" (2005, p. 477). Perhaps the distinction in emphasis between our understandings of individual clinical practices and those of community health agendas is that community health targets whole populations, or communities within larger populations, and they do so through emphasis on the role of social and environmental determinants of health (Scaffa & Brownson, 2005, p. 478).

> Such ongoing community programs in the Los Angeles area that target childhood obesity, breathing disorders, and delinquency are greatly influenced in assessment of need by social and environmental determinants of health. In these examples, health and well-being are advanced or prevented by complex interactions between the total environment (physical, social, and economic) and the resultant individual and community response. Researchers at the University of Southern California (USC) have identified a link between childhood asthma and living within the boundaries of a major freeway or street. Clearly a program targeting only the child with asthma would not alter the significance of the problem. This provides a good example of communities as complex systems. In a community health approach, all concerns must be addressed and included in the intervention. These would include socioeconomic concerns, establishing neighborhoods, air quality, and perhaps agendas for a safe distance from heavily trafficked roadways, or efforts to provide more public transportation or cleaner fuel. All are of interest and concern to the coalitions and partnering of community practitioners in this example (USC, 2005).

Brownson (2001) recognizes the multiple factors affecting health. The previous example demonstrates these in identifying a socioecological approach to improving health. Brownson recognizes a further layer of complexity demonstrated by the influence of the political environment, which may include regulation, legislation, and policy. Interventions within the realm of community health are intended to decrease the incidence rates of disease, disability, and death through preventive activities by reducing the impact of the disease through early detection and treatment. Such community health initiatives may include both public and private efforts to promote, protect, and preserve the physical, mental, social, and spiritual health of those in a community (McKenzie & Smeltzer 1997).

COMPREHENSIVE MODELS FOR COMMUNITY-BASED INTERVENTION

Occupational therapists may be most comfortable with entering the community in the interests of those with disabilities. We have a strong information and skill base that prepares us for this kind of service, and we can recognize both strengths and areas of need in our populations. McColl et al. (1997) discuss several models of practice from a disability perspective that we can expand for community use to include multiple roles of prevention, restoration, maintenance of function, and remediation (McColl, 1998). The first model, the **client-centered rehabilitation model**, is one in which clients engage therapists to help them solve the problems they encounter as they seek to achieve their goals (McColl et al., 1997, pp. 511-513). The client is in charge of his or her life and seeks the therapist's expertise only in order to obtain information and guidance. Of course this is an oversimplification of the process, but it serves to emphasize the importance of a client-driven goal structure. This model recognizes and encourages autonomy and places the therapist in the critical role of facilitator, instructor, advocate, and guide. These roles are becoming ever more important to the community development work today that is being practiced to encourage sustainability through the recognition of strengths in the community. In the context of community, the therapist may provide the map, or interpret the map, that will help the client to proceed on his or her way toward a meaningful, self-selected place in the community. The therapist helps "clear the way" and also provides direction and instruction when it is needed. The therapist does not do the work of the client, but instead guides and facilitates the work the client chooses to do. Lifestyle redesign programs may be considered in this way.

The second model discussed by McColl et al. (1997) emphasizes the social origins of issues relating to disability (pp. 513-515). As we have learned through our earlier discussion in Chapter 1, this particular model defines *community* as geographical, referring to a particular area or locality, but it also recognizes community to be relational, referring to a group with shared interests and values, mutual obligations, a common history, or some other affinity. We are reminded by Kniepmann (1997) that community is always more than a geographic location for our practices; it also includes an "orientation to collective health, social priorities, and different modes for service provision" (p. 540). For the **community-based rehabilitation model,** the community is first that of persons who are disabled, but also, secondly, that of persons who are disabled within the context of the larger community.

Three assumptions are associated with the community-based rehabilitation model that are important to our multiple community roles. These include but extend beyond the community of the disabled. The first assumption recognizes that people with disabilities do not exist in isolation; rather, they are an integral part of the larger community, which also includes their families, friends, and neighbors. There is an assumed relationship; a "system is in place" that both supports clients in the community who are disabled and may also benefit from their contributions to the larger economic and social environment. We know from our earlier reading that although this "system" may appear to be open, it may, in many regards, also be closed to our clients.

The second and important assumption is that individuals and communities have available to them the resources needed to influence and enhance their own health, and it may be the practitioners' role to assist these individuals and communities in first identifying and then accessing these resources. The last assumption is that it is not only more possible but also perhaps more important to make small inroads of improvement to the quality of life for all people with disabilities in a community than to select out a few for the highest standard of care (McColl et al., 1997, pp. 513-514). Together, these assumptions provide us with an orientation for work in the community with all people, whether they are disabled or at risk for the onset of disabling conditions or not.

Another model of interest to occupation-centered community-based practice is that of **independent living**. Independent living is defined by Frieden and Cole (1985) as "control over one's life based on the choice of acceptable options that minimize reliance on others in making decisions and performing every day activities" (1985, p. 735). They go on to include "participation in day-to-day life in the community, and the opportunity to engage in a range of social roles" (1985, p. 735). The origins of the independent-living model developed out of a collective political movement of persons with disabilities (Cole, 1979; DeJong, 1979, 1993; Lysack & Kaufert, 1994; McColl et al., 1997). The independent living model continues to be an excellent example of the mobilization of politics and advocacy necessary to prevail and achieve one's goals; these are central concepts to occupation-centered practice in the community. Regardless of our client population or our clients' goals, we must be cognizant of the politics that influence the dissemination of resources and we, along with our clients, must assume the role and responsibility of advocacy.

Exercise 2-3

Do your programming ideas fit one or more of these community models? How can these models help you formulate programs that will meet the needs of your population and help them gain control over their own participation and engagement in their community?

_____

_____

_____

_____

THE COMMUNITY PRACTITIONER IN THE ROLES OF PREVENTION AND HEALTH PROMOTION

We have talked about **prevention** as one of the significant roles of community practice, and this is accurate for both the occupational therapist and the occupational therapy assistant. Prevention is described by Pickett and Hanlon (1990) as anticipatory action taken to reduce the possibility of an event or condition from occurring or developing, or to minimize the damage that may result if it does occur. Kniepmann (1997) discusses the prevention of disability and the maintenance of health from a number of perspectives. It is her contention that, as a profession, we must use the knowledge we have to help maintain health in prevention, health promotion, or building those characteristics we associate with the condition of wellness.

Health **promotion** includes any planned combination of educational, political, regulatory, environmental, and organizational supports of actions and conditions of living conducive to the health of individuals, groups, or communities (Green & Kreuter, 1991; Green & Ottoson, 1999). Green and Ottoson (1999) go on to define community health promotion as "any combination of educational and social supports for people taking greater control of, and improving their own or the health of a geographically defined area" (p. 729). In 2005, the World Health Organization (WHO) established the Commission on Social Determinants of Health (CSDH) to develop strategies for reducing health inequities. The CSDH concluded that health inequities are not inevitable; instead, they are mainly due to policy failures and inequities in daily living conditions, access to power, and participation in society. All of these areas are sensitive to health promotion efforts (WHO, 2008). Occupational therapists have been proponents for the profession's role as primary health promoters. Scriven and Atwal (2004) provide an assessment of opportunities for and the barriers to the adoption of a primary health promotion role by occupational therapists working in the United Kingdom. Tucker, Vanderloo, Irwin, Mandich, and Bossers (2014) point out the similarities between health promotion and occupational therapy. According to these authors, both are based on perspectives that share a goal of enabling individuals and populations to improve control over their health. Moll, Gewurtz, Krupa, and Law recommend the promotion of an occupational perspective in the public health arena. They see the value of occupation for health and well-being as fundamental to the profession, but that it is not well recognized in the field of public health. They believe this has to change and that occupational therapists (in Canada, specifically) can bring a unique and valuable perspective to the national dialogue on health promotion (Moll et al., 2013, 2015).

In community health practices, there are several ways one might work toward health promotion and the prevention of disability. Specifically, these routes toward prevention may be defined as **primary, secondary,** and **tertiary** (Joint Committee on Health Education and Promotion Terminology, 2001, p. 101; Kniepmann, 1997, pp. 532-534; Pickett & Hanlon, 1990, p. 81). A brief review of these potential options will be useful to expand our knowledge of practice in the community.

Primary prevention is directed toward the greater society. It focuses on healthy individuals who potentially could be at risk for a particular health problem. It is about reducing susceptibility. Bike and scooter helmets, seat belts, and healthy diets are examples. Efforts to avoid the onset of pathologies might work toward reducing susceptibility in a number of ways, including minimizing environmental factors that increase the risks of disease or injury (Tarlov & Pope, 1991). The spraying of wetlands to eradicate mosquitoes is another common example of primary prevention. The actions of the Representative Assembly of AOTA to mobilize occupational therapists to address the societal issues of obesity, stress, and violence, among others, also qualify as a call for primary prevention measures. Occupational therapy practitioners in the community are often instigators and promoters of efforts toward primary prevention. For example, they might consult to town planning boards about architectural barriers, work to lower speed limits in recreation areas where children play, support restrictions on unsafe toys, or see that gates and locks are on all swimming pool enclosures. There are many and varied ways in which we can engage in primary prevention.

Tarlov and Pope (1991) describe secondary prevention as efforts to target groups in the community who are thought to be "at risk," focusing on the detection and treatment of disease early in its preclinical or clinical stages. This can involve early detection of a potential health problem followed by appropriate interventions to halt, reverse, or slow its progression. Encouraging people to exercise more, for example, can help to control hypertension. Occupational therapy practitioners are certainly involved in secondary prevention, which can run the gamut from parenting classes for teens to the encouragement of condom use for those at risk of STDs. Teaching the well elderly how to access public transportation in an effort to widen their options for accessing meaningful occupations and thus maintain their health would also be considered secondary prevention.

The focus of tertiary prevention is to maximize function and minimize the detrimental effects of illness or injury (Kniepmann, 1997). Maximizing function and limiting disability are the goals. Although this is an area already very familiar to occupational therapy practitioners, we also want to emphasize efforts toward a focus on function, advocacy for social policy as it can influence one's health and ability to be independent, and the direct intervention concerns of the individual.

Most of the programs we discuss in this text that deal with prevention fall under the category of secondary prevention; however, some of our programming assumes elements of primary and tertiary prevention as well; often, it may be difficult to separate one from the other. Associated with prevention but with a different directive, health promotion has been the favored topic of many occupational therapists, including Madill, Townsend, and Schultz (1989) and McComas and Carswell (1994). For occupational therapy practitioners, health promotion or optimization is based in part on our basic belief that a balance of work, rest, self-care, and leisure/play is necessary for optimal health and well-being. Prompted by this belief, occupation is utilized to organize our daily rounds of activity in a way that will include this recommended balance. For many of our clients, guidance is needed in first recognizing deficits of balance; this is then followed by the offer of assistance in developing the skills, knowledge, and behaviors needed to engage in those self-selected activities that provide "meaningful" engagement. Lauckner, Krupa, and Paterson (2011) discuss the past 30-year history of health promotion, population health, and community participation in Canada. They describe community development (CD) as an approach within health promotion that is a "process of organizing and/or supporting community groups in identifying their health issues, planning and acting upon their strategies for social action/social change and gaining increased self-reliance and decision-making power as a result" (p. 260; Labonte, 2004, p. 90).

It is not realistic to think that we can separate the prevention of illness or trauma and the promotion of health and wellness; one is implied within the other. By providing those aspects of promotion that include information and resources geared to individual needs and wants and through orchestrated changes in behavior and motivation, we will reduce risk and thus help to prevent illness and accidents. Fuhrer (1994) talks of the feelings of elevated health and subjective well-being experienced by people who are engaged in activities they feel are health-promoting (p. 359). First, we must enlarge our own awareness of community resources as well as our own programs that promote health, whether these be options for education, medical care, or perhaps exercise/wellness classes. Our awareness of programs is then followed by the sharing of these resources with the client through well-articulated programming that is intended to bring about the desired directive of either prevention or promotion (Dyck, 1993; Finlayson & Edwards, 1995; Jaffe, 1986; Kniepmann, 1997).

Life change as a foundation for occupational therapy practice is realized through what Mandel, Jackson, Zemke, Nelson, and Clark describe as **lifestyle redesign** (1999, pp. 12-13). According to these authors, there are four core ideas of the occupational therapy profession that inform lifestyle redesign programs: "Occupation is life itself; occupation can create new visions of possible selves, occupation has a curative effect on physical and mental health and on a sense of life order and routine, and occupation has a place in preventive care" (Mandel et al., 1999, p. 13). Dieterle (2014) further elaborates on the elements of lifestyle. The term *lifestyle* refers to the daily choices we make; choices that may support health and well-being or hinder it. Lifestyle redesign provides an intervention when changes in lifestyle are merited to achieve balance and health (Dieterle, 2014, pp. 378-380). The USC Well Elderly Study is a prime example of the impact of the use of occupational lifestyle redesign to offer the well elderly a "customized routine of health promoting and meaningful daily activities" (Mandel et al., 1999, introduction).

Much of our work in the community is directed toward the promotion of health and well-being; however, we cannot assume that all of our clients will be equally engaged in the process, nor will all agree on the parameters of "health." Even though most people would support the idea of seeking better health, often the task of actually working toward the goal is received less enthusiastically. A review of those characteristics that influence learning and resulting behavior change will be helpful as you prepare to work in prevention and promotion. If you have previous clinical experience, this kind of practice may not be unlike intervention work that you have already accomplished in the institutional environments of emotional and physical rehabilitation. The teaching and acquisition of health-promoting behaviors is not simple, as anyone who has ever failed to maintain an exercise or weight loss program can attest. Understanding something of the building of self-efficacy and empowerment is critical to the success of this kind of programming. Kniepmann (1997) provides a useful summary of those constructs for behavioral change that will help in developing successful community programs to include the characteristics of social learning theory, self-efficacy, and perceptions of control as described in the research of Bandura (1977, 1982), Bandura and Walters (1963), and Rotter (1966). The work of these early theorists and researchers has helped to build ideas and strategies to understand the nature of change. Self-determination theory now elaborates on the nature of intrinsic motivation, social development, and well-being (Ryan & Deci, 2000; http://www.psych.rochester.edu/SDT/publications/pub_well.html) Motivational interviewing is gaining a wide and diverse audience of people interested in both understanding and facilitating change through the resolution of ambivalence (Miller & Rollnick, 2013). The reader is encouraged to pursue these resources. None of our practice and program participants are exempt from change, whether the change is desired or imposed by accident, illness, or circumstances of living.

Exercise 2-4

Is your proposed programming directed toward the prevention of disability or disease? Is it primary, secondary, tertiary, or a combination? Or would you say the emphasis is on health promotion?

_____

_____

_____

_____

_____

THE FUTURE OF OCCUPATION-CENTERED PRACTICE IN THE COMMUNITY

Trends in Health Care and in the Practices of Healthy Living

There is little doubt that health care is changing constantly and that, in response, occupational therapy is changing as well. In 1995, the American Occupational Therapy Association commissioned Health Policy Alternatives, Inc., to examine the future of health care and, particularly, occupational therapy's future within health care. This organization reported numerous markers of the rapid changes in America's health care system, most of them carrying negative implications, and they attributed these changes primarily to escalating costs and the lack of accompanying growth in the underlying economy in order to maintain a balance (Health Policy Alternatives, 1996, p. 1).

It has now been 20 years since this report was published, but it is well worth a revisit because of its continued relevance to the profession. We have witnessed many of its implications in our workplaces. First, there were reductions in institutional administrative structures, particularly in middle management; these were followed by reductions in treatment staff with resulting pressures on maintaining caseloads; and ultimately there were reductions in consumer access to health care and economic support for care. We now have managed care, a perceived restraint, but we also have primary care, and telehealth—new opportunities for the profession (Ciro, Randall, Robinson, Loring, & Shortridge, 2015). There will undoubtedly be other opportunities if we prepare ourselves to embrace them. The social, economic, and political worlds in which we live and practice have always encouraged, discouraged, or sometimes prevented how and where we choose to practice. Historically, there appears to be cyclical and necessary reversals in exchange systems—fat years and lean years. Restraint is the counterbalance of excess, but this most recent period of restraint shows no sign of ease.

Also, in 1996, the Pew Health Professions Commission predicted the pressures on physicians and nurses and also indicated that there would be pressures to consolidate the "allied" health professions. In its 1998 report, the Commission asked that health professionals "continue to consider, in fundamental ways how they best add value to the delivery of health services" (p. i). The Commission suggested that practitioners must contribute to the system in meaningful ways (that is, measure outcomes) or they would risk losing their autonomy. The impetus on evidence-based practice continues to grow in all of the health professions. There were messages to educators of future health care professionals as well, which included recommendations to stop preparing students for "yesterday's health care system" and to start preparing students for "emerging systems" (1998, p. iii). It was further suggested that this preparation should include broader education with regard to systems, organizational skills, and population skills. Emphasis on community practice in occupational therapy began to regain strength. Occupational therapists have been articulating these same messages. In 1997, Baum and Law described a changing health system paradigm that focused on (1) health rather than illness, (2) community approaches rather than medical interventions, (3) abilities and quality of life rather than deficits and survival, (4) personal versus professional control and responsibility, and (5) prevention rather than treatment (p. 280). Lifestyle redesign is an approach focusing on life quality and the belief that an individual may change the way he or she reacts to and interacts with the larger community. The coach/mentor/therapist provides the necessary information for the client to make informed choices in the redesign of his or her life to more effectively function in the world.

In a special issue of the *American Journal of Occupational Therapy,* Baum and Law called on the profession to be "responsive to the needs of our times" (1998, p. 7). There is little doubt that "the needs of our times" include all of society's ills: abuse, violence, joblessness, futility, and ignorance. In addition, there are new ills that result in increased stress, including competition for limited resources, pressure on family and other systems, and the loneliness and isolation that technology can produce. Baum and Law also reminded us that, in these troubled times, it is through engagement in occupation that people develop and maintain health (1998, p. 7). Additionally, it is also through membership in a shared, supportive community. In her presidential address to the American Occupational Therapy Association Annual Meeting, President Baum asked the profession what we must do now to position ourselves as the profession that works in both traditional and community health settings to enable occupations and remove barriers that limit participation. In her words, "Society is counting on our contribution" (Baum, 2005). The topic of a later address (Baum, 2006) was *Centennial Challenges, Millennium Opportunities.* The Centennial Vision for the profession was developed after many opportunities for feedback from shareholders, and it now offers a framework that we can use to guide practice regardless of context (Baum, 2006, p. 611).

Practice in the community that includes intervention, maintenance, and prevention is new for many health care providers, but for occupational therapy, it is a re-emerging practice arena. Appropriate to occupational therapy practitioners' renewed interests in community-based practice were other recommendations of the 1996 Pew Health Professions Commission to include (1) the encouragement of diversity to reflect the nation's population (i.e., our outreach programs to the inner city and ethnic urban population "pockets"); (2) the inclusion of interdisciplinary team competence (i.e., our expansion of teams to include both professional and layperson community members such as friends and neighbors); (3) efforts to continue to move toward ambulatory practice (i.e., our extensions of ambulatory practice to include not only intervention, but also maintenance of health and wellness and prevention of injury and illness); and (4) the encouragement of public service for all health professional students and graduates (i.e., our internships, fieldwork, residencies, and service learning opportunities in the community).

The Pew Health Professions Commission's (1998) fifth recommendation continues to be particularly significant to this text. Pertinent quotes from it are as follows:

- "Health professional programs should require a significant amount of work in community settings as a requirement for graduation. This work should be integrated into the curriculum."

- "Students should assist in the design and development of such programs."

- "Communities and the health agencies that serve them should actively participate in the partnerships through which these service programs can be built."

- "Existing programs of national service tied to debt forgiveness should be expanded and enlarged in order to incorporate more health professional graduates."

- "Professional associations should actively incorporate the idea of public service into regulation and professional development activity" (pp. iii-vi).

The Pew summary report, *Healthy America: Practitioners for 2005*, extended these directives to include prevention in its set of recommendations to educators. The report noted that the "largest share of our graduates will spend their careers in home- and community-based settings" (Pew Health Professions Commission, 1992, p. 5; Shugar, O'Neill, & Bader, 1991). The more recent national report, *Healthy People 2010*, echoes many of these ideas with its prevailing message of responsibility for health becoming the task of the individual (U.S. Department of Health and Human Services [U.S. DHHS], 1998, 2000). In 2010, the emphasis included an increase in quality and years of healthy life and the elimination of health disparities. *Healthy People 2020* (U.S. DHHS, 2010a) continues to focus on the elimination of health disparities and the achievement of health equity. Health disparities adversely affect groups of people who have systematically experienced greater obstacles to health (U.S. DHHS, 2010b, para. 6). However, we must ask how individuals will gain the necessary knowledge and skills to maintain and protect their health. In part, it is the responsibility of our profession, as well as others in health care, to close this potential gap.

One of our emerging roles in today's society will be to build healthy communities. Baum and Law (1997, 1998) suggest that occupational therapists must understand how people interpret and practice occupation, how they apply structure to their daily lives, and how they assign meaning. This can best be done in their natural, self-selected environments—in other words, in their communities. Community therapists, according to these authors, must be attuned not only to the interventional needs of their clients, but also to the ecological, physical, social, cultural, and health environments of the client's community in order to improve all available options for healthy living (Baum & Law, 1998, p. 8). Many of the program examples described in this text do just that; they are very responsive to environment. Some of them, such as the program embedded in the philosophies of the Jane Goodall Roots and Shoots Club, have preservation and protection of the environment as a central theme. See Chapter 19 for more information on these clubs. Baum and Christiansen (1997) refer to a changing paradigm in medicine and health care from a biomedical, acute-centered, and provider-driven approach to one that places more responsibility on the consumer (p. 31). We might conclude that this places more responsibility on us as occupational therapy practitioners to guide the consumer in ways of facilitating healthy habits and behaviors and in navigating community systems to obtain the information and services that they require.

Globalization of Occupation

Wilcock (1998) broadened our perspective of community to include global concerns in her call for occupational therapists to be responsive to the objectives of the WHO and potential roles in what she describes as the "new public health" (p. 221). She advocated for a strong foundation in occupation that would prepare the therapist for practices in wellness, preventive medicine, social equity, community development, and ecological sustainability. Her discussion included risk factors for **occupational dysfunction** (occupational imbalance, deprivation, and alienation). According to Wilcock (1998), **occupational imbalance** is a lack of balance between work, rest, self-care, and play/leisure that fails to meet an individual's unique physical, social, or mental health needs, thereby resulting in decreased health and well-being. **Occupational deprivation** may include circumstances or limitations that prevent a person from acquiring, engaging in, or enjoying his or her occupation. Such things as less-than-optimal health, isolation, poverty, and homelessness are examples. **Occupational alienation** represents a lack of satisfaction in one's occupations and a general sense of estrangement. Engagement in such tasks that the individual perceives as stressful or meaningless may result in occupational alienation. Bass-Haugen, Henderson, Larson, and Matuska (2005) added the following to these risk factors: occupational delay, occupational disparities, and occupational interruption. *Occupational delay* refers to occupational development that does not follow the typical schedule for the acquisition of occupational skills. *Occupational disparities* are inequalities of differences in occupational patterns among populations, often the result of occupational injustice. *Occupational interruption* is described as a temporary interference with occupational performance or participation as a result of a change in personal, social, or environmental factors.

Kronenberg, Algado, and Pollard (2005) are perhaps most representative of where occupational therapy can go in a humanistic mission to support social justice for all people. In 1997, Salvador Simo Algado launched the work of the Dolphin Association to help people who appeared to have been neglected or underserved by occupational therapy practitioners. Survivors of war, prisoners, immigrants, prostitutes, and people living with HIV/AIDS were all seen as part of this group (Kronenberg et al., 2005, preface). In 2002, the Dolphin Association was renamed Spirit of Survivors **Occupational Therapists Without Borders (SOS-OtwB)**. The global community representing both developed countries and developing countries is where dialogues and collaborations between occupational therapists and other professionals are encouraged. The authors view the SOS-OtwB as a catalyst for movement within the international community of occupational therapists. The goal is to "develop, implement and promote occupational therapy practice, education and research initiatives with marginalized people, inspired and guided by a vision of overcoming occupational apartheid and working toward **occupational justice**, while raising critical awareness about and facing up to the political nature of occupational therapy" (Durocher, Gibson, & Rappolt, 2013; Kronenberg et al., 2005, preface). **Occupational injustices** would then exist when participation is barred, confined, segregated, prohibited, undeveloped, disrupted, alienated, marginalized, exploited, or otherwise devalued (Townsend & Whiteford, 2005). Pollard, Sakellariou, and Kronenberg (2009) offer a definition of **occupational apartheid**: "Occupational apartheid is the segregation of groups of people through restriction or denial of access to dignified and meaningful participation in occupations of daily life on the basis of race, colour, disability, national origin, age, gender, sexual preferences, religion, political beliefs, status in society, or other characteristics" (p. 55). They propose the consideration of what they describe as transformational practice with the aim of effecting occupational justice and asserting new roles that are oriented to wider community needs. Many of the programs described in this text speak to occupational justice. In all of our communities, we have people in need for whom we can advocate and whom we can empower to advocate for themselves. Our urban and rural communities in the United States are home to children and adults who are disenfranchised or at great risk for becoming so. Global concerns are often first addressed in our own communities with the same energy and caring we would extend to others around the world.

Exercise 2-5

Occupational therapy students around the world have been instrumental in designing and, along with academic faculty and clinicians, implementing outreach programs and level I and II fieldwork experiences for populations in many underserved countries. Examples include the development of community playgrounds in Haiti and sensory stimulation and play programs for orphans in Ghana and Rumania.

Write down the ideas you may have for such programs, and discuss them with classmates and your instructors. Programs of this nature provide excellent opportunities for occupational therapy and occupational therapy assistant academic programs to work together on community program development. You may wish to further investigate some of the references mentioned in this section to expand your thinking regarding the globalization of occupation-centered practices.

_____

_____

_____

_____

_____

Since these recommendations and directives target all health care practitioners, we are not alone in considering new ways to practice in the community setting. However, occupational therapists have an ongoing history of practice in the community, with a body of published information to help those who may be new to explore their options. You should review the extensive list of publications at the close of this chapter and examine those that interest you. Many occupational therapists have always practiced with an awareness of the community or directly within it, and those who have done so know that it can be a significantly rewarding practice. It is virtually impossible to practice in the direct environment of the client—in the community system—without being aware of the need for maintenance of health, wellness, and prevention. The community system invites, and likely demands, a comprehensive array of services that includes all that we know and more. We must be practitioners, educators, skill builders, politicians, health promoters, and advocates—and probably a good deal more.

Our community practice history is an advantage as we prepare for return to the community, and our unifying belief and dedication to occupation as a way to orchestrate our practices is a substantial strength. Few professions have an agreed-upon belief system strong enough to organize their interventions without losing their sense of purpose in what can be a complex and demanding care environment—that of the community. It is our time to embrace the values and ideals of our founders and to meet the challenges of community head-on through our belief in the power of occupation.

SUMMARY

This chapter has introduced the term *occupation* as it has come to be used in occupational therapy theory and practice. Engagement in occupation centers our understanding of individuals and populations and helps us to frame their needs and assets. We have talked about the importance of systems, particularly as they inform our understanding of how communities do or do not work together. Terms used in community health models have been introduced to include the delivery systems of community-based and community-level interventions. We have compared primary, secondary, and tertiary models of prevention and looked at the ways in which occupation-centered practitioners might be involved in each of these. The chapter closed with a discussion of factors that may hold people back from occupational engagement: the various forms of occupational dysfunction. Finally, we have looked briefly at the global work that has added occupational justice and occupational apartheid to our awareness and understanding of opportunity and restriction in occupational engagement.

REFERENCES

Bandura, A. (1977). Self-efficacy: Toward a unifying theory of behavioral change. *Psychological Review, 84,* 191-215.

Bandura, A. (1982). Self-efficacy mechanism in human agency. *American Psychologist, 37,* 122-147.

Bandura, A., & Walters, R. H. (1963). *Social learning and personality development.* New York, NY: Holt, Rinehart, and Winston.

Bass-Haugen, H., Henderson, M. L., Larson, B. A., & Matuska, K. (2005). Occupational issues of concern in populations. In C. H. Christiansen, C. M. Baum, & J. Bass-Haugen (Eds.), *Occupational therapy: Performance, participation and well-being.* (3rd ed., pp. 28-36). Thorofare, NJ: SLACK Incorporated.

Baum, C. (2005). Harnessing opportunities and taking responsibility for our future. Presidential Address, American Occupational Therapy Association, 85th Annual Conference, May 9, 2005, Long Beach, CA.

Baum, C. (2006). Centennial challenges, millennium opportunities. *American Journal of Occupational Therapy, 60*(6), 609-616.

Baum, C., & Christiansen, C. (1997). The occupational therapy context: Philosophy, principles, practice. In C. H. Christiansen & C. M. Baum (Eds.), *Occupational therapy enabling functions and well-being* (pp. 28-43). Thorofare, NJ: SLACK Incorporated.

Baum, C., & Law, M. (1997). Occupational therapy practice: Focusing on occupational performance. *American Journal of Occupational Therapy, 51,* 277-288.

Baum, C., & Law, M. (1998). Nationally speaking: Community health: A responsibility, an opportunity, and a fit for occupational therapy. *American Journal of Occupational Therapy, 52*(1), 7-10.

Boulding, K. E. (1956). General systems theory: The skeleton of science. *Management Science, 2*(3), 197-208.

Brownson, C. (2001). Program development for community health: Planning, implementation, and evaluation strategies. In M. Scaffa (Ed.), *Occupational therapy in community-based practice settings* (pp. 95-134). Philadelphia, PA: Davis.

Ciro, C., Randall, K., Robinson, C., Loring, G., & Shortridge, A. (2015). Telehealth and interprofessional education. *OT Practice,* April 27, 7-10.

Clark, M. J. (2003). *Community health nursing: Caring for populations.* Upper Saddle River, NJ: Prentice Hall.

Clark, F., Wood, W., & Larson, E. (1998). Occupational science: Occupational therapy's legacy for the 21st century. In M. Neistadt & E. Crepeau (Eds.), *Willard and Spackman's occupational therapy* (9th ed., pp. 13-21). Philadelphia, PA: Lippincott.

Cole, J. A. (1979). What's new about independent living. *Archives of Physical Medicine and Rehabilitation, 60,* 458-461.

DeJong, G. (1979). Independent living: From social movement to analytic paradigm. *Archives of Physical Medicine and Rehabilitation, 60,* 435-446.

DeJong, G. (1993). Health care reform and disability: Affirming our commitment to the community. *Archives of Physical Medicine and Rehabilitation, 74,* 1017-1024.

Dieterle, C. (2014). Lifestyle redesign programs. In M. Scaffa & S. M. Reitz (Eds.), *Occupational therapy in community-based practice settings* (pp. 377-380). Philadelphia, PA: Davis.

Durocher, E., Gibson, B. E., & Rappolt, S. (2013). Occupational justice: A conceptual review. *Journal of Occupational Science, 21,* 418-430.

Dyck, I. (1993). Health promotion, occupational therapy and multiculturalism: Lessons from research. *Canadian Journal of Occupational Therapy, 60,* 120-129.

Engelhardt, H. T. (1977). Defining occupational therapy: The meaning of therapy and the virtues of occupation. *American Journal of Occupational Therapy, 31*(10), 666-672.

Finlayson, M., & Edwards, J. (1995). Integrating the concepts of health promotion and community into occupational therapy practice. *Canadian Journal of Occupational Therapy, 62,* 70-75.

Frieden, L., & Cole, J.A. (1985). Independence: The ultimate goal of rehabilitation of spinal cord injured persons. *American Journal of Occupational Therapy, 39,* 734-739.

Fuhrer, M. J. (1994). Subjective well-being: Implications for medical rehabilitation outcomes and models of disablement. *American Journal of Physical Medicine and Rehabilitation, 73,* 358-364.

Gray, J. M. (1998). Putting occupation into practice: Occupation as ends, occupation as means. *American Journal of Occupational Therapy, 52,* 354-364.

Gray, J. M., Kennedy, B. L., & Zemke, R. (1997). Application of dynamic systems theory to occupation. In R. Zemke & F. Clark (Eds.), *Occupational science: The evolving discipline* (pp. 309-324). Philadelphia, PA: F. A. Davis.

Green, G., & Haines, A. (2016). *Asset building and community development.* Los Angeles, CA; Sage.

Green, L. W., & Kreuter, M. W. (1991). *Health promotion planning: An educational and environmental approach* (2nd ed.). Mountainview, CA: Mayfield Press.

Green, L. W., & Ottoson, J. M. (1999). *Community and population health* (8th ed.). Boston, MA: McGraw-Hill.

Hall, E. T. (1969). *The silent language.* Greenwich, CT: Fawcett Publications.

Health Policy Alternatives. (1996, Nov.). *Health care and market reform: Workforce implications for occupational therapy.* Washington, DC: Limited Publication.

Jaffe, E. G. (1986). Nationally speaking: The role of occupational therapy in disease prevention and health promotion. *American Journal of Occupational Therapy, 40,* 749-752.

Joint Committee on Health Education and Promotion Terminology (2001). Report of the 2000 Joint Committee on health education and promotion terminology. *American Journal of Health Education, 32*(2), 90-103.

Kielhofner, G. (1985). *A model of human occupation: Theory and application.* Baltimore, MD: Williams & Wilkins.

Kielhofner, G. (1992). *Conceptual foundations of occupational therapy.* Philadelphia, PA: F. A. Davis.

Kielhofner, G. (1995). *A model of human occupation: Theory and application* (2nd ed.). Baltimore, MD: Lippincott, Williams and Wilkins.

Kniepmann, K. (1997). Prevention of disability and maintenance of health. In C. Christiansen & C. Baum (Eds.), *Occupational therapy enabling function and well-being* (pp. 531–553). Thorofare, NJ: SLACK Incorporated.

Kronenberg, F., Algado, S. & Pollard, N. (Eds). (2005). *Occupational therapy without borders: Learning from the spirit of survivors.* London, UK: Elsevier.

Labonte, R. (2004). Community, community development, and the forming of authentic partnerships: Some critical reflections. In M. Minkler (Ed.), *Community organizing and community building for health* (2nd ed.; pp. 88-102). New Brunswick, NJ: Rutgers.

Lauckner, H., Krupa, T., & Paterson, M. (2011). Conceptualizing community development: Occupational therapy practice at the intersection of health services and community. *Revie Canadienne d'Ergotherapie, 78*(4), 2011.

Lipman, M., & Mahan, L. (Directors). (1996). *Holding ground: The rebirth of Dudley Street.* United States: New Day Films.

Lysack, C., & Kaufert, J. (1994). Comparing the origins and ideologies of the independent living movement and community based rehabilitation. *International Journal of Rehabilitation Research, 17,* 231-240.

Madill, H., Townsend, E., & Schultz, P. (1989). Implementing a health promotion strategy in occupational therapy education and practice. *Canadian Journal of Occupational Therapy, 56,* 67-72.

Mandel, D., Jackson, J., Zemke, R., Nelson, L., & Clark, F. (1999). *Lifestyle redesign: Implementing the well-elderly program.* Bethesda, MD: American Occupational Therapy Association.

McColl, M. A. (1998). What do we need to know to practice occupational therapy in the community. *American Journal of Occupational Therapy, 52*(1), 11–18.

McColl, M. A., Gerein, N., & Valentine, F. (1997). Meeting the challenges of disability: Models for enabling function and well-being. In C. Christiansen & C. Baum (Eds.), *Occupational therapy enabling function and well-being* (pp. 509-527). Thorofare, NJ: SLACK Incorporated.

McComas, J., & Carswell, A. (1994). A model for action in health promotion: A community experience. *Canadian Journal of Rehabilitation, 7,* 257-265.

McKenzie, J., & Smeltzer, J. (1997). *Planning, implementation, and evaluating health promotion programs: A primer* (2nd ed.). Boston, MA: Allyn and Bacon.

Medoff, P., & Sklar, H. (1994). *Streets of hope: The fall and rise of an urban neighborhood.* Boston, MA: South End Press.

Miller, W., & Rollnick, S. (2013). Motivational interviewing: Helping people to change. (3rd ed.) New York, NY: Guilford Press.

Moll, S., Gewurtz, R., Krupa, T., Law, M., Lariviere, N., & Levasseur, M. (2015). "Do-Live-Well": A Canadian framework for promoting occupation, health, and well-being. *Canadian Journal of Occupational Therapy, 82*(1), 9-23.

Moll, S., Gewurtz, R., Krupa, T., & Law, M. (2013). Promoting an occupational perspective in public health. *Canadian Journal of Occupational Therapy, 80*(2), 111-119.

Nelson, D. (1977). Why the profession of occupational therapy will flourish in the 21st century, 1996 Eleanor Clarke Slagle lecture. *American Journal of Occupational Therapy, 51,* 11–24.

Nelson, D. (1988). Occupation: Form and performance. *American Journal of Occupational Therapy, 42,* 633-641.

Ohmer, M., & DeMasi, K. (2009). *Consensus organizing: A community development workbook.* Thousand Oaks, CA: Sage.

Pew Health Professions Commission. (1992). *Summary: Healthy America: Practitioners for 2005. A beginning dialogue for U.S. schools of allied health.* San Francisco, CA: The Center for the Health Professions, University of California.

Pew Health Professions Commission. (1996, November). *Critical challenges: Revitalizing the health professions for the twenty-first century. Third report, first release.* San Francisco, CA: The Center for the Health Professions, University of California.

Pew Health Professions Commission. (1998, December). *Recreating health professional practice for a new century. Fourth report.* San Francisco, CA: The Center for the Health Professions, University of California.

Pickett, G., & Hanlon, J. J. (1990). *Public health: Administration and practice.* St. Louis, MO: Times Mirror/Mosby.

Pollard, N., Sakellariou, D., & Kronenberg, F. (2009). *A political practice of occupational therapy.* London, UK: Churchill Livingston/Elsevier.

Reilly, M. (1962). Occupational therapy can be one of the great ideas of 20th century medicine. *American Journal of Occupational Therapy, 16,* 1–9.

Reilly, M. (1974). *Play as exploratory learning.* Beverly Hills, CA: Sage.

Rogers, J. (1983). The study of human occupation. In G. Kielhofner (Ed.), *Health through occupation: Theory and practice in occupational therapy* (pp. 93-124). Philadelphia, PA: F. A. Davis.

Rotter, J. B. (1966). Generalized expectancies for internal versus external control of reinforcement. *Psychological Monographs: General and Applied, 80,* 1-28.

Ryan, R. M., & Deci, E. L. (2000). Self determination theory and the facilitation of intrinsic motivation, social development, and well-being. *American Psychologist, 55,* 68-78.

Scaffa, M. (2014). Community-based practice: Occupation in context. In M. Scaffa, & S. M. Reitz (Eds.), *Occupational therapy in community-based practice settings* (2nd ed.). Philadelphia, PA: Davis.

Scaffa, M., & Brownson, C. (2005). Occupational therapy intervention: Community health approaches. In C. Christiansen, C. Baum, & J. Bass-Haugen (Eds.), *Occupational therapy: Performance, participation, and well-being* (3rd ed., pp. 478-492). Thorofare, NJ: SLACK Incorporated.

Scriven, A., & Atwal, A. (2004). Occupational therapists as primary health promoters: Opportunities and barriers. *British Journal of Occupational Therapy, 67*(10), 424-429.

Shannon, P. (1970). The work-play model: A basis for occupational therapy programming. *American Journal of Occupational Therapy, 24,* 215-218.

Shugar, D. A., O'Neill, E. H., & Bader, J. D. (Eds.). (1991). *Healthy America: Practitioners for 2005. An agenda for action for U.S. health professional schools.* Durham, NC: Pew Health Professions Commission.

Tarlov, A., & Pope, A. (1991). *Disability in America: Toward a national agenda for prevention.* Washington, DC: Institute of Medicine, National Academy Press.

Townsend, B. & Whiteford, A. (2005). A participatory occupational justice framework: population-based processes of practice. In F. Kronenberg, S. Algado, & N. Pollard (Eds.), *Occupational therapy without borders.* London, UK: Elsevier.

Tucker, P., Vanderloo, L., Irwin, J. Mandich, A., & Bossers, A. (2014). Exploring the nexus between health promotion and occupational therapy: Synergies and similarities. *Canadian Journal of Occupational Therapy, 81*(3), 183-193.

University of Southern California. (2005). *Research Agendas for the Community.* Los Angeles, CA: Author.

U.S. Department of Health and Human Services. (1998). *Healthy people 2010 objectives: Draft for public comment.* Washington, D.C.: U.S. Department of Health and Human Services.

U.S. Department of Health and Human Services. (2000). *Healthy people 2010* (2nd ed.). Washington, DC: U.S. Government Printing Office.

U.S. Department of Health and Human Services. (2010a). *Healthy People 2020.* (ODPHP Publication No. B0132). http://healthypeople.gov

U.S. Department of Health and Human Services. (2010b). *Implementing healthy people 2020.* http://healthypeople.gov/2020/implementing/default.aspx

von Bertalanffy, L. (1968). *General systems theory.* New York, NY: Braziller.

Wilcock, A. (1998). *An occupational perspective of health.* Thorofare, NJ: SLACK Incorporated.

World Health Organization. (2008). Commission on social determinants of health: report by the secretariat. http://www.euro.who.int/en/health-topics/health-determinants/social-determinants

Yerxa, E. J., Clark, F., Frank, G., Jackson, J., Parham, D., Pierce, D., . . . Zemke, R. (1990). An introduction to occupational science: A foundation for occupational therapy in the 21st century. *Occupational Therapy in Health Care, 6*(4), 1–17.

Suggested Reading

You may wish to review the following recommended occupational therapy literature describing earlier community-based programming of the 1960s, 1970s, and 1980s; the "needs" for many of the programs described here are still with us today.

Auerbach, E. (1974). Community involvement: The Bernal. *American Journal of Occupational Therapy, 28*(5), 272-273.

Bartlett, M. (1977). A community therapist in Alaska. *American Journal of Occupational Therapy, 31*(8), 485-487.

Braun, K. L., & Wake, W. (1988). Community long term care: PT/OT involvement in patient rehabilitation and maintenance. In E. Taira (Ed.), *Community programs for the health impaired elderly* (pp. 5-19). New York: The Haworth Press.

Broekema, M. C., Danz, K. H., & Schloemer, C. U. (1975). Occupational therapy in a community aftercare program. *American Journal of Occupational Therapy, 29*(1), 22–27.

Burnett, S., & Yerxa, E. (1980). Community-based and college-based needs assessment of physically disabled persons. *American Journal of Occupational Therapy, 34*(3), 201-207.

Cantwell, J. L. (1970). The community-junior college: Challenges to occupational therapy education. *American Journal of Occupational Therapy, XXIV*(8), 576-578.

Cermak, S. (1976). Community-based learning in occupational therapy. *American Journal of Occupational Therapy, 30*(3), 157-161.

Christiansen, C. H., & Davidson, D. A. (1974). A community health program with low achieving adolescents. *American Journal of Occupational Therapy, 28*(6), 346-350.

Coleman, W. (1975). Occupational therapy and child abuse. *American Journal of Occupational Therapy, 29*(7), 412-417.

Covey, S. (1970). Occupational therapy in the community. *American Journal of Occupational Therapy, XXIV*(7), 508-509.

Cromwell, F. S., & Kielhofner, G. (1976). An educational strategy for occupational therapy community service at the University of Southern California. *American Journal of Occupational Therapy, 30*(10), 629-633.

DeMars, P. K. (1975). Training adult retardates for private enterprise. *American Journal of Occupational Therapy, 29*(1), 39-42.

DePoy, E. (1987). Community-based occupational therapy with a head-injured adult. *American Journal of Occupational Therapy, 41*(7), 461-464.

Fazio, L. S. (1988). Sexuality and aging: A community wellness program. In E. Taira (Ed.), *Community programs for the health impaired elderly* (pp. 59-70). New York: The Haworth Press.

Finn, G. L. (1972). The occupational therapist in prevention programs. *American Journal of Occupational Therapy, 26*, 59-66.

Grossman, J. (1971). Community experience for students. *American Journal of Occupational Therapy, 28*(1), 589-591.

Grossman, J. (1977). Preventive health care and community programming. *American Journal of Occupational Therapy, 31*(6), 351-354.

Hasselkus, B. R., & Brown, M. (1983). Respite care for community elderly. *American Journal of Occupational Therapy, 37*(2), 83-88.

Hightower, M. (1974). A part of the community—rehabilitation—or apart from the community. *American Journal of Occupational Therapy, 28*(5), 296-298.

Hoff, S. (1988). The occupational therapist as case manager in an adult day healthcare setting. In E. Taira (Ed.), *Community programs for the health impaired elderly* (pp. 21-31). New York, NY: The Haworth Press.

Holmes, C., & Bauer, W. (1970). Establishing an occupational therapy department in a community hospital. *American Journal of Occupational Therapy, XXIV*(3), 219-221.

Howe, M., & Dippy, K. (1968). The role of occupational therapy in community mental health. *American Journal of Occupational Therapy, XXII*(6), 521-524.

Howe, M., Weaver, C., & Dulay, J. (1981). The development of a work-oriented day center program. *American Journal of Occupational Therapy, 35*(11), 711-718.

Hurff, J. M., Poulsen, M. K., Van Hoven, J., & Olson, S. (198). A library skills program serving adults with mental retardation: An interdisciplinary approach. *American Journal of Occupational Therapy, 39*(4), 233-239.

Johnson, J., & Smith, M. (1966). Changing concepts of occupational therapy in a community rehabilitation center. *American Journal of Occupational Therapy, XX*(6), pp. 267-273.

Laukaran, V. H. (1977). Toward a model of occupational therapy for community health. *American Journal of Occupational Therapy, 31*(2), 71-74.

Llorens, L. (1971). Occupational therapy in community child health. *American Journal of Occupational Therapy, XXV*(7), 335-339.

Magrun, W. M., & Tigges, K. N. (1982). A transdisciplinary mobile intervention program for rural areas. *American Journal of Occupational Therapy, 36*(2), 90-94.

Maguire, G. A. (1979). Volunteer program to assist the elderly to remain in home settings. *American Journal of Occupational Therapy, 33*(2), 98–101.

Maynard, M. (1986). Health promotion through employee assistance programs: A role for occupational therapists. *American Journal of Occupational Therapy, 40*(11), 771-776.

McColl, M., & Quinn, B. (1985). A quality assurance method for community occupational therapy. *American Journal of Occupational Therapy, 39*(9), 570-577.

Neistadt, M., & Marques, K. (1984). An independent living skills training program. *American Journal of Occupational Therapy, 38*(10), 671-676.

Neistadt, M., & O'Reilly, M. (1988). Independent living skills groups in a level 1 fieldwork experience. *American Journal of Occupational Therapy, 42*(12), 782-786.

Nochajski, S. B., & Gordon, C. Y. (1987). The use of Trivial Pursuit in teaching community living skills to adults with developmental disabilities. *American Journal of Occupational Therapy, 41*(1), 10-15.

Shalik, L. D., & Shalik, H. (1987). Cluster homes: A community for profoundly and severely retarded persons. *American Journal of Occupational Therapy, 41*(4), 222-226.

Stein, F. (1972). Community rehabilitation of disadvantaged youth. *American Journal of Occupational Therapy, 26*(6), 277-283.

Tickle, L. S., & Yerxa, E. (1981). Need satisfaction of older persons living in the community and in institutions, Part 1: the environment. *American Journal of Occupational Therapy, 35*(10), 644-649.

Tickle, L. S., & Yerxa, E. (1981). Need satisfaction of older persons living in the community and in institutions, Part 2: role of activity. *American Journal of Occupational Therapy, 35*(10), 650-655.

Walker, L. (1971). Occupational therapy in the well community. *American Journal of Occupational Therapy, XXV*(7), 345-347.

West, W. A. (1967). The occupational therapist's changing responsibility to the community. *American Journal of Occupational Therapy, XXI*(5), 312-316.

West, W. A. (1969). The growing importance of prevention. *American Journal of Occupational Therapy, 23*, 226-231.

Wiemer, R. B. (1972). Some concepts of prevention as an aspect of community health. *American Journal of Occupational Therapy, 26*(1), 1-9.

Wiemer, R. B., & West, W. A. (1970). Occupational therapy in community health care. *American Journal of Occupational Therapy, 24*(5), 323-328.

You may wish to review the following recommended readings relative to community-centered occupational therapy practice published in the 1990s:

Baum, C., & Law, M. (Eds.). (1998). Special issue on community health. *American Journal of Occupational Therapy, 52*(1), 7-77.

Brownson, C. A. (1998). Funding community practice: Stage 1. *American Journal of Occupational Therapy, 52*(1), 60-64.

Bumphrey, E. E. (1995). The role of occupational therapy in health promotion. In E. E. Bumphrey (Ed.), *Community practice: A text for occupational therapists and others involved in community care* (pp. 68-78). London, UK: Prentice Hall.

Burkhardt, A. (1997). Occupational therapy and wellness. *OT Practice, 2*(6), 28-35.

Camardese, M. B., & Youngman, D. (1996). H.O.P.E.: Education, employment, and people who are homeless and mentally ill. *Psychiatric Rehabilitation Journal, 19*(4), 45-56.

Crist, P., & Stoffel, V. (1992). The Americans with Disabilities Act of 1990 and employees with mental impairments: personal efficacy and the environment. *American Journal of Occupational Therapy, 46*(5), 434-443.

DeMaus, P. (1992). An occupational therapy life skills curriculum model for a Native American tribe: A health promotion program based on ethnographic field research. *American Journal of Occupational Therapy, 46*(8), 727-736.

Devereaux, E. (1991). The issue is: Community-based practice. *American Journal of Occupational Therapy, 45*(10), 944-946.

Dunn, W., Brown, C., & McGuigan, A. (1994). The ecology of human performance: A framework for considering the effect of context. *American Journal of Occupational Therapy, 48*, 595-607.

Gage, M., & Polatajko, H. (1994). Enhancing occupational performance through an understanding of perceived self-efficacy. *American Journal of Occupational Therapy, 48*(5), 452-461.

Giles, G. (1994). Editorial: Why provide community support for persons with brain injury? *American Journal of Occupational Therapy, 48*(4), 255-296.

Grady, A. P. (1995). Building inclusive community: A challenge for occupational therapy: 1994 Eleanor Clarke Slagle Lecture. *American Journal of Occupational Therapy, 49*, 300-310.

Greene, D. (1997). The use of service learning in client environments to enhance ethical reasoning in students. *American Journal of Occupational Therapy, 51*(10), 844-852.

Hurff, J. M., Lowe, H. E., Ho, B. J., & Hoffman, N. M. (1990). Networking: A successful linkage for community occupational therapists. *American Journal of Occupational Therapy, 44*(5), 424-430.

Ingstad, B. (1990). The disabled person in the community: Social and cultural perspectives. *International Journal of Rehabilitation Research, 13,* 187-194.

Kari, N., & Michels, P. (1991). The Lazarus Project: The politics of empowerment. *American Journal of Occupational Therapy, 45*(8), 719-725.

Lysack, C., Stadnyk, R., Paterson, M., McLeod, K., & Krefting, L. (1995). Professional expertise of occupational therapists in community practice: Results of an Ontario survey. *Canadian Journal of Occupational Therapy, 62,* 138-147.

Oliver, M. (1990). *The politics of disablement.* London, UK: MacMillan.

Parker, M. G., & Thorslund, M. (1991). The use of technical aids among community-based elderly. *American Journal of Occupational Therapy, 45*(8), 712-718.

Peloquin, S. M., & Christiansen, C. (Eds.). (1997). Special issue on occupation, spirituality, and life meaning. *American Journal of Occupational Therapy, 51*(3), 167-237.

Pizzi, M. (1992). Hospice: The creation of meaning for people with life threatening illness. *OT Practice, 4*(1), 1-7.

Reitz, S. M. (1992). A historical review of occupational therapy's role in preventive health and wellness. *American Journal of Occupational Therapy, 46,* 50-55.

Robnett, R. (1997). Paradigms of community practice. *OT Practice,* May, 30-35.

Ryan, S. (1993). The role of the COTA as an activities director. In S. Ryan (Ed.), *Practice issues in occupational therapy education* (pp. 193-204). Thorofare, NJ: SLACK Incorporated.

Schelly, C., Sample, P., & Spencer, K. (1992). The Americans With Disabilities Act of 1990 expands employment opportunities for persons with developmental disabilities. *American Journal of Occupational Therapy, 46*(5), 457-460.

Siebert, C. (1997). A description of fieldwork in the home care setting. *American Journal of Occupational Therapy, 51*(6), 423-429.

Spencer, J. (1991). An ethnographic study of independent living alternatives. *American Journal of Occupational Therapy, 45*(3), 243-250.

Vanier, C., & Hebert, M. (1995). An occupational therapy course on community practice. *Canadian Journal of Occupational Therapy, 62* 76-81.

Voas, R. (1997). Drinking and driving prevention in the community: Program planning and implementation. *Addiction, 92*(Suppl 2), S201-S219.

Welberding, D. (1991). The quarterway house: More than an alternative of care. *OT in Mental Health, 11*(1), 65-91.

Wood, W. (Ed.). (1998). Special issue on occupation-centered research. *American Journal of Occupational Therapy, 52*(6), 399-491.

3

Program Design and Development
What Skills Will I Need?

Fazio, L. S. *Developing Occupation-Centered Programs With the Community, Third Edition* (pp 41-58).
© 2017 Taylor & Francis Group.

KEY TERMS

1. Program/programming
2. Consensus organizing/community building
3. Communication
4. Effective/active listening
5. Mindfulness
6. Negotiation
7. Persuasion
8. Clinical reasoning
9. Partnering/collaboration
10. Leader/leadership
11. Leader/manager

This chapter focuses on learning to identify the skills and information the planner will need to design and develop a program. Youngstrom (1999) defines **program** as "a specifically designed service that is aimed toward a specific goal and is designed to achieve clearly defined outcomes or results" (p. 129). Specificity is important to this definition because, through specificity, we are able to produce program results that are clear and measurable. A program designed by an occupational therapy practitioner may take several directions. For example, it may be therapeutic in its intent—that is, designed to provide therapy for those in need of therapeutic intervention. This intervention, the provision of occupational therapy, may include identification of specific needs (or screening), assessment, treatment, and evaluation for individuals of any age. Of course, programming of this nature may be developed to provide a new service not offered previously, or it may be developed to extend service or fill a gap in services in an existing occupational therapy department. Extending new service for an existing program or enhancing present programming is often the first venture for new occupational therapists.

You will find the term **programming** commonly used in this text to denote the step-by-step orchestrated process of designing and developing a program; it may also be used to indicate the day-to-day format of service provision. Although occupation-centered programs may be intended to solve problems, the order followed in planning programs for people is not always linear and, at times, may seem less than logical. When an opportunity presents itself (such as a chance to meet with stakeholders), we do not say "no" even though our literature review is still to be completed.

Occupation-centered programs may also be developed for individuals who are not candidates for therapy as defined by the need for treatment of disability or disease. Rather, because of life circumstances largely beyond their control, they are considered to be at risk for developing destructive life patterns that may diminish their opportunities for quality experiences. Although programs for these populations may also involve screening and assessment, the intention is not to offer therapy. Screening and assessments are conducted to determine where the development of skills and the acquisition of knowledge and information will be required in order to reduce or diminish the potential for problems. Programs targeting the acquisition of skills, knowledge, and information neutralize risk. Whether our intentions are to provide therapy, to prevent problems by reducing risk, or to maintain health and wellness, the belief in occupation connects us.

Programs may also be designed to enhance and reinforce already present positive development. Because of occupational therapy practitioners' educational foundation and experience, programs can be carefully tailored to the specific needs of the individual. The understanding of occupation as an outcome of an intricate system comprising the individual's values, interests, needs, and wants offers a unique perspective to programming not found in other professions. An appreciation of the intricacies of occupation coupled with a practical foundation in the analysis of tasks permits the occupational therapy practitioner to match the teaching of skills with the acquisition of abilities for positive occupation-centered outcomes. An occupation-centered perspective offers a particularly unique contribution to the development of programming for "at-risk" populations as well as programs targeting the maintenance of health. Programs designed by those with education and experience in occupation-centered perspectives can then be successfully adapted to any population in need of services. Ohmer and DeMasi (2009) offer an additional option for programmers, and that is what they refer to as **consensus organizing** (pp. 13-16). Consensus organizing is one approach to community organizing. Community organizing is not a new way to work within communities. Saul Alinsky (1946, 1971) is likely the founder of community organizing, which was initiated with the primary goal of conflict organizing. The method was intended to empower a community through the development of "people's organizations" in which members of the community with similar interests would come together to confront and make demands on the existing power structure to create improvements for the whole community (Eichler, 2007). This kind of **community building** has as its primary intention the recognition of a community's assets and strengths, building toward empowerment, and connecting the community to outside resources to develop collaborative partnerships with neighborhood stakeholders (Ohmer & DeMasi, 2009). When we go into a community to design and develop a program, we may often find that community building is required to not only encourage participatory action from members, but also to ensure sustainability. Community building is discussed more fully in Chapter 9.

The actual process of program development is a bit like solving a puzzle: one piece placed at a time, and the placement of each piece demanding our knowledge, skill, and expertise. To help select the first piece of the puzzle, we might ask, "Just what do I need to know to begin the process of designing and developing a community program?" The answers are fairly simple. To begin, we need to know the following:

- How to communicate clearly and effectively
- How to listen
- How to collaborate and negotiate
- How to resolve conflict
- How to serve as a role model of occupational balance
- How to keep "occupation" as the core of our work
- How to provide leadership to empower others
- How to manage systems

To complete the package, we need the following:

- A solid occupational therapy professional education
- Strong professional and personal ethics
- Good common sense
- Energy and motivation to try something new

THE SKILL OF BECOMING AN EFFECTIVE COMMUNICATOR

The first skill—or perhaps we should say, the prerequisite skill—is to be an effective communicator. Most of us can communicate well enough to get the things we need and sometimes the things we want, but all of us can use some help in communicating effectively in many and varied situations. Effective **communication** is a skill to be learned, and we need to identify and practice the skills of finding and utilizing efficient and sufficient language to communicate our ideas with optimal results. This is the key to begin marketing our program. Sometimes we market/promote our ideas to the community itself and sometimes we first engage with representatives of the larger community through organizations or agencies. These various venues require different kinds of communication. Communication is a process. It is relational and heavily symbolic. To communicate effectively, it is necessary to understand the demands of both "sending" and "receiving" messages simultaneously (Adler, Elmhorst, & Lucas, 2013). The planner must be as competent as possible in all kinds of communication: dyadic, small-group, organizational, public, and sometimes mass. Understanding differences and similarities in the communication styles of cultures and cocultures and how to communicate in varying contexts is also critical to successful communication. An awareness of ethnicity and race, regional differences, sexual orientation and gender identity, religion, and ability/disability is foundational to effective communication or, at least, nonoffensive communication. The planner, from the beginning, is using communication to build and broker relationships. Every communication, large or small, is important.

Exercise 3-1

Practicing Communicating With the Listener: Your Definition of Occupation and Occupational Therapy

It is likely that, on many occasions, you will have to explain who you are and what you do as an occupational therapy practitioner. Perhaps you will explain this to those who you hope will welcome your programming ideas in their organization, and this may involve explaining your plans to other professionals. Somewhere in this process of introduction, you will explain to consumers. Although many of the people with whom you come in contact or wish to collaborate will have an idea of what occupational therapy is (perhaps from the roots of the words themselves or from personal experience), it is unlikely that many will appreciate the diversity in practice exhibited by the profession. This may particularly be the case if you choose to develop community-based programming targeting prevention or maintenance.

If one of your student experiences has provided the opportunity to explain occupational therapy to a group outside of the profession, you have a head start on this exercise. Experienced practitioners have likely developed their own definitions of occupational therapy; however, these definitions are usually tailored to a particular practice niche. If you, as the practitioner, are entertaining thoughts of designing and developing a program for a new niche, you may want to expand or change your definitions.

1. In your textbooks or the professional literature, find a definition or definitions of *occupation*. Write the definitions here (use additional paper if you need more space):

_____

_____

_____

_____

_____

Now do the same for *occupational therapy*:

_____

_____

_____

_____

_____

2. Using a highlighter, note key words that you find meaningful in the definitions of *occupation* and *occupational therapy*. Write those words:

_____

_____

_____

_____

_____

3. Review the key words you selected. You may have included words such as "participation" and "engagement." These are important considerations in community-based and community-centered practices. Use the words you have chosen to write your own definition of *occupational therapy*—a definition by which you, as a practitioner, would like to be identified. Remember to keep your definition broad and not specific to only one kind of practice or one kind of practitioner (e.g., occupational therapist or occupational therapy assistant). Write your definition here:

_____

_____

_____

_____

_____

4. Write your definition of what occupational therapists or occupational therapy assistants do (what you wish to do). Again, keep your perspective broad and avoid listing specific skills or roles. Begin to think of yourself as an occupation-centered practitioner. Write your definition here:

_____

_____

_____

_____

_____

5. Using the definition you developed, translate it to use in the following scenarios:
   (a) You wish to start a summer day camp for children who have been identified by parents and/or educators as emotionally or socially immature. It is not your expectation that any of the children will carry a diagnosis, but all may be seen to be "at risk." You have been asked by a mother, who is interested in your program, "What does an occupational therapist do?" and, "What can you do for my child?"
   (b) You have been asked by the pastor of your church to help start a program for young women who have come to the church's outreach center for sanctuary from human trafficking/prostitution. You believe an occupation-centered program may be an answer for these women.

In dyads or small groups, roleplay the two scenarios. Discuss and write your responses here. (You should also provide a verbal explanation. Remember to use the definition or definitions you developed in Question 4 to structure your answer to the question.)

_____

_____

_____

_____

_____

6. Continue the exercise by applying the following scenario:

You have at least partially won the trust of the mother in the first scenario, who now invites you to the Parent-Teacher Association meeting to talk about occupational therapy. You can assume that most of the audience will be interested in what occupational therapy can do for children, so you may wish to focus on this aspect. Consider how and why the children mentioned earlier may be at risk and what kinds of assistance your camp might offer. This is likely your first opportunity to begin marketing your proposed camp program for at-risk children to a large audience, so you might also wish to include how mothers might recognize whether their children would be good candidates for your camp. This one may be a bit challenging because there are several considerations that may be outside of your previous experience. You may wish to first discuss it with classmates. Share your earlier definitions. When you are ready, briefly write what you might say differently to this group and how your presentation style might be different. When you have written your responses, roleplay your brief presentation to the group.

_____

_____

_____

_____

_____

For scenario b, you have the opportunity to present your ideas to the pastor, the volunteers at the outreach center, and two influential members of the church congregation. Will you be able to articulate what you believe you can offer?

_____

_____

_____

_____

_____

7. Try different groups with different interests, and critique each other in your responses. Maintain the essence of what occupation and occupational therapy is and what occupation-centered practitioners do.

You may want to follow your preliminary response with some specific purposes related to the different groups you are targeting, but resist the temptation to drift into splintered definitions appropriate to only very specific populations. Rather, think about your definitions in a broad way: What does all of occupational therapy have in common? What do all occupational therapy practitioners strive to do regardless of their clientele? You may wish to direct some of your responses to the specific concerns of your audience; however, if you find yourself explaining how to evaluate joint range or reciting the basic tenets of sensory integration, start again! Use this space to make any notes you may need to structure your brief responses to new scenarios:

_____

_____

_____

_____

_____

Although critical, learning how to express our ideas and thoughts in a clear and succinct manner is only one aspect of communication. Often, when we are new to practice, we become so concerned with trying to communicate our ideas (particularly to patients, clients, and caregivers) that we forget to listen or are unable to do so.

THE POWER OF LISTENING

In *Effective Coaching*, Marshall J. Cook (1999) tells us that perhaps the best thing we can do for another person is to give that person our full undivided attention. We all have attempted to talk with someone who was shuffling through papers, talking to someone else, or gazing off somewhere. If you are unable to drop everything to listen to someone who needs your attention, it is best to be honest and ask that person to return when you are able to listen. It is a human tendency to engage in overlapping occupations, but the listening aspect of communication requires and deserves full attention, whether the speaker is a child, adult, client, coworker, or friend.

In his discussion of **effective listening,** Cook (1999) goes on to say that we must let the speaker finish before responding (pp. 70-77). It is easy to interrupt when we think we know the intent of the communication. In therapy environments, where we often hear similar questions and concerns from our patients/clients, the tendency to believe that we already know the outcome of a client's communication may be particularly troublesome. Often, we manipulate speakers when we interrupt or finish their sentences, particularly if they are not assertive enough to stop us. For many cultures, the therapist/professional represents a powerful authority position, and it would not be easy (and probably impossible) for the patient/client to redirect the communication. Of further note, listening to the needs of a "community" or population is critical to an effective assessment of programming need and successful outcomes. Individuals may reflect this information, but often the listener must be attuned to a larger, collective voice to ensure that all members are equally represented.

Adler and Elmhorst (2010) describe mindful and mindless listening. Mindless listening (reacting to messages automatically and routinely) can be efficient and useful at times, but mindful listening is needed in most of our communications. Jon Kabat-Zinn (2003) offers an operational working definition of mindfulness as "the awareness that emerges through paying attention on purpose, in the present moment, and nonjudgmentally to the unfolding of experience moment by moment (p. 144). In the context of listening, it is giving careful and thoughtful attention and responses to the messages we receive. **Mindfulness** is not a new concept. It is a meditation-based practice used to enhance the focus and general well-being of individuals. It can be used as a therapeutic tool as well as a personal growth experience. McKay, Wood, and Brantley (2007) devote several chapters of their *Dialectical Behavior Therapy Skills Workbook* to understanding and utilizing mindfulness skills. For a good, basic introduction, you may wish to read Langer's 1989 book titled *Mindfulness*. There is little doubt that being mindful will enhance your communication skills as a therapist and programmer. Your interviewing skills will also improve, as well as your ability to run a focus group as you develop your needs assessment process.

When you are using "listening" in your communications, be mindful and ask yourself, "Am I listening to understand the speaker (or) listening to critically evaluate the message that is being sent?" Covey (1989) tells us to first "seek to understand, then to be understood" (p. 235). Listen first, make sure you understand, then evaluate the message content. When you are listening to evaluate, analyze the speaker's evidence as well as his or her emotional appeals (Adler & Elmhorst, 2010, p. 85).

Other characteristics of effective listening include hearing, reflecting, and rephrasing. In the counseling professions, the term **active listening** (i.e., listening for the emotional/feeling content as well as the information that is being provided by the speaker) might be used to collectively describe these characteristics. Active listening might include the following:

- Hearing the actual words
- Talking and interrupting less than you might like
- Reflecting on and rephrasing what was communicated
- Paraphrasing/restating a speaker's ideas in your own words; content, intent, and feeling
- Asking sincere questions
- Hearing the emotional/feeling content as well as the information

If you would like to practice, there are many exercises to encourage active listening that your instructor may choose to provide, or these may be included in other aspects of your curriculum.

In summary, active listening describes the ability to hear and to mindfully listen with total consciousness to the words that are being spoken and also to the meaning and emotional content our speaker is expressing. This ability not only makes us good friends and desirable companions, but it is also absolutely critical to our varied roles as therapists and as programmers/planners.

Whether we are speaking to an employee, a consumer, the owner of a building we would like to lease for our program, or a granting agency board, we must express our ideas clearly and listen fully. It is a skill to be learned. In a global world where communications are often online, there are some additional considerations to employ: (1) if you receive a troublesome message, reread and share with someone you trust; (2) decide whether to respond; (3) do not respond right away; and (4) compose your reply offline (Adler, Rodman, & duPre, 2014).

USING YOUR COMMUNICATION SKILLS TO GET THINGS DONE

According to *International Webster New Encyclopedic Dictionary* (1975), to *negotiate* means "to confer or bargain, one with another, in order to reach an agreement." It is unlikely that you will move through your program design and development process without some **negotiation.** Negotiation does not necessarily mean compromise; it is important to keep this in mind as we develop our goals and objectives for programming. Our identified need for services and our related goals will continue to remind us of our directive to provide quality programming in ethical ways. If some compromise must occur, it will not be within these dimensions. Shapiro and Jankowski (1998), authors of *The Power of Nice*, put a bit of a spin on *Webster's* definition of negotiation by stating that "the best way to get what you want is to help the other side get what they want" (p. 3). The multiple levels of the needs assessment (discussed in Chapters 7 and 8) will give us at least the surface characteristics of what is "wanted" for our targeted population by the community, the organization, or the facility for which we may provide service, and the various stakeholders, including those who will actually receive the services. Our ability to actively and effectively listen will allow us to identify the more subtle wants that may not necessarily be articulated by these groups.

Jay Conger (1998) adds another characteristic of communication to the negotiation mix—the art of **persuasion.** He states that effective persuasion "is the ability to present a message in a way that leads others to support it" (p. 25). Adler and Elmhorst (2010) talk about the need for ethical persuasion. According to these authors, ethical persuasion is the act of motivating an audience, through effective communication, to voluntarily change a particular belief, attitude, or behavior. They go on to say that those who wish to "persuade" are encouraged to maximize their credibility (this is the persuasive force that comes from the audience's belief in and respect for the speaker).

How do we, as programmers, build credibility? Just like anyone else who wishes to persuade, we demonstrate our competence, know our subject, earn the trust of our audience through honesty, and emphasize our similarity to the audience (most particularly in our commitment to shared goals) (Adler & Elmhorst, 2010, p. 413). How do we prepare for audience persuasion? Whether you are speaking to a group of stakeholders, the city council, potential funders, or all of these, there are some very practical things you can do to ensure your effectiveness. First, know that some anxiety is a given and that you may feel more relaxed if you walk around before the presentation. Also, do not eat just before speaking, and avoid both alcohol and caffeine. Choose comfortable and familiar clothing that makes you feel and look good. Rehearse in front of friends or colleagues and make bullet points to follow, but do not write down every word. Look up and make occasional eye contact with friendly faces. Last, you are sharing what you know with people who want to know it too, and you believe in the importance of what you are sharing (Adler & Elmhorst, 2010, p. 393).

In seeking to persuade others, it is in our interest to first influence and then to convince them to support our ideas and plans for a community program. We also do not want to lose sight of the fact that our ideas and plans have been, in part, generated directly from our needs assessment so that we will be on target with what our shareholders want and expect.

Interestingly enough, as we expand our ideas regarding negotiation in the design and development of community programs, we are also talking about the skills that are relevant, even critical, to our clinical relationships with clients/patients. This refers to a therapist's abilities to negotiate the selection of treatment goals with the client/patient, or what in the past we may have referred to as *motivating* the recipient of services. We probably cannot truly motivate patients/clients because they must do that for themselves; rather, we negotiate and persuade and do so within carefully structured environments that are motivating.

Mattingly and Fleming (1994) provide another window of understanding for this intricate and delicate client/patient/therapist negotiation in what they describe as *interactive reasoning,* or collaborating with the person. They provide numerous examples of how therapists demonstrate skill in learning to interact with their clients/patients (i.e., how they "collaborate"). The therapist's ability to interpret what a person wants from therapy and the meaning that person attaches to the progress he or she wishes to make is perhaps the highest level of communication-based negotiation we could identify in our therapy process, and it is significant in our understanding of what Mattingly and Fleming describe as **clinical reasoning.** Clinical reasoning is a complex process involving at least three approaches: procedural reasoning, interactive reasoning, and conditional reasoning. Fleming (1994) collectively refers to the mobilization of these processes in collaboration and treatment as the "therapist with the three-track mind" (p. 119). As mentioned previously, it is likely interactive reasoning that best engages the therapist and the patient/client in the negotiation process through a true collaboration. Successful collaboration is at the root of effective intervention, whether with one person or many.

Partnering: Developing Collaborative Relationships

We know that collaborating with other professionals, agencies, organizations, and community members strengthens our ability to provide programming that is relevant, efficient, and effective; however, in today's climate, that may not be enough. The term **partnering** better describes what must occur in order to work effectively and to obtain funding. Karsh and Fox (2003) tell us that, to turn a good idea into a winning program (that will be funded), the right partners must be actively involved (p. 150). **Collaboration** is a term that we are all familiar with, but in reality, it is a concept and set of behaviors that most of us find quite difficult. In his book, *No More Teams!*, Schrage (1989) suggests that most Americans support the idea of being a team player, but they often prefer to be the captain. Rugged individualism begins, for most of us, in kindergarten. Very few people have much experience at true collaboration (i.e., sitting down with the intent of working with others [individuals, groups, organizations] and making a commitment to finding the best possible solution to the problem). However, the more that people with expertise and varying points of view are sincerely committed to developing a solution to a pressing problem, the more likely it is that the solution (the programming) will be developed and developed with quality. In community programming, our partners may include other health care practitioners, teachers, school administrators, universities, museums, city parks and recreation, the police department, the fire department, the chamber of commerce, parents, and consumers, to name a few. Negotiating collaborations and partnerships will likely challenge our communication styles, our ability to listen, and our knowledge base, but the rewards will be well worth the extra effort.

This may be a good place to introduce something that often occurs when we want to collaborate—namely conflicts. Conflicts are inevitable no matter how carefully we craft our needs assessment. In fact, the conduct and results of the "on-the-ground" needs assessment are most often where we begin to identify conflicts that may arise, and we can be prepared for them. Here, we return to our earlier look at negotiation. Fisher and Ury (1981) tell us that handling conflicts constructively is a negotiation where two or more parties or groups discuss specific proposals to find a mutually acceptable agreement or outcome. Of course, what we want for the protection of communities is a ""win-win" situation, where everyone is satisfied (Fisher & Ury, 1981, p. 143). Katz and Lawyer (1994) suggest that conflicts may occur at several places in a negotiation: over the topic at hand (what to do), the process (how to do it), relational issues (how parties will work together and how they want to be treated by one another), and ego/identity issues (perceived competence, honesty, commitment and fairness) (p. 137).

If conflicts are inevitable, then managing conflicts and negotiating successful working relationships is another addition to our skill set. How do we respond to conflicts? We can "avoid" them. Katz and Lawyer (1994) and Fisher and Ury (1981) suggest that sometimes the issue may be simply too trivial to deal with or the gains too small and short-term. We may decide to accommodate to build social credits when harmony and stability are more important than our "being right," or "getting what we want at the time." If a quick, decisive action is needed (in a situation that, if ignored, would lead to an emergency), we may do what is described as "competitive competing" and take the action or make the decision (Katz & Lawyer, 1994, p. 141).

We have talked about collaborating, and this may be seen as the best action; particularly if we can assume that it is possible to meet most of the expressed needs. "Compromise" often has to occur in collaborations, and this is when parties involved give up something that they had hoped to attain. With stakeholders in community programming, this is often a difficult agreement for the programmer to negotiate and may take the services of additional conflict managers/negotiators to resolve.

PREPARING TO NEGOTIATE

When you are ready to negotiate, it is often best to focus on the means (ways of achieving your goals) rather than ends (the goals or outcomes that you want). Fisher and Ury (1981) list the following for the negotiator to consider:

- Clarify the interests and needs of all parties
- Consider the best time to raise the issues
- Consider differences between the parties involved, including culture
- Encourage all parties to prepare statements outlining what they want to achieve from the negotiation

In actually conducting the negotiation, consider the following:

- Identify the ends all parties are seeking
- Together, brainstorm a list of possible solutions
- Evaluate alternative solutions together
- Implement and follow up on the solutions; try them out

Exercise 3-2

Practicing Negotiation

1. In small groups, try your hand at negotiation. Two people will roleplay something in their lives that is causing a conflict or potential conflict (it can be something as seemingly simple as which housemate/roommate will cook and which one will clean up). Use the structure suggested earlier, and all members of the group can contribute. The structure of this negotiation will not be unlike what you may do in the future when you are negotiating programming and outcomes with and between stakeholders.

_____

_____

_____

_____

_____

LEADING AND MANAGING

All of the previously mentioned skills come together in helping us to identify ourselves as **leaders** and **managers**—two qualities significant to the role of community program planner and facilitator. We will first examine your present management skills and your potential to become a manager. The first task of good managers is to manage themselves and their own round of daily occupations.

Managing "Yourself" First

Do you currently represent yourself as a model for a healthy balance of occupations? Take a moment to reflect on your response and perhaps those of your classmates or colleagues. In particular, students are likely to say that they do not have enough time in the day or week and that they find themselves studying to the exclusion of leisure and self-care. Time, of course, is not infinite. It is likely that we do not manage time; rather, time manages us, but we are not victims. If we begin by making a daily, weekly, or monthly map of the way we spend our time, then we can learn to manage ourselves within the time we have available. These skills need to be learned as students. If we do not manage to balance our occupations today, it is not likely that we will later, and our future as managers may be in jeopardy.

Mapping Time for Engagement in Daily/Weekly Occupations

On a separate piece of paper, using the pie in Figure 3-1 to represent the time available to you in a day or a week and using colored markers or pencils to separate work/productive activity, play/leisure, and self-care, draw a slice in the pie to represent the percentage of time you require for each of these categories.

Figure 3-1. Pie graph of daily occupations.

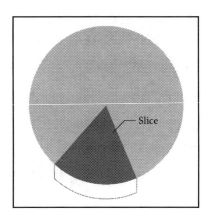

We have not attempted to define meaning in daily occupations, but this is implicit as we move on with this exercise. What occupations/activities have meaning for you, and which ones do not? It is likely that we feel more balanced when we have a distribution of meaningful and meaningless activities in our day. After all, most of us cannot attend to a totally meaningful existence. It would be exhausting!

What about play/leisure? Is it important to you to play every day? Do you need that balance? It does not matter what activity you choose to represent play; that will depend on your values and interests and how you establish meaning in your life. Play may mean tossing a ball against a wall or rolling it to your cat; perhaps play means running three miles, engaging in sex, cooking, or another activity of choice. According to Sutton-Smith (1997) adult play may take many forms to include fantasy ventures celebrated in games of chance, war games, and fantasy festivals. Many people today enjoy dressing up as movie, TV, or gaming characters. This is termed cos- (costume-) play. You may want to dust off your light saber and Jedi robe and make your way to WonderCon.

Although it commonly may be considered self-care, taking a bath or a shower uninterrupted is pure leisure for some, particularly for those with small children. If it is important in order for you to feel balanced, then draw in the time you spend doing it. If it is not important, if it does not hold meaning for you, or if you do not consider it true play/leisure, then leave it out of your map under this category. After all, one person's play may be another person's work or self-care. In mapping time for work, again, it is important to recognize how much overlap plays a part in assigning meaning to occupations. For many people, their work is also their play, and even though to others they appear to work to the exclusion of play, in reality, they may feel quite balanced.

Review your "pie" and take a careful look at what you have. Is there any activity in which you regularly engage that is missing? Is there anything you deem to be truly meaningful missing? Critically evaluate your map. You probably look more balanced in your daily/weekly occupations than you might have expected, and you probably have some empty space to use as you choose (play, self-care, and/or work). The human animal is fairly self-protective. We are skilled at balancing our occupations even when, at times, we believe ourselves to be balance-impoverished.

Remember this exercise and complete it whenever you feel unsettled regarding your balance of occupation(s). You may need to re-examine your priorities. Priorities change frequently when we are goal directed and as we move from one context to another. Are your priorities appropriate to what you wish to achieve? Do you have enough "good" stress in your life (stress that you can successfully manage)? We need good, manageable stress to build efficacy, but not relentless stress that is out of our control. This kind of stress makes us sick and shortens our lives.

Now that you have completed the previous exercises, you should have a better sense of your *priorities* and how these priorities influence your personal balance of occupations. You have identified your communication strengths as well as those areas where you may need to do a little work on your communication skills. You now have a much better grasp of what it means to manage yourself.

THE CHARACTERISTICS OF A MANAGER/DIRECTOR

There are many resources available to you for the fundamentals of management (such as budgets, staffing, billing, and daily operations), and you will find them referenced in Part III of this text. If you are aspiring to start a community program and to manage/direct operations, then you either must be familiar with all of the expected operations of an occupational therapy department or you must have access to the services of someone who does. If you are a student, then this book is intended as a supplement to an occupational therapy professional education management and supervision course or courses rather than as a replacement for such courses.

If you are a professional but have not had the opportunity to manage a department or program, then taking the time to closely observe the manager of your place of practice is strongly recommended. Also, if possible, spend time with a mentor who is successfully operating a program such as the one you are contemplating, with the goal of understanding the management of day-to-day operations. Arranging an additional internship or externship in management would be beneficial to students who are seriously considering developing and managing programs. Of course, the intent of a community program is to offer a service or services to a targeted population. The skills involved in delivering an occupation-centered service are implicit in your professional education and any advanced coursework, specialty practice, and/or credentials you may have earned beyond your professional courses and fieldwork.

Management involves managing complex whole systems of both things and functions, but often, those who are considered to be the best managers are known for their demonstrated abilities in the management of people. In his book, *Winning 'Em Over,* Jay Conger (1998) talks about the revolution in management that was occurring in the business world at the time. This revolution was marked by a shift from a management model strongly anchored in the power of authority and hierarchy to one of persuasion and teamwork. Shapiro and Jankowski (1998) echoed those thoughts in their book, *The Power of Nice.* At this writing, we still see indicators of attention to the needs of workers in the workplace. Perhaps most publicized have been the "worker-friendly" environments of organizations such as Google, Facebook, and the California-based outdoor gear clothing manufacturer, Patagonia. The dress code at Patagonia does not even require shoes and employees can surf during the work day (Chouinard, 2016). Has a shift actually occurred in the world of business and in the business of health care? It seems likely that the upper tiers of health care management, the tiers that represent the transition to business and corporate influence, may be struggling with the shift from power-dominated authority to a friendlier model. Although these shifts are probably not entirely voluntary, Conger and others would suggest that Generation X was a strong part of the mix, forcing a more interactive management style. Members of Generation Y have their own views regarding work, among other things. Sometimes called the "Net Generation" and the "First Globals," they were born between 1982 and 1991. They are technologically adept and like to learn by doing. They like multitasking and may ignore what does not interest them, sometimes at the expense of their work (Adler & Elmhorst, 2010; Adler et al., 2013). Members of the present "hipster" generation, however, expect moral and ethical investment for themselves and others.

As mentioned earlier, in his discussions, Conger (1998) elaborates on persuasion as a central concept for managers in developing relationships with their personnel/teams. He feels that the components of successful persuasion include "building your credibility; finding the common ground; developing compelling positions and evidence; and connecting emotionally" (pp. 43-46).

We might propose the question, "Who knows more about persuasion than the occupational therapy practitioner?" These concepts are also core to successful therapy, and the core skills we use as therapists are central to our abilities as managers, directors, and leaders. The same is true of teamwork and collaboration; occupational therapy practitioners have always seen themselves as participants in teams. For the students, working in groups represents the beginnings of the belief in teamwork as the most effective way "to get the job done." Therefore, the profession of occupational therapy has already acknowledged the importance of management by persuasion, teamwork, and collaboration.

THE CHARACTERISTICS OF A LEADER

In his discussion of **leadership**, Townsend tells us that "leadership is unique to each person" and that in his estimation, "leadership is a matter of character" (Bennis and Townsend, 1995, p. 13). Both Townsend and Bennis delineated the qualities of a good **leader** to include controlled personal ambition, intelligence, and a clear and well-articulated communication style. Many writers on leadership and management styles agree with these characteristics, particularly those centered on effective communication (Bennis & Goldsmith, 1997; Capodagli & Jackson, 1999; Conger, 1998; Cook, 1999; Shapiro & Jankowski, 1998). Writing about leadership from an occupational therapy perspective, Gilkeson (1997) described the successful leader as someone who is unique. She also noted that common traits that all leaders possess are "values, vision, communication skills, persistence, self-confidence, optimism, empathy, and observation" (1997, pp. 3-4).

Drawing a distinction between leaders and **managers**, Bennis and Goldsmith (1997) noted that "managing is about efficiency," and "leadership is about innovating and initiating" (p. 4). In their words, "leaders conquer the context" (p. 4), and the context of concern to occupational therapy practitioners—the environment of health care and health maintenance—is most certainly a flying carpet these days. To conquer it, a leader must be agile, visible, and clever.

Can the leader and the manager exist in one person? Perhaps, but it is more likely that the most comprehensive leadership is produced by a team. This team must include a charismatic and visionary leader and managers who are effective and efficient in the understanding and control of multiple systems. The team members must be ethical, loyal to their cause, skilled, and above reproach. Bennis and Goldsmith (1997) noted that the profound difference between a manager and a leader is that a "good manager does things right and a leader does the right things" (p. 4).

In some circumstances, the development of a community program may pose a risk for the developer. The luxury of taking such a risk alongside a good manager may not be financially realistic. Therefore, the programmer often must acquire the skill sets of both a leader and a manager, at least in the beginning. Certainly, the programmer is a leader; starting a new programming venture in the community, whether for profit or not for profit, would not likely occur to anyone else, but often the skills needed to manage the developing program have to be learned. Perhaps the true leader and the true manager cannot ever really exist in one person; the personalities, the ways of being and the ways of thinking, are likely different. The wise leader, though, will certainly appreciate the intricacies of management. If not able to employ a management team early on, he or she will at least consult with one as development occurs.

Early in this chapter, we discussed the importance of clear and efficient communication. The first task of the leader is to sell him- or herself as well as the proposed program, which requires the ability to engage others in the venture. Most likely, the planner/leader will need to obtain support for his or her potential program from those outside of occupational therapy, beginning the processes of collaboration and partnering. The nature of these early communications may be different from those that will follow. Soon after, though, the planner must engage the support of a team that will be carrying out the programming. The planner must gain the team members' trust and must encourage them to share in the excitement that comes with such an undertaking. The task of the leader/manager is first to recognize and then to supervise and manage the knowledge and skills of others in such a way as to form a successful and productive goal-directed team. A leader must clearly communicate his or her goals for a program and accompanying expectations for the performance of employees and others who will take responsibility. It is also critical that a leader provide honest, direct, and open feedback regarding performance and participation while not losing sight of the larger goals. A successful communicator will be able to provide honest and supportive feedback that will strengthen and empower the employee and the program. It will also be the programmer's responsibility to recognize leadership potential in others and offer encouragement and skill building. Leadership development in our communities is important to building community assets and capacity and is critical to programs that are sustainable (Green & Haines, 2016). How can we do this without some comfort with leadership ourselves?

Exercise 3-3

Reinventing Yourself as a Leader

Now that you are on your way to becoming a more effective communicator and you are developing an awareness of what skills are necessary to be an effective manager/director, you must begin the process of reinventing yourself as a leader. If you consider yourself to be a leader now, look at strengthening your capacities. Young, less experienced leaders are likely to have difficulty in delegating responsibility to a team. Not trusting anyone but yourself to do a job will lead to rapid burnout and, eventually, failure. In community programming, sustainability is achieved only when we involve the community in all aspects of the design and development process from beginning to end. We bring substantial expertise, but in most cases, the program belongs to the community. The following exercise to help you recognize and develop leadership qualities is adapted from Bennis and Goldsmith (1997):

1. What do you personally consider to be the qualities, attitudes, and behaviors of a leader? You may wish to think of those people who are considered to be leaders. List the characteristics here, and note your skills and/or attributes beside each one in that particular area:

Qualities	
(e.g., personal honesty)	Your Qualities
Attitudes	
(e.g., open/friendly)	Your Attitudes
Behaviors	
(e.g., working hard)	Your Behaviors

Carefully assess your strengths with regard to these issues. Do you have leadership qualities that will assist you in the development of new occupation-centered programs? You may wish to discuss the results of your personal assessment with others. Most people have trouble identifying their own leadership qualities and tend to minimize their strengths in this area. Your friends, colleagues, and family may be able to help.

WHAT KNOWLEDGE AND SKILLS WILL I NEED?

We have discussed ways to develop our abilities to communicate clearly and effectively, how to identify daily and weekly time use in prioritizing for occupational balance, and how to recognize and develop the characteristics that make a good leader and manager, but there is one more thing we must do. We must recognize that what we must know (knowledge) and what we must do (skills) are the foundation upon which leadership and management develop; without them we have little about which to communicate. Although we have briefly touched on the importance of meeting the needs of our targeted community population, it is imperative that we avoid soliciting needs and wants that we cannot realistically hope to satisfy. Not only would this be unethical, but it would also be enormously stressful and foolish. Experienced professionals have a good idea of their knowledge base and their skills but often still need to do some self-assessment homework in regard to the information and skills necessary to successfully design and develop a community program. This does not mean that if you identify a need in your target population but find yourself lacking in knowledge or skills that you must give up the idea for the program. What it does mean is that you must acquire the knowledge and skills yourself (mentorships/continuing self-instruction/education) or that you must engage the services of other professionals, paraprofessionals, and volunteers/community members. Identifying and encouraging expertise in your community of stakeholders will be one of your significant tasks.

Students bring a variety of skills, expertise, and experience to the learning environment, and these skills need to be identified. For students, prior experience and resulting knowledge and skills are the foundation upon which occupational therapy principles, philosophy, and practice will be placed. Unique skills, expertise, and experience often produce the entrepreneur.

Occupational therapy practitioners as well as students may over- or underestimate their expertise and may often fail to anticipate the need for adequate resources. Thus, before you initiate program design and planning, complete the following checklist. This exercise will be helpful in achieving a good sense of what you can offer to any potential program. As you develop your ideas for specific programming, it will help you to identify areas where you may need some assistance.

Exercise 3-4

Self-Assessment of Knowledge and Skills Relevant to Designing and Developing Community Programs

1. Assessing what you know: your present knowledge base
   a. Your academic knowledge base: Consider what you have studied, including your professional occupational therapy education and other disciplines you might have studied previous to or following occupational therapy that you think might assist you in designing, developing, and working in occupation-centered community practice. Highlight your academic knowledge base here:

   _____

   _____

   _____

   _____

   b. Your experiential knowledge base: Consider any previous or present experience that contributed to your present knowledge base that might assist you in designing, developing, and working in occupation-centered community practice. Such experience might include clinical practice, outcome/evaluation research, sales, managing, marketing, interacting with communities, or other areas. Highlight your knowledge gained through experience here:

   _____

   _____

   _____

   _____

2. Assessing your skills

Consider what you can do. Do you have expertise with particular modalities, tools, equipment, or assessments used in occupational therapy practice or other clinical practices? Consider any particular credentials you may have earned, certifications, and, for the practicing occupational therapy assistant, service competencies. Do you have particular expertise with arts and crafts? A sport? Music? Do you have any other skills that may not be directly related to clinical practice but that might be useful when working in the community? Remember that we are also interested in prevention of disease and disability and the maintenance of health and well-being. (*Note:* Of course the previously mentioned skills are interrelated with knowledge, but for the purposes of this exercise, we will separate them.) Highlight any skills you may have here:

_____

_____

_____

_____

_____

In later chapters, when you have selected your target population and have begun to discuss the needs they may have and the kinds of programming that will help you meet those needs, you will want to revisit these earlier lists of knowledge and skills in view of your new perspective. Remember that your programming will likely be successful only if you identify and build the skills and knowledge (assets) of your community members as well as your own.

In conclusion, when you have selected your target population and know its needs, you will do the following:

- Determine the knowledge and skills required to successfully meet the needs of the target population
- Revisit the knowledge and skills of the planner and others (to include the community) that may be involved in developing the program

The difference between these two items will tell you where you must acquire additional knowledge/skills (if realistic and if time permits) or find others to partner with (professionals, paraprofessionals, volunteers, and community members).

SUMMARY

To return to our original question, we must ask ourselves, "What do I need to know to develop a community program?" Throughout the course of this chapter, we have identified the following areas of personal responsibility in preparing the foundation for program development:

- Using clear, mindful, and effective communication styles
- Knowing how to effectively and actively listen to others
- Developing the skills of collaboration, conflict management, and negotiation
- Recognizing the responsibility to serve as a role model of occupational balance
- Knowing how to provide occupation-centered services for our patients/clients/consumers
- Knowing how to provide leadership and how to encourage it in others
- Knowing how to manage and direct systems

These characteristics, which are established on a firm base of professional ethics and personal integrity as well as sound occupation-centered practice knowledge and skills, will provide a foundation for the continued development of any additional expertise that may be needed to become an insightful and effective planner, leader, manager, and director. The resulting "package" will not be difficult to market.

REFERENCES

Adler, R., Elmhorst, J., & Lucas, K. (2013). *Communicating at work: Strategies for success in business and the professions* (11th ed.). New York, NY: McGraw Hill.

Adler, R., & Elmhorst, J. (2010). *Communicating at work: Strategies for success in business and the professions* (10th ed.). New York, NY: McGraw Hill.

Adler, R., Rodman, G., & duPre, A. (2014). *Understanding human communication* (12th ed.). New York, NY: Oxford University Press.

Alinsky, S. (1946). *Reveille for radicals.* New York, NY: Vintage Books.

Alinsky, S. (1971). *Rules for radicals.* New York, NY: McGraw Hill.

Bennis, W., & Goldsmith, J. (1997). *Learning to lead: A workbook on becoming a leader.* Reading, MA: Addison-Wesley.

Bennis, W., & Townsend, R. (1995). *Reinventing leadership: Strategies to empower the organization* New York, NY: William Morrow.

Capodagli, B., & Jackson, L. (1999). *The Disney way.* New York, NY: McGraw-Hill.

Chouinard, Y. (2016). *Let my people go surfing: The education of a reluctant businessman* (2nd ed.). New York, NY: Random House.

Conger, J. (1998). *Winning 'em over: A new model for management in the age of persuasion.* New York, NY: Simon and Schuster.

Cook, M. (1999). *Effective coaching.* New York, NY: McGraw-Hill.

Covey, S. (1989). *The seven habits of highly effective people.* New York, NY: Fireside-Simon and Schuster.

Eichler, M. (2007). *Consensus organizing: Building communities of mutual self-interest.* Thousand Oaks, CA: Sage.

Fisher, R., & Ury, W. (1981). *Getting to yes.* New York, NY: Penguin Books.

Fleming, M. (1994). Therapist with the three-track mind. In C. Mattingly & M. Fleming, *Clinical reasoning: Forms of inquiry in a therapeutic practice* (pp. 119-136). Philadelphia, PA: F. A. Davis.

Gilkeson, G. (1997). *Occupational therapy leadership: Marketing yourself, your profession, and your organization.* Philadelphia, PA: F. A. Davis.

Green, G., & Haines, A. (2016). *Asset building and community development.* Los Angeles, CA: Sage.

Kabat-Zinn, J. (2003). Mindfulness-based interventions in context: Past, present, and future. *Clinical psychology: Science and practice, 10*(2), 144-156.

International Webster new encyclopedic dictionary. (1975). Chicago, IL: The Language Institute of America.

Karsh, E., & Fox, A. (2003). *The only grant-writing book you'll ever need.* New York, NY: Carroll and Graf.

Katz, N., & Lawyer, J. (1994). *Resolving conflict successfully.* Thousand Oaks, CA: Corvin Press.

Langer, E. (1989). *Mindfulness.* Cambridge, MA: Perseus Books.

Mattingly, C., & Fleming, M. (1994). *Clinical reasoning: Forms of inquiry in a therapeutic practice.* Philadelphia, PA: F. A. Davis.

McKay, M., Wood, J., & Brantley, J. (2007). *Dialectical behavior therapy skills workbook.* Oakland, CA: New Harbinger.

Ohmer, M., & DeMasi, K. (2009). *Consensus organizing.* Thousand Oaks, CA: Sage.

Schrage, M. (1989). *No more teams! Mastering the dynamics of creative collaboration.* New York, NY: Doubleday.

Shapiro, R., & Jankowski, M. (1998). *The power of nice: How to negotiate so everyone wins—especially you.* Hoboken, NJ: John Wiley and Sons.

Sutton-Smith, B. (1997). *The ambiguity of play.* Cambridge, MA: Harvard University Press.

Youngstrom, M. J. (1999). Developing a new occupational therapy program. In K. Jacobs & M. Logigian (Eds.), *Functions of a manager in occupational therapy* (3rd ed., pp. 129–142). Thorofare, NJ: SLACK Incorporated.

4

Getting Started
Where Do Ideas Come From?
Selecting a Population for Programming

LEARNING OBJECTIVES

1. To explore ideas for occupation-centered programs
2. To explore a variety of avenues for developing programs
3. To select a population and a condition/problem for your programming
4. To explore planning models to help organize your selection of population and your identification of early programming goals and outcome
5. To initiate a logic model for planning your program

KEY TERMS

1. Program
2. *Walking* and *Windshield* surveys
3. Community profile
4. Consensus organizing and building
5. Capacity building
6. Target population
7. Condition/problem
8. Member/client/consumer
9. Advocacy groups
10. Logic models

Fazio, L. S. *Developing Occupation-Centered Programs With the Community, Third Edition* (pp 59-74).
© 2017 Taylor & Francis Group.

SCENARIOS FOR POTENTIAL PROGRAM DESIGNS

A successful program utilizing the occupation of gardening could begin with any one of the following scenarios:

1. Recent trends in the professional and community-oriented literature suggest that there is considerable interest in—and civic and government funding for—programs to assist persons with severe and persistent mental illness to find a productive niche in their local communities. A further review of the pertinent literature finds evidence to support gardening as a suitable prevocational venue to establish long-term skills for continued employment in the community. A specific profile, needs assessment, and asset assessment of the planner's local community will help to determine whether local demographics and needs are reflective of the larger trends.

2. "I love to work outdoors, and I think gardening is very therapeutic, so I'd like to start a gardening program for persons with severe and persistent mental illness who reside in the community or are homeless. I'd like to staff it myself [an occupational therapist or an occupational therapy assistant] but might want to include the assistance of retired volunteer gardeners. I would also collaborate with the local garden club and members of the community. All would help to raise vegetables, herbs, and flowers for local restaurants, and maybe someday we would have a food truck at least partly supplied from the garden."

3. A group of advocates for young adults with developmental disability, living in a community group home in a small rural town, is seeking someone with knowledge of prevocational/job skill development and vocational/job services and resources to help these young adults find a productive niche in their community. The tasks involved in maintaining the group home may include carpentry, painting, landscaping, and gardening as well as the daily and weekly household tasks. A planner who has familiarity with task/activity analysis, developmental disabilities, and prevocational and vocational skills is needed.

4. The management of a day-treatment facility for older adults with varying stages of dementia wishes to expand programming to include use of adjoining property or perhaps the facility's rooftop. Suggestions for additional programming have included an aviary, care of small animals, a garden, and other similar suggestions for outdoor occupations geared to the interests and abilities of the clients. The programmer is a consultant to the facility and will be responsible for the development of the new and expanded programs.

These brief illustrations suggest several avenues for potential programmers that will lead to the design, development, and implementation of a program with these communities. The success of all of these will ultimately be based on the match between the needs of a population, the needs of the general community, the strengths and assets of the population, and the assets and resources of the community. The interest and expertise of the programmer will be required in bringing together partnerships, collaborations, resources, and effective programming for the participants. One may begin with personal interest and expertise followed by the search for a population that can benefit from a comprehensive assessment of needs and assets and perhaps some asset building. Alternatively, the programmer may first identify a population with need and match this need to his or her interest and expertise. The beginnings may differ, but the process of development, implementation, and evaluation will remain largely the same. The goal will be planning and organizing that involves the population and the community from the beginning and results in a program that is sustainable.

GETTING STARTED

Just how do we begin establishing an occupation-centered program? We might start by asking why programs are needed in the first place. In reply, we would suggest that a program is responsive to need. **Programs** are designed to clearly focus effort and activity in meeting the needs of an identified group. For us, as occupation-centered practitioners, these needs may be to develop knowledge and to provide information and skills in order to help our clients/patients/members/consumers first identify and then engage in meaningful occupations. These are our areas of expertise.

Ideas for programming are seldom spontaneous. As the aforementioned examples illustrate, the impetus for new or expanded programs come from a number of sources that may include (1) other occupational therapists, such as the manager of your department (e.g., the need for an extension of services or to fill a service gap when an outpatient clinic for pain management clients is needed; or a summer camp for children who are receiving school-based services); (2) patients and their families (e.g., Parkinson's patients and spouses requesting an exercise program that they can enjoy together); (3) other health care providers/professionals (e.g., dentists/orthodontists who wish to help their patients manage temporomandibular joint pain or to meet the dental needs of children on the autism spectrum); (4) advocates for populations in need of services (e.g., engagement in work or balanced occupations); and (5) perhaps most importantly, the community itself when they need assistance in program planning or consensus and asset/capacity building. In addition to the sources listed previously, the changing health care environment itself may be the impetus for ideas (e.g., postsurgical hand therapy clinics or cardiac maintenance and wellness programs) as well as changes in funding for health care (e.g., managed care directives that have pushed for service continuation in other areas). Finally, the recognized need to bring together services for clients in a new or more efficient way that is more readily understood and accessed by the community may generate ideas for new programs (e.g., child day care and therapeutic programming for children with disabilities coordinated with child day care for siblings, or intergenerational programs coupling retirement facilities and schools or community centers). Certainly, new programs may come as the result of a structured marketing plan originated by the insightful leader/planner. In all cases, you will go to the literature to find information on your targeted population and on your potential programming/intervention, and you will obtain evidence to support the use of gardening for your population or similar populations.

An example of sources for programming ideas can be seen in the parent-child program, to be introduced later, which came about as a result of networking with other professionals (teachers and education coordinators) who were familiar with other occupation-centered after-school programs originated by occupational therapy students. The expressed need was for some kind of programming that would strengthen parents' involvement in their children's educational pursuits, particularly in science. It was clear that the need was strongly occupation-centered and appropriate to our interests and abilities.

When we come up with ideas ourselves, most often they are based on something that we enjoy or care deeply about. The gardening program is a clear example of this kind of motivation, but the interest and accompanying skills motivating the development of a program could just as easily be horseback riding, keeping and caring for pets, dance, music, drama, arts and crafts, river rafting, surfing, scuba diving, or anything else for which we feel a profound affection. We also must harbor a belief in the activity's potential as therapy or as prevention. Israel "Izzy" Paskowitz's successful surfing program for children with autism was initiated through an intense love of surfing as a sport, a belief in the healing power of the ocean and love for his own son with autism (http://www.surfershealing.org). Carly Rogers also expresses a strong belief in the healing power of the ocean, and this belief is a significant thread in her surfing programs for children and for combat soldiers (Rogers, 2015; Rogers, Mallinson, & Peppers, 2014).

As a psychologist, Jolkowski (1998) speaks of the power of utilizing our interests in developing and marketing programs. He encourages the exploration of what he describes as niche markets. In his case, he extended his personal interest in music to develop group programming for musicians who were experiencing performance anxiety (Jolkowski, 1998, p. 5). Occupational therapy practitioners interested in music can develop similar programming but could instead target musicians with stress-related hand injuries or those musicians who wished to prevent hand injuries. Clearly an understanding of occupation and the meaning invested in such an occupation as that practiced by the professional musician would place the occupation-centered practitioner firmly in the marketplace. In the same article, Phillips (also a psychologist) found his particular niche in the sport of golf, but the programming was similar in that it targeted performance anxiety (Jolkowski, 1998, p. 5). Again, for occupation-centered practitioners, the niche might be expanded to help golfers avoid or treat golf-induced or golf-related injuries. Personal interest and skill in the occupation of golfing must certainly be advantageous in developing such a practice.

As mentioned earlier, a need might be expressed by persons in the community, an advocate or advocacy group, a family member, or sometimes by a potential client or groups of clients. If we think we can fill that need, the beginnings of a new program may emerge. You could also generate an idea because you recognize what may become a lucrative endeavor, which may be one of the seminal ideas for a private practice; however, an idea alone is not enough for the design of a program that will achieve results. Meticulous research and continued work will be necessary to ensure a successful program in the present and over time.

In summary, ideas for programs may come from the following:

- Other occupational therapy practitioners
- Patients/clients and/or their families
- Other health care providers/professionals
- Advocates or advocacy groups
- The community itself
- Stakeholders from all of these groups and more
- The changing health care environment
- The program developer's interests and skills

REVISITING SCENARIO 2: THE COMMUNITY GARDEN EXAMPLE

Let us return to the idea of a community garden for persons with severe and persistent mental illness who are homeless. What happens next? Even if gardening is not new to our experience, there is still research to be done. Since community gardening is an idea that has come to fruition in many and varied ways, there are resources available to you. The occupational therapy–managed horticulture program at the Veteran's Administration Medical Center in Brentwood, Los Angeles, referred to as the *vet's garden*, is one of the longest-running and most successful ventures of its kind (Strege, Molina, & Jewell, 1991). Gardening as a prevocational and vocational skill and knowledge set is utilized in this program. Substantial information describing horticulture therapy and the therapeutic aspects of gardening is available on the Internet and in print. There are also many resources for the occupation of gardening in general. *Country Gardens* magazine now includes a special section, "Breaking Ground," that showcases gardening projects for populations in need of nutritional resources as well as physical and psychological sustenance (Martin, 2015). A cursory search of *OT Practice* reveals "OT Goes Green" programs for sustainability that include OT programming utilizing plants and plant-related materials (Wagenfeld, 2013). Another *OT Practice* article from 2012 focuses on ergonomic gardening (Wagenfeld & Buresh, 2012). Melinda Suto, an occupational therapist from the University of British Columbia, and her colleagues are focusing on community gardening in the study of psychosocial issues and bipolar disorder, as reported in CTV News (2015). We have some literature to support our idea, and we likely can glean an "expert" or two for an interview from this group. See the close of this chapter for websites offering additional gardening information and resources. Regardless of your selected modality, you can further your research at the library or on the Internet. The Internet has made the process of program development much more efficient than it was even a few years ago.

It is important to note that, although our second community garden scenario was greatly influenced by personal interest in gardening as therapy, we will discover that it was also facilitated by the concerns of stakeholder/citizens who felt that persons with severe and persistent mental illness (certainly, "idle" and homeless persons with severe and persistent mental illness) present problems for the city. Perhaps this interpretation seems a bit brutal, but there are many and varied motives for the practice of good works, and the astute planner will stay abreast of these motives, mobilizing them toward positive outcomes for the clients.

In Part V of this text, we describe some of the characteristics of urban homeless, and we know that persons with severe and persistent mental illness are a large part of this group. The development of programming for this population is challenging even to the most experienced therapist. Clients are extremely varied in their interests, values, and skills, and it is not easy to find meaningful occupations for them.

The idea of a community garden in our example may be a possible solution. Our task, then, may be not only to develop a garden in the community, but also to build a community around a garden.

WHERE DO YOU LOCATE A GARDENING PROGRAM?

To expand on our second scenario, the location of the targeted population was an urban downtown setting. The planning process was initiated by exploring the ways in which people could garden in a large city, assuming that they had no property of their own. This exploration can be facilitated by contacting the botanical gardens, the city's department of parks and recreation, or local nurseries. In some cities, community gardens are sponsored by a university cooperative extension division of agricultural sciences. All of these resources offer potential for future partnering. To find a site for your program, you also can do the following:

- Contact city or regional agencies for collaborative ventures
- Contact the chamber of commerce, churches, or local businesses
- Go to the telephone book, the library, and/or the Internet
- Check posted notices at the local market or town hall
- Ask people in the community

An extremely helpful resource for planning, enhancing, and sustaining a community gardening project is the *Community Gardening Toolkit* available from the University of Missouri Extension. This guide covers everything from the history of community gardening to "how to make one happen." The section on "finding a site" and "obtaining it" offers information not easily found elsewhere (McKelvey, 2015). In addition, do not forget to look up Eagle Street Rooftop Farm established by Annie Novak in Brooklyn, New York, where the ground soil it too toxic to farm (something you may want to consider) (Novak, 2016).

Finally, another way to find a site is to simply walk around the neighborhood where you wish to provide your program. Ohmer and DeMasi (2009) refer to this method of gathering information as a **windshield survey** (pp. 141-143). Whether you walk or drive, this is an important part of what we describe as developing the **community profile,** or getting to know as much as possible about the community/neighborhood where your program is expected to take place.

If most of the people you plan to serve reside in apartments or public housing, there is likely some empty (and neglected) lot that could be set aside for a garden or an empty lot that could be developed in that way. Some urban garden sites are quite restrictive, and of course the garden site in our example needed to be where the population to be served was located. It was not likely that the client/members would board a city bus and travel to the garden daily (although once the garden was established, perhaps they would). This ability to navigate the community, in fact, could have been one of the goals of the program.

As we think about our program participants at this stage of the planning process, we must clarify the rather liberal use of terms we have used to describe them. During our planning process and before they actually become participants, we refer to them as our **target population,** or those we have targeted to receive our services. When the members of our target population become involved in our program, we may refer to them in several ways. In general, those participants who are not paying for services (that is, community gardeners) prefer to be referred to as **members,** and a club structure designating membership may be useful for many types of community programs. Although the term *outpatient* may be used in some cases, the more medical term *patient* is less used in community settings. **Client** and **consumer** are the common terms used to designate the participant of services for prevention, maintenance, and general wellness programs. Third-party payers may have a preferred terminology that you will certainly want to use if you are relying on them for reimbursement. Finally, when in doubt, ask the consumers how they prefer to be known. Often, it may just be a term such as *camper, gardener,* or *craftsman.* Today, we find the term *maker* to be a generic name that many creative people like to use (American Craft Council, 2015).

After Identifying a Population, Locating a Community, and Doing Some Literature Review, What Comes Next?

Planning in a Nutshell

If you are planning a gardening program such as the one described, some negotiation will likely occur as you select and organize a site. From the beginning, you are identifying and communicating with members of the community, building relationships, and identifying partners. In most circumstances, even before visiting the community, you have researched existing programs and have found evidence that they are successful using the parameters for measurement that you have selected (your early ideas and tentative goals/outcome). Initial need has been established by others, but you have verified that need through your literature reviews. In your planning, you may want to think about locating a farmer's market in or near your site in the future. This would provide an excellent bridge between your population and the larger community. If you have not already located it, you have a good idea what kind of site/location you require (e.g., slope, sun, shade, water, accessibility, and so on), how large it should be, and zoning requirements. You have honed your communication/negotiation skills and have begun to get to know the community (in person). You may have developed a preliminary list for what equipment/supplies will be needed to begin and an estimate of what they will cost. Certainly your supply and equipment list, staffing, and client/member selection will require additional work, but that can come later.

You might encounter the scenario, as in our case example, where urban leaders/stakeholders want something done but do not want to spend any money to do it. In addition, you might not know how much they will provide until you have presented your proposal. Thus, it might be advisable to identify some potential small, private granting organizations (such as garden clubs or family sponsors of local gardens and parks). These private granting organizations can be delegated to a secondary plan to be identified if you are not able to get the monies you need from your first organization. At this stage, you are not expected to have well-developed plans for the program; you have ideas, certainly, but now you are focused on building your profiles and getting to know people.

Attracting the Volunteers/Community Residents

A significant challenge for a project such as the one we are describing is in attracting the potential client/members to the site to begin the work of gardening and to get the volunteer help that will be needed to develop the program. You may have already contacted the local gardening clubs (or maybe a local nursery where the community buys gardening supplies) to solicit the assistance of volunteers who have a strong commitment to gardening (this was included in the draft plan to the city or other decision-making group). It is important for your volunteers to be part of the community and to be invested in it; sustainable projects do not happen if you have volunteers who are only "doing for others" and then go home to another community. Members of the community are identified and provided with resources from the beginning. They must believe in the work and believe that it is "their work." Perhaps you also have access to local students. Although they might not be gardeners, their enthusiasm would be an equally strong attribute, and many schools offer service learning credits that can be an incentive.

While the process of accessing volunteers to supervise the gardening seems simple enough, helping them to feel comfortable with the client/member population used in this example may not be so easy. You will need to know the needs of both groups. You will also need to know the configuration of this community. Does it include your targeted population, or are they considered to be interlopers (members of an entirely different community)? If they are not considered part of the community, building consensus may be an important part of what you will be doing. Basically, **consensus organizing and building** involves parallel organizing, in which community organizers/planners mobilize and bring together interests within the community as well as the political, economic, and social power structure outside of the community (Chaskin, Brown, Venkatesh, & Vidal, 2001; Ohmer & DeMasi, 2009). We will return to consensus organizing and building later; for now, suffice it to say that we, as beginning programmers, need to be aware of what this means and alert to opportunities, and this often involves a larger agenda than what we can accomplish. We can and do, however, build **capacity** and **assets** within our communities alongside our programming.

For our population example, you will need to explore any preconceptions your potential volunteers might have regarding persons with severe and persistent mental illness and the homeless. You will need to know how to present factual information so that it will be heard in the most productive way. Although statistics regarding this population (i.e., how many persons with severe and persistent mental illness who are homeless populate the city) will be critical in establishing need, it will not necessarily be convincing information for this group. An **advocacy group** can provide a strong incentive to your potential volunteers based on realistic information and an emotional investment. These are groups of persons who advocate for a particular group of people—generally people with disabilities and/or those with special needs. Advocates may be persons who are disabled themselves, relatives or friends of these persons, and professionals. You might wish to contact local advocacy organizations such as the National Alliance for Mental Illness or other advocacy groups with similar interests. Utilize community resources such as directories of social services for your city or county to find the groups that might be best able to assist you.

You may have years of experience working with persons who have various forms of mental illness, or you may have little or no experience, but a critical skill in working with nonprofessionals is to understand their experience and their views and to not minimize either. The average person knows about mental illness from the media or from brief personal encounters with a delusional and hallucinating person living on the streets. Neither image presents all there is to know, but your task is to skillfully distinguish between the realities and the myths. Further, you must provide an incentive that is meaningful to your volunteers. Assuming you accepted this challenge because it has meaning for you, sharing your commitment to this venture with your volunteers should not be difficult. If you accepted the challenge with little real interest, then it is doubtful that you will be able to mobilize the help you need.

Attracting Your Clients/Members

Once you have your cadre of motivated volunteers and perhaps a staff member or two, you can begin recruiting client/members from your targeted population. You may want to arrange for a van or truck to drive around and encourage people to come with you. If you have homeless shelters or missions in the community (and you probably do), solicit their assistance in providing transportation for your clients/members. If homeless persons with severe and persistent mental illness are indeed a problem for the city/community, then the police or volunteer police organizations might assist in spreading the word about your program and in transporting potential members to your garden. Another option is to solicit the assistance of churches or other volunteer groups working in the area. There is some caution necessary when working with this population. You want to offer programming opportunities, but you probably do not want to encourage an encampment. The local law enforcement may be a critical group for you to contact early on to help you maintain the needed boundaries. It would likely be best to locate your garden near supported housing and appeal to that population rather than those who are currently living in parks or on the street. However, it may be your goal to build a self-sufficient village—something to think about.

Once your clients/members have arrived, they will be kept there by the enthusiasm, care, skills, and knowledge that you, your staff, and your volunteers can contribute. It is important for your first group of participants to be involved in the actual building of the garden plots and in the initial development of the gardens because this group will become your future supervisors, perhaps your board members, and your strongest advocates. This garden will be sustained by building the members' loyalty and commitment to this community while also enhancing their knowledge and skills.

Although our case example was designed for an urban area, you can do the same thing in a suburban or rural area. In these locales, you might not find a large population of homeless persons with severe and persistent mental illness or adolescents who are delinquent youth offenders, but you can apply a similar concept with other groups in need. Gardening on a smaller scale—even in pots or on rooftops, patios, or windowsills—has been very successful in nursing rehabilitation facilities, in residential facilities for persons who are developmentally delayed, and in numerous school-based facilities.

If we expand our ideas to residential housing for the well elderly or adults who are developmentally disabled or on the autistic spectrum living in the community, then a shared community garden will be an excellent way to keep these populations connected to their neighborhoods/communities and to meaningful participation. In addition, the grouping of clients/members of different ages and abilities together with volunteers of different ages and abilities will help to create community—something we should facilitate at every opportunity.

Whereas suburban and rural areas often have fewer restrictions on establishing gardens and selling their produce than urban areas do, finding small granting agencies or donations in these areas may be more difficult than in the city. These are reasonable tradeoffs in many ways, and the opportunities to make the garden a "paying proposition" with the therapeutic rewards of sharing dividends may outweigh the opportunity for donations. However, do not automatically assume that grants and donations are not available in rural areas; startup monies, in fact, are likely to be there as well.

BEGINNING TO THINK ABOUT "YOUR" POPULATION, ITS CONDITIONS/PROBLEMS, AND TENTATIVE GOALS FOR PROGRAMMING

Through our garden example, you see how an idea takes shape and grows into a program step by step. You are likely going to begin with the choice of a population and/or an accompanying condition/problem. It is difficult to think of conditions and problems separately. Our targeted population and the conditions/problems they are experiencing forms the foundation of our program; from these, we will begin to develop the first of our profiles. Sometimes problems and conditions are intertwined, and sometimes they are separate. For example, we may have become aware of the growing numbers of children who are diagnosed with juvenile type II diabetes (a diagnosis and what we will describe as a **condition**). These children can be said to have **problems**. The literature will tell you how researchers, doctors, and parents describe the problems that encourage and/or exacerbate the condition of diabetes. I would also include a review of popular media as part of your research—these resources are fast and generally accurate. They also put you in touch with what members of the public think and know (or believe). You can and should back this up with published research/evidence, which, however, is slower in coming to print. The next chapter in this text will provide information on trends, and it is frequently through the popular literature that trends and trending issues first present themselves.

In both juvenile and adult-onset diabetes, obesity is first identified as the most significant problem, and it may be related to diet and inactivity. You may choose to have your programming/intervention directed to both of the latter. Throughout the course of planning, it is wise to continue to return to our earliest intention—what we believe is our purpose in planning this particular program/intervention—and to ask the following questions:

- Why is a program needed? Are there multiple reasons?
- Why this program? How is it occupation-centered?
- How will this program have meaning for the client/member? For the community?
- Will it strengthen the community? Build relationships?
- What do we expect will be the outcomes of the program? What will it achieve now and in the future?
- Is it sustainable? Will it remain strong after we leave?

When we begin to define our purpose and think about outcomes (or what we expect will happen), we are beginning to develop the goal or goals that we will use to guide the programming toward outcomes and ultimate impact. For now, these are early, tentative goals to provide direction as we proceed in the planning process. These goals are not intended to be fully developed, and they may not yet be accompanied by measurable objectives—that will come later. For now, they serve to define and structure our purpose/intent. They keep us focused, ultimately on outcomes and the larger impact.

In our community garden case example, the central idea or tentative goal based on what was perceived to be the need was to establish a community for homeless persons and others with severe and persistent mental illness living in the city and to help this community become interdependent with the surrounding communities. Second, another tentative goal was to provide a variety of meaningful choices of occupation for those involved in the program and to build their knowledge and skills (their assets). At this point in the process, these goals are very vague statements, and it might be difficult to write objectives that would be measurable or outcome based. They do, however, define our purpose, and they provide a good foundation for the more formal goals and objectives that will follow.

Exercise 4-1

Trying Out Your Ideas

Now that you have a general understanding of what is involved, try brainstorming some programming ideas of your own. At this point, the ideas do not necessarily need to be practical and you do not need to know exactly how you will carry them out. You may have an idea of a potential need in mind already and, as in some of our early scenarios, that need may be specific. If so, tailor your ideas to those needs.

1. Write your ideas here:

_____

_____

_____

_____

_____

2. What is your target population? What special needs does this population have that must be considered in your planning? Do you need to do some additional research? In our program development courses at the Chan Division of Occupational Science and Occupational Therapy at the University of Southern California, we have found it useful to use the Centennial Vision Statement of the American Occupational Therapy Association (Baum, 2006) to help students determine populations of interest to them. The population categories are children and youth; disabilities and participation; health and wellness; productive aging; and rehabilitation, work, and industry. This approach not only helps students to define their populations of interest, but also serves the aims and needs of the profession in meeting agendas for the future.

What population or agenda does the Centennial Vision Statement propose that you find most interesting at this early stage of your planning? Or, is there another population you are considering? Make some notes about the need or needs of such a population here:

_____

_____

_____

_____

_____

In our community garden example, the population consists of homeless men and women with severe and persistent mental illness, and there is the possibility of children accompanying their parents. In our parent-child example to be introduced a bit later, the population comprises inner-city fourth- and fifth-grade boys and girls and their parent (mother, father, or other home-care provider). When, as occupational therapy students and practitioners, we think of "special needs," we often think of physically, emotionally, or cognitively disabling conditions. Certainly these things must be considered in our work in the community; however, we must also consider the "special needs" prompted by socioeconomic circumstances. The clues to these considerations in our present example are "homelessness" and "the inner city." Both of these considerations will require our attention as we address the needs of our case example populations and develop their service profiles.

Persons who are homeless owing to severe and persistent mental illness must not only deal with the repercussions of their particular illness, but also develop their own adaptive survival measures to remain safe and nourished. The adaptive strategies that permit survival on the street must be understood and appreciated by planners if community programs of this nature are to be successful.

The first "special need" noted by the parent-child program planners was, in fact, their own. To be responsive to several of the participants, it was necessary for some of the planners to speak both Spanish and English; the need to translate the written materials into Spanish was also quickly apparent. There were also other concerns prompted by the inner-city public school environment and the multicultural considerations of the children and parents.

3. Have the earlier scenarios and the gardening example prompted your consideration of any other needs your targeted population may have that will influence your program planning? If so, note those needs here:

_____

_____

_____

_____

_____

4. If you have identified additional needs, what will they require of you and of your program? Will you require new knowledge? Expertise?

_____

_____

_____

_____

_____

5. Stop and ask yourself the following questions, and note your responses in the space provided. Why this program?

_____

_____

_____

_____

_____

How is it occupation-centered?

_____

_____

_____

_____

_____

How will it have meaning for the client/member/participant? Will this program build assets for the population; for the community?

_____

_____

_____

_____

_____

What will be the purpose? What do we want the outcomes to be? Remember these are outcomes for the program—the collective outcome for all of the participants.

_____

_____

_____

_____

_____

What might be a tentative goal or goals relative to the purpose for all participants in your program? What do you want to accomplish for all participants? Note that, with the community garden example, we stated that the primary purpose, or tentative goal, was to establish community for all of the participants and to help this community mesh and become interdependent with other communities. Later, you will find that, for the parent-child program, the purpose or tentative goal is to build parent-child teams toward a more sustainable present and future education for the children.

_____

_____

_____

_____

_____

6. What are your ideas for where the programming that you are proposing might be accomplished? Do you already have a community in mind or will you locate one?

_____

_____

_____

_____

_____

The process of locating a community and a site within the community may be very different from one program to the next. In our gardening example, the idea was developed before actually locating the specific population or the site. The program held certain advantages for the city and, in fact, when the plan was proposed, assistance was offered in finding a suitable garden site, without cost, adjacent to an established community garden.

The location of a site for the parent-child program took several turns before resolution. In the early planning stages, where you are now, it seemed obvious that the program should be held at the school. Before actually completing the profiles and needs assessment, it was believed that the program would be conducted immediately after school and that the children would be joined in one of the classrooms by their parents. This also seemed to be a convenient place and time for the occupational therapy coordinator and students who would be conducting the program to get together. Most of the activities were appropriate to the tables, chairs, and desks of the classroom, so it seemed the perfect place. In fact, much of this early brainstorming was on target; however, a detailed series of profiles and assessments of need helped the planners to design a program much more appropriate to the concerns of the participants and, therefore, much more successful.

Planning Models to Guide Programming

This may be a good place to talk about suggested models to help you as you continue to develop your ideas. You have already generated enough information to begin to structure your continued work; however, in the early stages of program planning, it can be difficult to visualize the big picture (although this kind of vision is necessary to maintain focus and to avoid getting lost in detail too early in the process). A **logic model** can be an extremely useful tool from the beginning to the end of your programming.

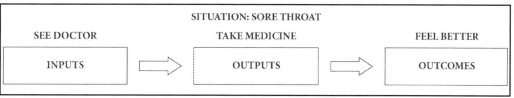

Figure 4-1. Common example of a logic model. (Adapted from University of Wisconsin Extension. (2008). *Logic model development: teaching and training guide*. Madison, WI: Author.)

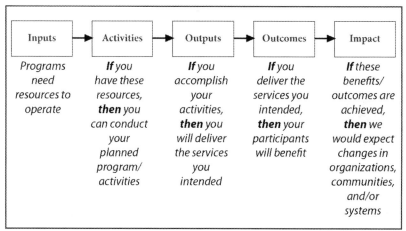

Figure 4-2. Logic model example: the "if–then" relationship. (Adapted from W. K. Kellogg Foundation. (2004). *Using logic models to bring together planning, evaluation, and action: Logic model development guide.* Battle Creek, MI: Author.)

In its simplest form, the logic model begins with a picture of your program (the multiple profiles you will accomplish, the structure of the programming, evaluation, and anticipated outcome). It represents a sequence of "if–then" relationships and may be considered the core of planning as well as evaluation (University of Wisconsin Extension, 2008).

Most likely you will find logic models discussed in guidelines provided by grant funders for the development of frameworks for mapping out the grant program. According to the W. K. Kellogg Foundation, logic models are a "systematic and visual way to present and share your understanding of the relationships among the resources you have to operate your program, the activities you plan, and the changes or results you hope to achieve" (W. K. Kellogg Foundation, 2004, preface). Logic models give grant reviewers a visual of the whole program in flowchart format. Logic models can be a valuable method for establishing program planning, an implementation plan, and the program evaluation plan. They have several components, including inputs, processes, outputs, and outcomes.

A logic model is a depiction of a program showing what the program will do and what it is expected to accomplish. In its simplest form, the logic model begins with a picture of your program (i.e., the multiple profiles you will accomplish, the structure of the actual programming, evaluation methods, and anticipated outcomes). It represents a sequence of "if–then" relationships. If the series of "if–then" relationships is implemented as intended, the desired outcomes will be achieved. It is a framework for describing the relationships between investments, activities, and results, and it may be considered the core of planning as well as evaluation (University of Wisconsin Extension, 2008). Figure 4-1 shows a common example of how the "if–then" relationship leads to outcomes.

Underlying all logic models is a programs's theory of change. *If* we do this, *then* we can expect a certain thing to happen. This is exemplified in Figure 4-2.

Most likely, you will find logic models discussed in guidelines provided by grant funders for the development of frameworks for mapping out the grant program. According to the W. K. Kellogg Foundation, logic models are a "systematic and visual way to present and share your understanding of the relationships among the resources you have to operate your program, the activities you plan, and the changes or results you hope to achieve" (2004, preface). Logic models give grant reviewers a visual of the whole program in flowchart format. For the planner, logic models can be a valuable method for establishing program planning, an implementation plan, and the program evaluation plan. Logic models have several components in common, including inputs (what resources you have to operate your program), processes (your planned activities), outputs (the product and/or service that you intended), outcomes (how your participants will benefit), and impact (changes in organizations, communities, or systems) (see Figure 4-2).

Visit both the W. K. Kellogg Foundation website (http://www.wkkf.org) as well as the University of Wisconsin Extension website (fyi.uwex.edu/programdevelopment/logic models) for additional information and examples as you prepare your own logic model in Exercise 4-2.

Exercise 4-2

After you have visited the websites and see what the model can look like and how it works, try drafting your present ideas in this format (or another of your choice). You can use a graphic display of boxes, as has been shown, or other shapes (circles, storyboards, etc.). It is important to retain arrows and the relationships between inputs, outputs, and outcomes, but how you choose to do that is up to you. You will not have all of the information to finish your model until you have completed your program proposal; it will be your working document, which will develop as you add your ideas and plans.

At this point in your work, it may be useful to present your idea or the idea of your working group in a brief proposal to classmates. If you are a professional or are working independently, present your idea to colleagues or others who might provide constructive feedback. Have their suggestions caused you to alter your initial plan? If so, in what way? (*Note*: It is almost always necessary to make alterations in your initial plan during the development process, but this should not mean compromising your initial idea.) Note your response here:

_____

_____

_____

_____

_____

If classmates or others found your idea amusing, remember that all great leaders and planners were probably ridiculed at least once. Observers of a young midwestern artist in 1923 struggling to start a filmmaking business based on a "mouse" must have laughed long and hard, but, undoubtedly, their grandchildren visited Disneyland and certainly recognized Mickey Mouse (Capodagli & Jackson, 1999). Most observers told Mrs. Fields that she could never survive "just selling cookies." She now not only survives, but has over 650 domestic locations and 65 international locations in 11 countries (http://www.mrsfields.com/the story/story-bottom.html).

If your idea is larger than your present abilities can handle, save it for the future. This reveals an important point. Begin now to keep a journal or file of ideas for programs. Many great ideas were probably first recorded on cocktail napkins; the same can hold true for great ideas in occupation-centered programming. Your occupational therapy professors and instructors and your colleagues drop interesting ideas for practice and program development all of the time. Occupational therapy journals and publications frequently highlight entrepreneurial practices, as do the journals and newsletters of other helping professions. An idea does not have to be yours alone to be successful.

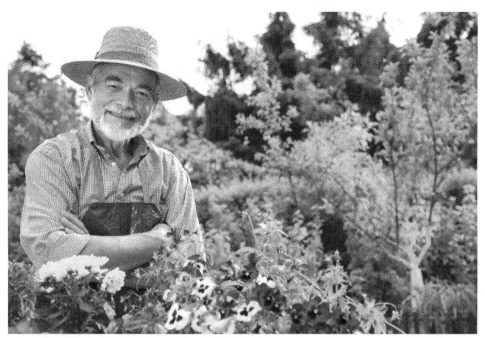

Sustaining people and the planet: organic landscapes.

Consider all of these ideas to be "pearls of programming wisdom" and write them down to stimulate your future program-planning ventures.

In a few years, when your practical wisdom and experience match your present creativity, intellect, and enthusiasm, pull out the journal or file and see what interests you. If you are already a practitioner, you probably have lots of ideas; nevertheless, still take the time to organize them in a file, and when you feel the need for a change, page through the file and take a good look around you. You will most likely find opportunities just waiting to be discovered. I have found that former students frequently contact me a few years into their careers, now ready to "get serious" about that program, practice, or nonprofit they designed as students. Keep that proposal where you can revisit!

SUMMARY

This chapter proposes that you begin your programming with an idea—yours or someone else's—but an idea that interests you and hopefully one that you are passionate about. Your first interest may involve only the population with no clear idea of programming, or it may be the program idea that stimulates you while you have not yet decided on a population.

Since we started talking about community programming in occupational therapy, our awareness and accompanying agendas have grown. Needs assessments are now accompanied by asset identification, and our profiles are more sophisticated. We talk about asset development and capacity building. We have learned that helping a community build knowledge and skills contributes to strengths, independence—or interdependence—and sustainability. We now have stakeholders, collaborators, and partners. Our roles as programmers are changing and becoming more complex. Our understanding of "community" is also changing, and while this helps us to expand our programming ideas and venues, it also makes accountability and outcome/impact measurement even more critical. The one thing that has not changed is the need for careful and detailed planning that includes asking lots of questions and pursuing the answers in the community and through our growing resources within and outside of the profession. In the communities we serve, there has never been a reduction in needs, and now we are better prepared than ever to understand and help meet those needs.

REFERENCES

American Crafts Council. (2015). *Website*. http://www.craftcouncil.org

Baum, M. C. (2006). Presidential address, 2006 centennial challenges, millennium opportunities. *American Journal of Occupational Therapy, 60*(6), 609-616.

Capodagli, B., & Jackson, L. (1999). *The Disney way*. New York, NY: McGraw-Hill.

Chaskin, R. J., Brown, P., Venkatesh, S., & Vidal, A. (2001). *Building community capacity*. New York, NY: Aldine DeGruyter.

CTV News (2015). http://www.ctvnews.ca/health/sowing-the-seeds-of-change-b-c-urban-gardens-help-those-with-mental-illness-1.2604209

Jolkowski, M. (1998). *Practice strategies: A business guide for behavioral healthcare providers*. Washington, DC: American Association for Marriage and Family Therapy.

Martin, T. (2015). Breaking ground. *Country Gardens, 24*(4), 27-29.

McKelvey, B. (2015). *Community gardening toolkit*. Columbia, MO: University of Missouri Extension.

Novak, A. (2016). *The rooftop growing guide: How to transform your roof into a vegetable garden or farm*. New York, NY: Ten Speed Press.

Ohmer, M., & DeMasi, K. (2009). *Consensus organizing: A community development workbook*. Thousand Oaks, CA: Sage.

Rogers, C. (2015). Surfing as healing: Ocean therapy [lecture, July 23, 2015]. Los Angeles, CA: Chan Division of Occupational Science and Occupational Therapy, University of Southern California.

Rogers, C., Mallinson, T., & Peppers, D. (2014). High-intensity sports for posttraumatic stress disorder and depression: Feasibility study of ocean therapy with veterans of operation enduring freedom and operation Iraqi freedom. *The American Journal of Occupational Therapy, 68*(4) 395-404.

Strege, M., Molina, M., & Jewell, J. (1991). Vets' gardeners reap a full harvest. *Advance for Occupational Therapists, 5*(31), 6-8.

University of Wisconsin Extension. (2008). *Logic model development: teaching and training guide*. Madison, WI: Author.

Wagenfeld, A. (2013). Nature: An environment for health. *OT Practice, 17*(18), 15-19.

Wagenfeld, A., & Buresh, B. (2012). Ergonomic gardening. *OT Practice, 17*(9), 8-11.

W. K. Kellogg Foundation. (2004, 2001, 1998). *Using logic models to bring together planning, evaluation, and action: Logic model development guide*. Battle Creek, MI: Author.

Suggested Internet Resources

Children's gardening and community gardening grants (including opportunities for free seed, tools, plants, garden products, and assistance), ideas, projects, products, books, and manuals:

> http://www.hort.vt.edu/human/CGgrants.html
>
> http://www.hort.vt.edu/human/commgrants.html
>
> http://www.hort.vt.edu/human/CGmoreres.html
>
> http://www.hort.vt.edu/human/CGbooks.html

Community Gardening: The American Community Gardening Association provides links to university and college horticultural extension programs; community gardening specific to states and locales, and general community gardening information, including getting started, organizations to assist, and funding. You can contact this association at http://www.communitygarden.org/links/index.html

Israel "Izzy" Paskowitz: www.surfershealing.org

Mrs. Fields Cookie Company: http://www.mrsfields.com/the_story/story-bottom.html

Top 10 Gardening Apps You Need Now: Gardenista: http://www.gardenista.com/posts/the-top-ten-gardening-apps-you-need-now

University of Wisconsin Extension: fyi.uwex.edu/programdevelopment/logic models

W. K. Kellogg Foundation: http://www.wkkf.org

5

Identifying Trends and Forecasting Futures

LEARNING OBJECTIVES

1. To learn how to identify current events reported in the media and in professional literature that may affect you and your potential program

2. To explore how historical events and eras have affected health care and the occupational therapy profession

3. To analyze trends to make forecasts regarding the potential success of your planned program

KEY TERMS

1. Trends
2. Forecasts

Fazio, L. S. *Developing Occupation-Centered Programs With the Community, Third Edition* (pp 75-87).
© 2017 Taylor & Francis Group.

Ohmer and DeMasi (2009) strongly suggest that those working in the community, particularly those who have community organizing as their agenda, must grasp the "big picture" in order to understand what is happening locally in communities. For these authors, understanding the big picture involves analyzing current political, economic, and social trends and their potential impact on communities (Ohmer & DeMasi, 2009), particularly the impact on low-income communities—where many of the needs we are responsive to as programmers—arise. For example, changing policies on immigration in the United States have resulted in the influx of increasing numbers of people and increasing demands for social services, affordable housing, and education in local communities all over the country. Global and national thinking is required to act locally (Ohmer & DeMasi, 2009).

Weil (1996) states that there is a growing assumption that private nonprofit organizations can respond better and more cheaply to social problems in low-income communities than public services can. Shifting responsibility from the federal government to state and local governments and nonprofits has resulted in decreased public funding for social and human services, the growth of managed care, and outsourcing to for-profit organizations. These changes have often resulted in declining resources for low-income communities and the individuals who live in them (Weil, 1996). Much of our occupation-centered programming occurs in these communities, and our partners are often nonprofits. It is imperative that we stay current in all of these arenas that can and will impact our programs.

As programmers, we must also access the national and local political climate and how it affects our communities of interest. Federal changes in housing policies, the way welfare benefits are distributed, and other policy changes that generally give more freedom to local governments who may or may not be prepared for it can affect our programming positively or negatively. Economic changes over the last several years have affected our local communities in different ways. Corporate downsizing, shifting companies and jobs overseas, job loss, and displacement have all influenced our communities (Ohmer & DeMasi, 2009; Weil, 1996). When jobs leave communities, many of the other small businesses and services leave as well. Empty storefronts, abandoned homes, and empty lots are only some of the changes that result.

In 1987, Wilson's research reported that the base of stable working- and middle-class families in low-income communities eroded throughout the mid- to late-twentieth century. As a result, local institutions were weakened (e.g., churches, businesses, and schools), and the sense of community was diminished. We are again reminded of Putnam's (2000) words, discussed in Chapter 2 of this text and captured so well in the title of his book, *Bowling Alone: The Collapse and Revival of American Community*. Areas where there is concentrated poverty (e.g., census tracts where 40% or more of residents are poor) have many challenging problems accompanying poverty: poor education, declining mental health, increased teen pregnancy, delinquency, and crime (Bishaw, 2005; Leventhal & Brooks-Gunn, 2000). We all appreciate these poverty-associated problems; they often represent the needs of many within our programming populations.

This is but a small window into the interconnections between systems affecting our programming populations and their communities. What are we describing? The impact of past, present, and future trends—and that is the point of this chapter. As programmers, we have to be apprised of trends in multiple areas of interest: economics, politics, social arenas/public attitudes, education, medicine and health, and perhaps more.

A PROGRAMMING SCENARIO

A community program can be designed to encourage positive parent-child communication through activities and experiences that focus on shared occupations. Such a program may bring a family closer together in their combined efforts to prepare the child for a successful academic future. The planning and funding of such a program may be greatly

(continued)

influenced by current trends in public sentiment prompted by real and threatened public and unprovoked bombings and shootings; some of them occurring in elementary and middle school, as well as a general media concern for an increase in violent acts. This results in a resurgence of parental concern regarding children's safety and the lack of positive parent-child experiences. A later example of a parent-child community program will help to demonstrate how an issue impact tree can be used to forecast possible futures for a potential program to address some of these trending issues.

Stated quite simply, our question is what is happening in the community, region, state, country, and world today that will impact us and our ideas and plans for the future? As we venture into the design and development of new programming, the practice of following trends must become a part of our daily and weekly routines. This is not to suggest that each of us should construct a sophisticated statistical trends analysis; rather, we should use the existing information in the literature and the media to chart the direction in which things will likely go (**trends**). According to Celente (1991), a "trend is a definite, predictable direction or sequence of events," and "tracking trends shows us how we got here, where we are, and where we're going" (pp. 4-5). We then should use these trends to make forecasts. These **forecasts,** or scenarios of the probable future, will permit us to make more critical judgments regarding our own futures relative to practice and, particularly, to new or continued community programming.

In fact, today we really do not have much choice in the matter of considering and responding to trends. In the preface to the original edition of *The Temporary Society,* Bennis and Slater (1968) commented that to engage in the forecasting of social trends "in a world of unprecedented complexity during changes of unparalleled rapidity" is probably as absurd as it is necessary.

At least on a weekly basis (and preferably daily), web-based news and/or major newspapers should be read to ferret out events that may affect us as we practice "occupation-centered" interventions. For example, what are the current political events at both the international, national, and state levels? By perusing current events and headlines, we can determine where the public sentiments lie and where the state and federal dollars are going; thus we may be able to forecast where these funds are likely to go in the future. Wars, political intrigues, and adolescent or young adult fads may appear to be vastly remote from our concerns regarding therapy, wellness, and health. If we remain alert, these things can and likely will affect the programming we might propose and the funding available to make it possible.

Issel (2014) refers to "trigger events," such as awareness of a problem, a periodic strategic planning effort, or newly available funds for a health-related program. The trigger event leads the planner to collect data about the health problem, the characteristics of the people affected, and their perceptions of the problem. These data, along with additional data on available resources, constitute an assessment of a community's needs and assets (Issel, 2014, pp. 14-15).

ANALYZING TRENDS BY REVIEWING HISTORY

Our analysis of current and developing trends must also include our awareness of history. We all know of the tremendous impact that World Wars I and II had on the history of occupational therapy. The first clinic-community program developed by the author of this text was for veterans of Vietnam. Although this programming was in response to numbers and need, it unfortunately was initiated with inadequate preparation. An earlier event/trends review might have ensured a better result for this program. The programming met the immediate need in something of a crisis mode, but it could have been more proactive had the insights and advanced preparation from an analysis of trends been utilized. An analysis or analyses of the social trends and the characteristics of the developing counterculture might have encouraged the design of programming that would have helped Vietnam veterans re-enter the community and avoid the emotional trauma that many encountered. This would be true of any programming designed to meet the needs of persons experiencing crisis situations and programming designed to assist in the process of cultural/environmental assimilation (as for refugees). Programming for veterans and military personnel today, in many ways, reflects similar needs experienced by combat soldiers and veterans of the unpopular past wars. Trends helped us predict what the outcomes might be: post-traumatic stress (e.g., shell shock, combat fatigue), displacement from employment and suitable housing, or traumatic relationships and failed marriages. Unfortunately, our previous experiences have not helped very much in the prevention of these problems when trends predicted that they accompany most wars, particularly those not supported by the majority of the population.

Current best-selling books and film in the popular marketplace give us information regarding the interests, needs, and wants of the public—the public that we, too, are a part of and seek to serve. Often, novelists of both fiction and nonfiction, screenwriters, songwriters, and other representatives of popular culture can provide a window to trends or perhaps even set them.

FINDING TRENDS IN THE PROFESSIONAL LITERATURE

Certainly, we must read our own professional literature and that of other health care practitioners, but program descriptions likely will be responding to trends rather than setting them. Those who are setting trends probably will not know it for some time, and even then they may not make a publishable record of such events. We must, however, remain aware of the actions our professional organization is taking at both the state and national levels with regard to the requirements for education and practice. Many of our leaders have been and are courageous trendsetters, but the profession of occupational therapy historically has been conservative; it has moved toward the future tentatively, avoiding uncharted territories. Whatever stance you prefer, our professional affiliations offer us both freedoms and restraints, and neither can be ignored.

Practice in the community does not mean practice outside of our discipline or our profession, but it in many ways requires an even closer relationship to our values and ethics than in the more institutional-based environments. We may find it difficult at first to open our thinking to entertain innovative arenas from which practice may originate. Legislative decisions; public laws and reforms; and national, state, and local budgeting are factors that may specifically influence our practices, but we most likely learn of these while we are feeling their effects. Our reactions are often prompted either by not being prepared (and "missing the boat" while another more savvy provider steps in) or, sadly, by preparing and investing in a rigid service model that is rapidly becoming obsolete.

Global Trends

Tracking global trends will strengthen your perception of need and help establish the parameters of your program. The World Health Organization's (WHO) website (http://www.whol.int/en/) can provide statistics and information for countries around the world. WHOLIS is the WHO library database, from which you can search any country or topic; for example, *Health Topics: Obesity*. You may then access articles of interest free of charge. Accessing the *World Health Report* can provide information on such topics as "life expectancy," which will offer charts for most countries with figures for birth rates, variations in life expectancy for males and females, population figures, and so on. Global trends are particularly useful to validate the need for both domestic and international programs in the area of primary prevention.

THE IMPACT OF TRENDS:
GENERATING QUESTIONS TO CONSIDER

Sometimes events, perhaps predictive of trends, appear to have little to do with us and are ignored. No one can doubt that health care in the United States has been and is changing rapidly. Could these changes have been predicted? An analysis of the large expenditures incurred in the therapy provisions of the 1980s and 1990s likely would have at least partially predicted the inevitable downsizing we are presently experiencing. Even now there are regional changes that are predictive of changes that have occurred or will occur across the country. What are professionals doing to prepare for the changes that may occur? This prompts some interesting questions. Should health care providers seek more or less regulation? With what disciplines should we form alliances? Is it time for new liaisons?

Occupational therapy educators and practitioners are responding to the recent trends denoting policy and funding shifts affecting medical care. Preparing for roles in primary care is one example of occupational therapists, as well as other health care providers, following a trend by preparing themselves with new skills and knowledge (Hart & Parsons, 2015; Metzler, Hartmann, & Lowenthal, 2012, 2014; Muir, 2012; Waite, 2014). Preparation will also require forming new professional and lay partnerships and coalitions. We will need to involve our communities at all levels.

Telehealth has also been identified by the American Occupational Therapy Association (AOTA) as integral to health care reform and accompanying trends and trending issues in the delivery of medical services. According to Cason (2015), programs and concepts included in the Patient Protection and Affordable Care Act of 2010 are expected to transform health care in the United States from a volume-based health system to a value-based health system with increased emphasis on prevention and health promotion. Cason proposes that telehealth will be one way to improve the health care experience, the health of populations, and the affordability of care; she wants occupational therapists to be prepared for this opportunity.

It would certainly appear that people are becoming more responsible for the state of their health. At least we can concur that they are generally more aware and likely worry more about it. Is this a trend? Did the changes in the perceived quality of health care prompted by the corporate entry into an arena thought to be humanistic cause us to become responsive to the need to care for ourselves? Are young adults learning to place their trust exclusively in their own actions? Will the next generation be even more self-determined and internally controlled than the last one? How will they prepare for shrinking resources and diminished health care and retirement dollars? There is little doubt that they will live longer than their predecessors. Grasping control of your health and life without sacrificing quality and meaning requires skills. Who will provide those skills? Will the trend become a frenzied desire to protect your physical and emotional health and the health of your children in order not to use resources for illness, or will there be a growing number of drug, alcohol, and accident victims? Will the rich expect to pay for their own services, and will everyone else then be without access to services? All of these are questions that may be answered by awareness of trends.

Therapists entering the workforce in the 1950s, 1960s, and 1970s witnessed the ebb-and-flow cycling of reimbursement and salaries, programming styles, and resources; in response, they have had several turns at reinventing the profession. It would appear that the time is right for yet another such reinvention.

What about the so-called Generation X or Y? Apparently, these groups are already engaged in the quest for meaning outside of the traditional domains of institutional prerogative. What better groups are there to engage in the health care practices of tomorrow, both as givers and receivers? Will these groups require new modes of skill and information provision?

The foregoing discussion comprises a series of questions prompted by a cursory review of trends—trends that promote forecasts and trends that, assuming we listen, will help us to outline future practices.

The following exercises will help you learn the initial steps to the process of forecasting the direction of future practice.

Exercise 5-1

Identifying Trends by Tracing History

1. To begin this exercise, review your knowledge of history, including occupational therapy history. Under the categories provided, note those things and occurrences that have affected the nature of our profession (think broadly, and add categories if you choose). You may wish to go to the Internet to obtain the information or use other references of your choice. You will discover that, in some eras, you will find more outstanding events of a political nature (i.e., wars, notable presidential elections), with philosophies that may accompany such political events (i.e., optimism for the economy or lack of it); attitudes may, as well, be optimistic, pessimistic, or uncaring (i.e., anti-government/establishment views in the 1960s and in the present). Research agendas that have affected life-threatening diseases through medication, surgeries, and vaccinations are present in some degree in all of these time frames and may be marked by significant events and/or technological advances. Last, technology as a category has evolved from the telegraph and light bulb to the almost daily changes in telecommunications we currently experience.

   You may also wish to consider the transfer of this grid to a flipchart or to the board to facilitate group work.

	Events	Philosophies	Attitudes	Technology
Pre-1930				
1930-1950				
1950-1970				
1970-1990				
1990-present				

   From your position in the present, review the previous exercise and highlight those things/events that have, in your observation, had a positive impact on the profession of occupational therapy and those things/events that may have had a negative impact.

   Is there anything happening in the profession today that your analyses of events might have predicted with regard to practice, legislation, education, or reimbursement?

   If you wish, discuss this with your classmates, colleagues, or others, and note your comments here:

   _____

   _____

   _____

   _____

   _____

   _____

METHODS FOR TRENDS TRACKING

Today there are multiple sources from which to gather current global and national trends. For gathering information on political, economic, and social trends, Ohmer and DeMasi (2009) recommend the following: mass media including local and national newspapers; library resources and databases (books and journals); and the Internet to access such resources as local, state, and federal nonprofits, foundations, and organizations focusing on low-income communities; websites for think tanks and other research organizations. See list of helpful web resources at the end of this chapter.

Of course, our professional organizations are critical in helping us to determine what trends may impact our practice areas. The AOTA tracks trending issues to help members know what to anticipate in all practice areas defined by the Centennial Vision process: children and youth; mental health; rehabilitation, disability, and participation; health and wellness; productive aging; and work and industry. Yamkovenko (2015) provides this window into present and future practices in *The Emerging Niche: What's Next in Your Practice* (AOTA, 2015).

Exercise 5-2

Identifying Recent Trends

1. Since identifying trends may be a new process for you, it may be helpful to do a sorting activity to begin. Either by placing labels on a large table or by writing on a board, note the following categories of events (local, regional, national, and international) that may be responsive to trends:

   a. Events reflective of economics

   b. Events reflective of politics

   c. Events reflective of public interests and attitudes

   d. Events in education

   e. Events in medicine and health

   f. Events in scientific research

   Provide yourself with not only your local newspaper, but also copies of such newspapers as the *Washington Post, New York Times, Wall Street Journal,* and any others that you believe will help you create a view of the future. What is happening in Europe, for example, may be significant. Look at the impact the English had on the history of American rock and roll. However, these newspapers will likely highlight events for you that may be of significance. Watch local and national news programs for at least 1 week before you begin this exercise. Also, use the Internet to determine what people are interested in and what they are talking about. Of course not everything you see on the Internet is factual. Although fiction can tell us a lot when we are looking for trends, we must learn early on to separate fact from fiction or conjecture, particularly in doing research (Garretson, 1997). In terms of social media, the AOTA offers ongoing help to occupational therapy practitioners, educators, and students with navigating this world, including recommendations for how to use social media to enhance your practice, as well as ideas for those using Twitter, Facebook, and LinkedIn (social@aota.org).

2. As you go through your newspapers, news journals, and notes gleaned from newscasts and the Internet, highlight or clip those you have selected and place them under the categories noted previously. If this is done as part of a class exercise, do it first without discussion. When everyone is finished, discuss your findings. Is there agreement? Disagreement? While this is an equally valid exercise when done alone, having other opinions and perspectives broadens your observations.

3. As a class or with colleagues, review your selections and separate out those you think may represent a trend that could affect occupation-centered intervention, either therapy-based or models that promote health-wellness. Remove all of the news items that you decide are not likely to impact occupation-centered programming.

4. Working with those items remaining, separate out your selections to make two categories—one comprising those trend predictors that may have a positive impact on occupation-centered intervention, and another for those that may have a negative impact.

Steps to Identifying Trends and Forecasting Futures

The following list summarizes the steps you will take to identifying trends and forecasting futures:

- Find resources such as newspapers, news journals, websites, and others.

- Retrieve pertinent articles and notes and place them under one of the identified eight categories.

- Review your categories and clippings.

- Remove any news items that you feel will not be likely to affect the practice of occupation-centered interventions.

- Make two categories of those items remaining—one category of items that may have a positive impact and one category of those that may have a negative impact on occupation-centered programs.

- Review your categories and try some forecasting. What is likely to happen next?

From the identification of trends come forecasts. Forecasts are what you might anticipate or predict will come of the reviewed trends. Forecasts can supply answers to questions such as, "What impact will these apparent trends have on you professionally and personally?"

From the work you have completed in the previous exercises, can you make forecasts or predictions about how those things you have identified will likely have an impact on present and/or future occupation-centered interventions, either therapy-based or health mainte-nance/promotion/wellness practices? How will they affect you personally? How will they affect your professional expectations? If you wish, you may use the six broad categories of practice identified by the Centennial Vision to help you organize your forecasts/predictions: children and youth; mental health; rehabilitation, disability, and participation; health and wellness; productive aging; and work and industry (AOTA, 2007).

5. Note your forecasts or predictions here:

_____

_____

_____

_____

_____

    a. What do you anticipate will be the effect of your forecasts or predictions on occupation-centered intervention in general?

_____

_____

_____

_____

_____

b. What do you anticipate will be the effect on you personally and professionally?

_____

_____

_____

_____

_____

6. Considering what you have found, note here any identified trends/forecasts that may influence your interests in community programming (either positively or negatively).

a. At present, my community programming interests are:

_____

_____

_____

_____

_____

b. Trends that may have a positive impact:

_____

_____

_____

_____

_____

c. Trends that may have a negative impact:

_____

_____

_____

_____

Remember that even if you identify negative trends, this does not necessarily mean that you give up your ideas; rather, it means that you use the present information to make adaptations to your future plans or at least to develop contingency plans.

7. If you have identified negative trends in the previous exercise, how might you wish to adapt your planning, or what contingency plans will you adopt in order to be better prepared for your future?

Continue to be aware of events and trends, and continue to make forecasts. You may wish to begin charting your forecasts to see how accurate you are. Organize a file that categorizes your interests; when you see something (such as a newspaper article or a news story), retrieve and/or clip it and drop it in your file. Review the contents periodically, and examine for developing trends. Always look for social, economic, and political significance. Keep separate categories for things dealing specifically with occupational therapy and other health professions.

Ramsey and Robertson (1993) suggest the use of an "issue impact tree" to help in the identification of trends. The following exercise is an adaptation of their work and may be helpful as you organize your thoughts about the impact of trends on the planning of your programs.

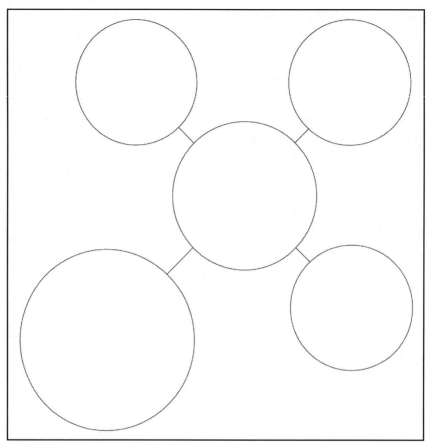

Figure 5-1. Issue impact tree. (Adapted from Ramsey, D., & Robertson, S. (1993). *Breaking into new markets: Expanding roles in mental health. Workshop resource book.* Bethesda, MD: American Occupational Therapy Association.)

8. Select an issue that may be reflective of a trend, such as technology-based distance education, reductions in medical-based health care financing, affordable home–based technology, or another of your choice; it does not necessarily need to be related to health care or practice. Write the issue you have selected in the largest of the circles represented in Figure 5-1. Working alone or with a group, brainstorm on what you think may be major implications of this issue. Write these implications in the next larger circle immediately adjacent to the largest one.

   Now, think about second-level implications that may grow from the first level. Place these in the next group of circles. Either alone or as a group, come to a consensus to determine which of the implications you believe are most likely to occur.

   Score them as follows:

   1 = Most likely to occur

   2 = Might occur

   3 = Least likely to occur

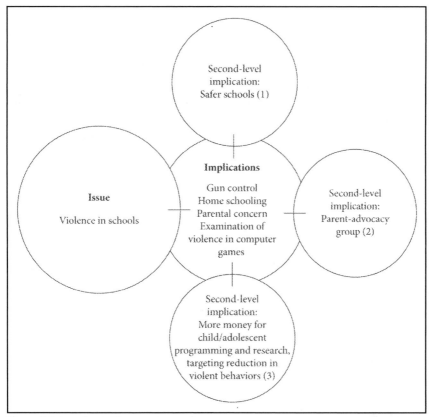

Figure 5-2. Issue impact tree, case example.

RESULTING IMPLICATIONS FOR FUTURE OCCUPATION-CENTERED PROGRAMMING

The parent-child community program case introduced earlier will help to demonstrate how an issue impact tree can be used to forecast possible futures for a program. As you review Figure 5-2, you will see that the primary issue—real and threatened violence in schools—has a number of primary and several second-level implications that may be reflected in the development of future programming.

It is likely that the current and next few years will welcome community- and school-based prevention programming and research in relation to (1) violent behavior exhibited by children and adolescents, (2) the nature of and time spent on computer games by children, and (3) the nature of parent-child communications and time spent in shared activities.

As we develop this scenario and others in later chapters, you will see how we continue to return to the information provided by trends analyses and the resulting future forecasts and predictions.

SUMMARY

The planning of occupation-centered programs does not occur in a vacuum. An identification of trends based on past and present information will encourage the planner to anticipate the future and make forecasts regarding the potential successes of his or her proposed programming. Envisioning the future will prompt the planner to be prepared for changes in population, funding, and market demands.

It is intended that you use the results of the previous exercises to help you plan your future programs. As a practitioner and program development specialist, you will find it critical to your progress to continue some ongoing analysis of trends. As a leader and manager, you may wish to place futures forecasting on a yearly retreat agenda; without it, an organization cannot successfully complete five- to ten-year planning. Skillful and sometimes intuitive futures forecasting can place you and your organization in the position of setting trends and designing futures rather than scrambling to keep up with those that are occurring. Begin now to establish habits that will place you in the forefront of futures forecasting.

REFERENCES

American Occupational Therapy Association. (2007). AOTA's centennial vision and executive summary. *American Journal of Occupational Therapy, 61,* 613-614.

American Occupational Therapy Association. (2013). Engaged in ongoing effort to promote role of occupational therapy in primary care. http://www.aota.org/Publications-News/AOTANews/2013/Primary-Care-Promote.aspx

Bennis, W., & Slater, P. (1968). *The temporary society.* San Francisco, CA: Jossey-Bass.

Bishaw, A. (2005). *Areas of concentrated poverty: 1999.* Washington, DC: U.S. Department of Commerce: Economics and Statistics Administration, U.S. Census Bureau.

Cason, J. (2015). Telehealth and occupational therapy: Integral to the triple aim of health care reform. *American Journal of Occupational Therapy, 69*(2),

Celente, G. (1991). *Trend tracking.* New York, NY: Warner Books.

Garretson, C. H. (1997). *Factors affecting Webmasters' sense of responsibility for information accuracy.* Unpublished thesis. Statesboro, GA: Georgia Southern University.

Hart, E., & Parsons, H. (2015). *Occupational therapy: Cost-effective solutions for a changing health system.* Bethesda, MD: American Occupational Therapy Association.

Issel, L. M. (2014). *Health program planning and evaluation.* Burlington, MA: Jones and Bartlett.

Leventhal, T., & Brooks-Gunn, J. (2000). The neighborhoods they live in: The effects of neighborhood residence on child and adolescent outcomes. *Psychological Bulletin, 126*(2), 309-337.

Metzler, C., Hartmann, K., & Lowenthal, L. (2012). Defining primary care: Envisioning the role of occupational therapy. *American Journal of Occupational Therapy, 66*(3), 266-270.

Metzler, C., Hartmann, K., & Lowenthal, L. (2014). Role of occupational therapy in primary care. *American Journal of Occupational Therapy, 68*(Suppl 3), 25-32.

Muir, S. (2012). Occupational therapy in primary health care: We should be there. *American Journal of Occupational Therapy, 66*(5), 506-510.

Ohmer, M., & DeMasi, K. (2009). *Consensus organizing: A community development workbook.* Thousand Oaks, CA: Sage.

Putnam, R. (2000). *Bowling alone: The collapse and revival of American community.* New York, NY: Simon and Schuster.

Ramsey, D., & Robertson, S. (1993). *Breaking into new markets: Expanding roles in mental health. Workshop resource book.* Bethesda, MD: American Occupational Therapy Association.

Waite, A. (2014). Prime models: Showcasing occupational therapies' role on primary care teams. *OT Practice, 19*(7), 8-10.

Weil, M. O. (1996). Community building: Building community practice. *Social Work, 41*(5), 481-499.

Wilson, W. J. (1987). *The truly disadvantaged.* Chicago, IL: University of Chicago Press.

Yamkovenko. (2015). The emerging niche: What's next in your practice. http://www.aota.org/Practice/manage/niche.aspx

Additional Websites

AOTA: http://www.aota.org/Practice/Manage/Social-Media/social-media-goals.aspx. (social@aota.org)
World Health Organization (WHO): http://www.who.int/en/

Federal Government Websites

Federal Bureau of Investigation (FBI): Crime Reports: http://www.fbi.gov/ucr/ucr.htm
HOME program: http://www.hud.gov/offices/cpd/affordablehousing/index.cfm
U.S. Census Bureau: Data on Poverty: http://www.census.gov/hhes/www/poverty/poverty.html
U.S. Department of Education: No Child Left Behind: http://www.ed.gov/nclb/landing.jhtml
U.S. Department of Housing and Urban Development (HUD): http://www.hud.gov/

National Political Parties

Democratic Party: http://www.democrat.org/
Republican National Committee: http://www.gop.com/

Think Tanks and Research Institutes

Center for American Progress: Domestic and Economy: http://www.americanprogress.org/issues/domestic Economic
    Policy Institute: http://www.epinet.org/
The Heritage Foundation: http://www.heritage.org/
The Urban Institute: www.urban.org
Urban Institute Research on Affordable Housing: Housing America's Low-Income Families: http://www.urban.org/
    toolkit/issues/housing.cfm
United Nations Development Programme: http://www.undp.org

Public Radio and Broadcasting

National Public Radio: Economy: http://www.npr.org/templates/topics/topic.php?topicld+1017
Public Broadcasting Service: NOW—Global Inequality: http://www.pbs.org/now/politics/income.html
Public Broadcasting Service: NOW—Understanding Globalization: http://www.pbs.org/now/politics/globaldebate.html

Federal Legislation: Tracking

Tracking Legislation on the Internet: Use this site to find out about new, changing, and proposed federal legislation:
    http://www.pbs.org/now/politics/legislation.htm.

II

Developing Your Program
Design and Planning Phase

6

Developing a Timeline for Program Design, Planning, Preparation, Implementation, and Evaluation

---

LEARNING OBJECTIVES

1. To appreciate the importance of maintaining a timeline in the accomplishment of program design, implementation, and review/evaluation

2. To understand and implement positive elements of time management

3. To explore various formats for organizing and displaying timelines

4. To define the three phases of efficient program development: (1) the design and planning phase, (2) the preparation and implementation phase, and (3) the review and evaluation phase

5. To identify tasks associated with each phase of the program development process and to develop a timeline to reflect these tasks

---

KEY TERMS

1. Timeline

2. Time and business management

3. Design and planning phase

4. Preparation and implementation phase

5. Review and evaluation phase

Fazio, L. S. *Developing Occupation-Centered Programs With the Community, Third Edition* (pp 91-96).
© 2017 Taylor & Francis Group.

One of the first critical steps of the program design and development process is to establish a firm calendar of what is to be done. This will help accomplish the program's goals and determine when each step must be taken in order to initiate the work at the anticipated time. This calendar, or **timeline,** ensures that nothing will be forgotten and that there will be no surprises that cost time and often add expense.

There are many ways to develop a timeline; much of the design and detail depends on the organizational style of the individual. For planners who are sufficiently organized in their work routines, a sketchy timeline is generally enough to permit them to maintain a schedule; those individuals who are less organized, on the other hand, will need to include all of the steps.

We discussed managing personal time in Chapter 3, and that information becomes even more critical as we begin what may appear to be the daunting task of designing, planning, preparing, implementing, and evaluating a program. Covey (1989, 2004) has long been a leader in identifying the elements of effective **time and business management**. In his 1989 text, Covey describes a "time management matrix" that is organized according to those activities that are deemed urgent/not urgent and those that are considered important/not important (pp. 146-182). Organizing in this way helps the planner prioritize tasks and spend time wisely. Other business and personal planners have offered strategies for organizing and staying on task. Glei (2013) describes elements that are necessary to build a routine and to sharpen your creativity. Smith (2016) provides time management assistance to manage procrastination, reduce stress, and increase productivity—all necessary to assist planners as they not only develop programming, but manage all of the other demands of family, personal needs, school, and often other employment. Allen and Fallows (2003) are also interested in being productive and in doing so without stress. In their analysis, anxiety is caused by a lack of control, organization, and preparation. Focusing on outcomes is necessary but can cause distress if preparations are delayed or dismissed. You may wish to review some of these recommendations and strategies for managing the several phases of getting from "idea" to program outcomes.

DESIGNS FOR TIMELINES

Timelines may be organized according to the full process of designing, developing and evaluating a program. For example, one might prefer to develop the timeline according to the three phases of program development outlined in this text:

1. Design and planning phase

2. Preparation and implementation phase

3. Program review and evaluation phase

Whatever approach you choose, it is often helpful to have a template, or several, to choose from to help structure your work. You can build these to stand alone, or you may wish to coordinate a template with your logic model. There are multiple online sources for the creation of organizational templates.

SmartDraw permits you to input your information into the template you choose, and it will align and space events and milestones automatically as you enter your information (https://www.smartdraw.com). Another source, from https://www.bing.com/images (type "timeline templates" in the search bar), provides multiple designs for timeline templates, both for working and for presentations. Granting agencies also offer recommendations for preferred templates for specific sections of the timeline that deal with funding proposals. Others are not specific to a particular granting agency, such as https://www.grantstation.com/includes/tracks/grant_proposal/writing-timeline.pdf.

The Design and Planning Phase

The **design and planning phase** may include the following: (1) identifying trends and needs to develop and support program ideas; (2) research of established and existing programs similar to the one you are designing or expanding; (3) researching and developing the community profiles to include identification of a community's assets and strengths; (4) researching and developing the service population profile; (5) identifying a potential partnering organization and stakeholders; (6) conducting the assessment of need; (7) consideration of an organizing theory to guide programming choices; (8) identifying program impact, outcomes, and tentative goals for the program; (9) determining program objectives and the general structure of the program to be offered; and (10) beginning the plan for sustainability.

This preliminary phase would include the detailed template/calendar for interviews and on-site visits to build a collaborative relationship with the proposed partnering organization. Such information can be obtained previous to your visit to determine an early match with your purpose. Information such as the mission and philosophy of the sponsoring organization, data for the community profile, and the needs assessment can likely be obtained from the organization's website. You should also block out time for the research that will be needed to develop the service population profile, to explore other established and existing programs that may be similar to the one you are designing, and to obtain evidence that similar programming is effective. When you have obtained data regarding the community's assets, particularly the "people assets," you will want to anticipate time to determine how best to train staff and volunteers. In addition, scheduled time to review and chart trends on a daily or weekly basis would help to ensure that this program will likely be viable now and in the future. If you are a practicing clinician and you find that you will need to obtain new practice skills or knowledge, you must anticipate this on your timeline as well. For those working in a group or as part of a team of collaborators, a coordinated timeline/calendar will balance the workload.

The Preparation and Implementation Phase

The **preparation phase** will include the following: (1) review of all data collected in the preliminary phase; (2) establishment of a theory to guide programming choices; (3) firm goals and accompanying objectives that will lead you to outcome and impact measurement; (4) development of detailed, day-to-day program plans to enable goal achievement; (5) matching of potential staff, furnishings, equipment, supplies, and space to the goal and objectives; (6) specifying a budget of needed funds; (7) identifying potential funding sources, their specific timelines, and securing the funding; (8) selection of program evaluation methods; and (9) continuation of planning for sustainability. If you have identified a potential funding/granting agency, this would be the time to become familiar with their requirements and their application process. Work toward the submission of an application will be blended with your timeline.

Although there may be some blurring between the preparation phase and the **implementation phase,** once we know that some of the planning has already occurred, our timeline for the implementation phase will include the following: (1) more detailed and specific budgeting related to actual acquisition of funds; (2) hiring and training of staff; (3) acquisition of all equipment and supplies; and (4) active marketing. The completion of this phase would then signal actual startup and continuation of the programming.

The Program Review and Evaluation Phase

The program **review and evaluation phase** would be initiated with the process evaluation to determine if your program is doing what you think it is and whether changes are needed. Such a review and evaluation and the formative evaluation of objectives can be conducted on a weekly basis or at the end of a programming cycle. This information will assist in fine-tuning goals, objectives, programming details, and longer-term evaluation measures. This first phase of evaluation would establish the foundation for the measurement of longer-term outcomes, perhaps measured in 6 months, after 1 year, or continued for several years toward a measurement of impact. This early phase would include a critical review of all data collected, including data provided by any individual assessments that may have been done as well as any formative or summative data that have been collected. As mentioned previously, such data would then be evaluated against the program's goal or goals and objectives. The results of these evaluations would prompt the examination of program content and mode of delivery to determine if either or both would require change to better meet the goals. Finally, resultant changes might be initiated in the actual measurement of the goal(s), and objectives might be altered (we would assume goals would not be changed, since their relationship to outcomes and impact had already been established). Finally, the programming content or delivery might be changed. Progress toward sustaining the program—including building community assets and capacity—is monitored.

At the 1-year review is when you will revisit staff and volunteers to see if more or different training is needed. This is part of the process or formative evaluation. At this review, it would be appropriate to again review the ongoing collection of trends, to update the community profile, and perhaps to revisit the assessment of needs. At earlier intervals—perhaps monthly and certainly at 3-month intervals—the budget, staffing, furnishings, equipment, supplies, space, and marketing would require scrutiny.

For this phase of planning, some program planners prefer to move from the template to a large lined calendar or white board where they can record what has to be done each month and each week of the month for the full length of the process. Access to the progress of this schedule is important when there is a team working together. If they were also the recipients of grant or foundation funding, they would include any reporting and resubmission deadlines on this calendar as well as the collection dates for required program data. It should be noted that your funding sources may require program evaluation and review on differing schedules.

Other planners who may not require a detailed calendar might prefer to develop lists of what must occur each month. For example, if a planner wishes to establish a private practice, a monthly list calendar might look something like the following:

- Month 1:
  - Investigate trends.
  - Meet with a financial planner and/or small-business attorney.
  - Conduct a market analysis.
  - Complete community profiles.
- Month 2:
  - Investigate site location.
  - Network the professional community; perhaps seek partners and collaborators.
  - Initiate an early needs assessment with the professional community.

Although the format and style you choose in creating a timeline will depend on personal preference, some form of time mapping must be included to ensure that no detail is forgotten. Some sites and many insurers will require inspections by fire and safety personnel or perhaps licensure or credentialing before a program is permitted to open. Both of these requirements could take months, so they must be anticipated. Another consideration is equipment, which could arrive in a matter of days but can sometimes take months. If it takes only a few days for delivery, it cannot be ordered until you have a space for it. Finally, ask yourself the following questions as you continue to develop your timeline. If you're remodeling space, what is the projected time for completion? If remodeling or building is initiated in the winter or spring, how will weather affect your projected opening? When will you hire staff? How will the staff be paid before you generate revenue or receive funding? In anticipating responses to all of these questions, it is far better to be proactive than reactive; answers to these questions are necessary and must be represented on your timeline.

Exercise 6-1

Establishing Your Timeline

Choose a template and/or other format for development of your timeline of tasks. As you anticipate your full program plan, group the tasks to be completed according to the three phases discussed on the previous pages. As you continue to work on your programming, through the chapters of this text, you will provide more detail for the timeline.

1. Design and planning phase:

_____

_____

_____

_____

_____

2. Preparation and implementation phase:

_____

_____

_____

_____

_____

3. Program review and evaluation phase:

_____

_____

_____

_____

_____

If you are designing and planning a program as a student group, then your template/calendar will reflect the tasks that must be completed to develop your proposal over the course of your academic semester, quarter, or year. However, you will still develop the full timeline for the remainder of the tasks, even though you may not actually be implementing the program as part of your assignment. If you are implementing the program, your timeline will be expanded, as recommended here.

4. When you have completed the outlined exercises and have defined all of the tasks that will be necessary to take your program from initial design through implementation to review and evaluation, transfer the specific tasks to a calendar of your choice. The timeline is a work in progress and will need to be revisited frequently as you continue your work.

SUMMARY

Regardless of the style or format, developing and following a timeline is the key to accomplishing all of the tasks of program development in a timely and efficient manner. Several recommendations have been made for ways to develop your timeline calendar; Part III of this text includes additional examples. Organizing your timeline around the three phases of program development has been identified as a preferred method of organization. These phases include (1) the design and planning phase, (2) the preparation and implementation phase, and (3) the program review and evaluation phase.

It will be important to make your calendar as functional as you can. Devising a method to note when a task has been completed can be encouraging and will keep you motivated during the months when things may slow down more than you would like. A wipe-off calendar that you can post on the wall is another option, since you may have to frequently move things around (for example, acquisition of funding or a loan, staff hiring, arrival of equipment, and progress on developing a space). An electronic calendar can work as well as long as a group/team can work collaboratively.

REFERENCES

Allen, D., & Fallows, J. (2003). *Getting things done: The art of stress-free productivity.* New York, NY: Penguin Books.

Covey, S. (1989). *The seven habits of highly effective people.* New York, NY: Simon and Schuster.

Covey, S. (2004). *The eighth habit.* New York, NY: Free Press.

Glei, J. (2013). *Manage your day-to-day: Build your routine, find your focus, and sharpen your creative mind.* Las Vegas, NV: Amazon Publishing.

Smith, J. (2016). *Time management: Simple and effective time management techniques to manage procrastination, reduce stress, increase productivity plus get more out of your day.* CreateSpace Independent Publishing Platform.

7

Developing the Profiles of Your Population and the Community, Researching the Supporting Literature, Finding Evidence, and Identifying Experts

The Beginning of the Assessment of "Need"

LEARNING OBJECTIVES

1. To recognize the layers of inquiry necessary to determine the services needed by a population

2. To learn how to profile a community for information to support the need for services

3. To understand the characteristics of the service profile as it is used to support the need for specific targeted population services

4. To develop a comprehensive profile of your selected population and community

5. To thoroughly investigate relevant research literature to support the need for a program

6. To identify and locate evidence that supports the effectiveness of programs such as the one being proposed (evidence-based practice)

7. To appreciate the art of practice and the value of a judgment-based practice

8. To identify those individuals who may be able to validate our early ideas for a program and our anticipated goals (expert opinion)

Fazio, L. S. *Developing Occupation-Centered Programs With the Community, Third Edition* (pp 97-118).
© 2017 Taylor & Francis Group.

KEY TERMS

1. Layers of inquiry
2. Community profile
3. Population
4. Census data/U.S. Census Bureau
5. Centers for Disease Control and Prevention (CDC)
6. Condition
7. Context
8. Service profile
9. Evidence
10. Evidence-based planning
11. Translation/implementation science
12. Clinical decision making
13. Systematic reviews
14. Critically appraised papers (CAPs)
15. Synthesis matrix
16. Expert opinion
17. Judgment-based practices of care

Several **layers of inquiry** are necessary to determine what programming services are needed by a population. We initiate the investigation of these layers of inquiry first at our desks, then we will continue in the community itself. These layers include knowing the community where you will provide services, including the assets of the community; knowing the targeted population that will receive services; and, if you anticipate working with an agency/facility, knowing what that administration wants for its clients/patients and what the clients/patients want for themselves. You must also determine the needs of your stakeholders. Some of your stakeholders are likely included in these groups, but there may be others. If any of these areas are neglected in the early stages of planning, it is likely that you will not be as successful as you could be.

In summary, layers of inquiry to determine what programming services you will provide are as follows:

- Know the community where you will provide services, including knowing the assets and capacities of the community
- Know the targeted population who will receive services
- Know what services the agency/facility administration wants for the clients/patients
- Know your stakeholders and their needs for your population
- Know what the clients/patients want for themselves

One other "layer" we want to include in our list was discussed in Chapter 3; the various ways to ascertain your present foundation of personal and professional knowledge and skills (i.e., knowing your potential for providing services). If you participated in the exercises provided, you have a good sense of what you can offer a potential program. It is important to remember, regardless of where you are in your occupational therapy program of study or in your career, that you do possess a considerable amount of both knowledge and skills. Many, if not all students today have had previous work, family/home, and academic experience. Often, these are the experiences that bring a unique perspective to your practice, particularly in the less proscriptive environment of the community. In the context of community, we are truly defining and creating a new practice—not only for the community and the population residing within it or transitioning through it, but also for ourselves as practitioners. Whether the particular practice has occurred previously, this community coupled with the uniqueness of the programmer sculpts a totally new practice that cannot be duplicated in other settings.

What Are Community Profiles?

As discussed earlier in this text, community is a complex concept and one that the potential programmer must explore at many levels. By examining one level at a time, we will investigate the community broadly to create a description of what factors exist that may impact our developing plans. We are referring to this description or brief picture as the **community profile.**

Community profiling was, early on, developed as a tool for community development (Baldock, 1974; Henderson & Thomas 1987). During the 1980s and 1990s, a group of related techniques—needs assessments and social audits—were revived. *Social audit* is a term that was used to describe studies that sought to demonstrate the impact on communities of changes in public policy or of major factory closures that were occurring in the United States in the 1970s and 1980s. In 1985, global concerns for community development were reflected in the Archbishop of Canterbury's report titled *Faith in the City*, which suggested that inner-city churches might undertake parish audits as a means of reassessing their role in urban communities. This was a turning point in an ongoing examination of the role of the church in offering help and support specific to the "needs" of a community.

More recently, many local authorities have harnessed new and evolving technology to produce statistical profiles and maps that identify areas with particular problems such as high levels of crime, educational underachievement, poverty, or disadvantage. Their aim has primarily been to target resources more effectively. In addition, community profiles have been used as one element in the development of strategies to bring decision making and service delivery to the neighborhood level. Communities, community groups, and voluntary organizations have also initiated or conducted community profiling exercises as a means of demonstrating to statutory service providers that they are not receiving an adequate level of services or that they have needs that are not currently being met. Community profiles may cover both needs and resources of a wide range of issues affecting a community.

For our purposes in occupation-centered community program development, we will define a community profile in this way: "A community profile is a comprehensive description (of the needs and resources, assets and capacities) of a population that is defined, or defines itself, as a community. The comprehensive profile includes our selected population, or populations, and the community where we find them." Our purpose, ultimately, is to improve the quality of life for the individual and for the community.

Developing a series of profiles that will offer a comprehensive view of the multiple issues a population faces everyday will prevent us from developing programming for isolated issues that are, in fact, only part of very complex pictures. Issues such as poverty, housing, employment, and health are interrelated and must be considered in any program development and planning. Certainly, we cannot attend to everything, but we must be sure we are aware that our programs are "bricks" in a very large "house." As we have mentioned previously, resources/assets might include housing, parks, hospitals, clinics, community centers, churches, and schools, but they should also include the "time" people may have and the expertise they can make available to others. Each of these areas of resources/assets may also include areas of need. However, for our purposes as beginning programmers, we are separating the assessment of need and assets from the profiles. As you continue to program in the future, you may choose to combine this work.

We know that resources/assets can be tangible and that they often are, but they can also be intangible, such as formal and informal skills of members of the community and informal and formal networks of support, such as families, households, neighbors, congregations, and community organizations. What of the "qualities" a community represents? Communities may represent themselves as resilient, determined, and trusting or perhaps just the opposite. These things have been identified as components of social capital and can be influenced and developed.

PROFILING THE COMMUNITY

In creating the community profile, the Aspen Reference Group suggests that the planner contribute equal attention to both the community demographics (that is, age, sex, ethnicity education, and so on) and to the social demographics, or those community social and medical services that currently exist as well as those that are lacking (what we have called *assets and resources/capacities and needs*) (DiLima & Schust, 1997, pp. 73-74). The addition of social demographics will help the planner know not only whether his or her services are needed, but also what services are needed to complement those that may already exist. This is important information in identifying partners and forming coalitions. Forming complementary services to those that are currently being provided is often the best way to enter a community. Collecting demographics that include service dimensions for the community will help us to determine whether our proposed programming is already being offered; perhaps with further investigation we could know whether additional services are warranted, possibly with alternative methods of delivery. The sum of all of the observations and research we conduct will result in a description, or profile, of the community or communities where our targeted **population** resides and engages in occupation (and the community, if different, where we will provide services).

> In many instances, the programmer may feel some familiarity with the larger community. Perhaps, for example, he or she has lived in the community such as suburban Denver, Colorado, for some time, but if programming is being considered in a downtown Denver sanctuary for runaway teenagers, the programmer must explore and understand the specific community—in our example, downtown urban Denver. The next level to be considered is the community of the homeless in urban Denver and the community of runaway homeless teens, which is perhaps similar in some ways but likely very different in others. Of course, communities are made up of individuals. Each homeless teen in our example brings with him or her the remnants of the cultures and communities from which he or she may have recently sought exit. These multiple layers of community always exist and must be explored and understood in order to define and develop the most effective programming possible. Thus, as part of our community profile, we include a thorough analysis of our population, their condition, and the context where we find them. Together, this forms our service profile (see Figure 7-1).

Developing the Profile of Your Selected Community: How Is It Done?

For most of our program designs and plans, we will seek the support of an agency/facility in order to assist us with our work. This does not preclude the possibility that programs can develop without such agency/facility support or sanction (e.g., private practices, not-for-profits). However, it is strongly recommended that initial student learning experiences be structured to include work with an agency/facility. By doing so, you have already identified an ally/friend who has done the preliminary groundwork at establishing his or her identity as a community asset. You may have

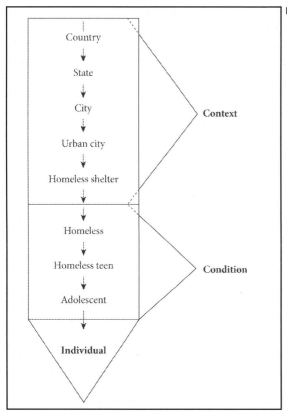

Figure 7-1. Layers of community.

identified a partnering agency alongside your interest in a population. This partnering agency may be a nonprofit you have worked with before, a Level I Fieldwork site, or another organization where you have volunteered. When you make your choice of a population, you will determine where to find them (the context/community). As you develop these profiles, you will determine the population's network, its assets and resources, and any agencies it is presently involved with; this will likely lead you to a partnering agency if you have not already identified one. First, identify the location of your agency and the neighborhood/community where your targeted population resides. This may be the same community where the agency is located or it may be different (e.g., a detention center population may come from many communities within an urban city or the state). At this point, it is back to the computer to collect as much demographic information as you can.

Collecting Data to Help You Understand Your Population and Its Community: Census and CDC Data

Census data are often the place to begin to establish a foundation for understanding the community or communities. If you have not already done so, you can obtain such data from the **U.S. Census Bureau's** website: http://www/census.gov. It will lead you to various resources for demographics to help you understand your population and the relevant community. Ohmer and DeMasi (2009) encourage the use of census data to obtain the overall demographic characteristics of the neighborhood, and social, economic, and housing characteristics. The Census Bureau can offer such information as the general demographics of a community (i.e., total population and growth rate, gender, age, race/ethnicity, households by type and family size); social characteristics (i.e., school enrollment, educational attainment, marital status, fertility, grandparents, language spoken at home); economic characteristics (i.e., employment status of individuals aged 18 years and over, occupations of the employed labor force, commuters, income, and poverty status); and housing characteristics (i.e., occupancy, how long residing at an address, occupants per room, housing and rental values). We can learn a great deal about our population and the community from census data, but perhaps of equal importance as we develop the profile of our population are the **Centers for Disease Control and Prevention (CDC)**. The CDC can offer significant information about the conditions and diseases experienced by our population in addition to what we can obtain from the Census Bureau and perhaps other city, regional, and state data collection agencies. In addition, the CDC offers information to aid in the prevention of illness and disease. For example, the CDC website (http://www.cdc.gov) includes information (under "Healthy Living—Health Topics") on adolescent and school health, food safety, healthy weight, overweight and obesity, smoking and tobacco use, and vaccines and immunization.

Once you have demographics and background, locate the community where your agency is situated and the community where your targeted population resides if different. Mapping will give you a sense of where your selected community is located with respect to adjacent communities. The location of landmarks, public buildings, and public services will be useful as you begin to develop specific objectives for the program and identify partners and collaborators. As you develop your program, you may find that you will rely heavily on public services; if this is the case, you will want to obtain more specific and detailed maps such as those of transportation networks and public services. Determining the boundaries of ethnic neighborhoods and accompanying services adjacent to your selected community may be useful information. While these boundaries sometimes are fluid, permitting easy passage of persons and things from one neighborhood or community to another, they also can be fixed by language, social custom, and culture. This may affect your targeted population and the range of services your program will provide.

Considering the information provided to structure the dimensions of a community profile, think about how you will develop the profile of the community or communities where your anticipated population resides as well as where the agency/facility is located. As suggested earlier, begin by locating the agency/facility on a map. In the following exercise, note any generic information the map might provide, such as landmarks, public facilities, and so on. Also determine what route you might wish to take when you make your first visit to the site. Locate a route that will provide you with optimal observational information to assist you as you develop your profile. Even if you are already familiar with the location, locate it on a map to visually center it with regard to surrounding communities. If your participants will rely on public transportation, you will want to check it out later. This careful and detailed mapping of communities is likely of greater importance to those who establish programs in large urban areas; however, smaller communities may hold isolated cultures or socioeconomic groupings with whom the programmer is equally unfamiliar.

Exercise 7-1

Initiating the Profile of Your Selected Community

1. Using a highlighter, draw what you presently perceive to be the boundaries of your selected community on a map. Note surrounding communities, locations of freeways, and other points of interest.
2. Record here any information you are able to glean from your map review, including landmarks and public facilities (libraries, parks, and so on). If you are already familiar with the location, use what you know to supplement the map review.

_____

_____

_____

_____

_____

3. Develop a brief profile of the community you have selected using demographic information from the census bureau or other resources of your choice. This profile should provide you with a foundation from which you can extend your research as you continue to investigate the community. Record your responses in the space provided.

a. Socioeconomic data:

_____

_____

_____

_____

_____

b. Level of education:

_____

_____

_____

_____

_____

c. Nature of family households (that is, single-parent, extended, and so on):

_____

_____

_____

_____

_____

d. Ethnicity and religion:

_____

_____

_____

_____

_____

e. Other data you may wish to collect:

_____

_____

_____

_____

4. List potential partners in the community who may be able to collaborate in your programming efforts; consider clergy, law enforcement personnel, shop owners, schools, service organizations, and others:

_____

_____

_____

_____

Profiling Our Population in Anticipation of Programming

As a student, when you are preparing to select an agency/facility for which you wish to design and plan a community program, you are informed of the population that agency serves. Experienced therapists most often wish to expand or extend programming within their area of experience and expertise (i.e., public school therapists may wish to extend programming to after-school clubs or day camps; acute care therapists may wish to develop outpatient services). In these examples, the therapist may wish to solicit the assistance of an agency/facility with which he or she is already affiliated. In many instances, the therapist may seek referrals from other agencies as well. In expanding or extending services, conducting an investigation of the services already available, as mentioned earlier, would be important.

It is also important to remember that seeking support from an agency/facility is a different relationship than one where a program is developed "for" an agency/facility. The latter circumstance is suggested as a good first student experience. Of course, students may not have had sufficient experience to develop expertise with a particular population, as we might expect from a practicing therapist. However, selecting a population on the basis of interest and sometimes previous experience in a different context is an equally valid way to begin programming.

Although the potential population cannot be fully explored and understood outside of the context of the specific community, we can and should carefully research both before developing an interview format and instrument to facilitate the on-site assessment of needs. As we have suggested with the early development of the community profile, it is best to begin with a map or maps. By gathering necessary demographic data, we can also "map" our expected population by finding out all we can before going on site. With some preliminary information about the community and about the expected population, we will be prepared to ask the most useful and focused questions when we first meet the administrator or professional who will contribute to the needs assessment.

To return to our earlier Denver example, at the core of the potential program in downtown Denver and composing one level of community is the adolescent. Our first challenge will be to understand the developmental characteristics of adolescence. Only later, after reviewing what we know of adolescents, do we consider the needs imposed by the complex layers of community. In our example, homelessness may be the next characteristic to investigate. Homeless, runaway teens may or may not be the same homeless, runaway teen in New York City, Denver, Las Vegas, or Los Angeles. While knowing something about one community will likely tell us something about the others, it will not tell us everything. We may know statistically that, nationwide, runaway teens are likely to have attempted suicide, have been abused, and are addicted to drugs and/or alcohol (see Part V of this text). But those characteristics may or may not be present to the same degree in every community of runaway teens. To continue our understanding we must learn something about shelters, sanctuaries, and transitional centers. These settings may provide the context for programming and are, in themselves, yet another layer of community. This community is sometimes self-selected by the homeless teen; but often it is imposed by social services or the police. Therefore the population of one shelter-community may represent programming needs differing from another based on whether it was chosen by the teen or ascribed by authorities.

As you can see from the previous example, before even going to a specific site, we have at least three or more areas to research if we anticipate program development to meet the needs of homeless teens. We must develop a profile of the population—in our example, adolescence (see Figure 7-1).

POPULATION, CONDITION, AND CONTEXT = SERVICE PROFILE

Figure 7-2. Service profile.

We know that the population cannot be fully explored and understood outside of the context of the specific community, but we also know that the previous information will be adequate to assist us as we prepare more targeted questions to ask when we go on site to first visit with those persons (i.e., administrators, other professionals, service providers, and additional stakeholders) who will help us as we continue to develop our program design. We have mentioned credibility as one of the prerequisites for developing a successful working relationship with the agency, others who may assist us, or future collaborators. A carefully researched and insightfully prepared community profile and anticipated service profile will go a long way toward establishing your credibility. If your anticipated population comprises individuals with disabilities, you must include this in your research of conditions. It is suggested that many homeless teens have been unsuccessful in school. They may be experiencing difficulties with learning and/or social bullying. These may be additional conditions to be explored with our earlier example. Remember that we are developing a service profile for the population, which is simply a place to begin. Certainly not all adolescents, or all adolescents who are homeless, or all adolescents who are substance abusers exhibit the same individual profiles, nor do they have the same needs. However, they have many characteristics in common, and those are what we hope to identify with this early research. Later, when we meet them, we will determine where the needs of our specific population may differ from those of the general population.

It may be useful to mention that the experienced therapist who is considering developing a new program but is not yet ready to target a specific site may wish to postpone the community profile, first observing and researching service populations similar to what is anticipated. The community selected for observation may be different from the one where programming will eventually be developed, but there is useful information to be gained. By understanding the general needs of the population—developmentally, clinically, and socially—you can develop the community profile when the site has been selected. You will know the parameters of your profiles and you will know how your knowledge base and skills are matched to what the anticipated need will be. You will also have a much more realistic idea of the resources that will be needed, whether you gain the expertise to supply these or you glean them from partners and collaborators in the community.

We must learn all we can about the **condition** of homelessness and particularly about homelessness during adolescence. We have also mentioned the conditions of substance abuse and abuse by others. Learning what we can about these conditions will further strengthen our profile, and offer assistance as we develop relevant programming. We must also investigate the **context** for services: shelters, sanctuaries, and transitional centers. The sum of this information will provide us with the profile of anticipated community-based services for this population, our **service profile** (Figure 7-2).

Exercise 7-2

Developing the Service Profile

The following are examples of populations for whom occupation-centered, community-based programs have been designed; use them to practice identifying the population, the conditions, and the context to develop a service profile. You will likely discover some overlap in examining population and condition.

Population, Condition, and Context

1. Junior high school adolescent girls between the ages of 12 and 15 years who are pregnant or raising an infant while attending school
2. Well elderly men and women between the ages of 65 and 94 years who are living in a low- to moderate-income, inner-city, transitional apartment complex
3. Young adults with low vision who are living at home and working in the community
4. Adults on the autistic spectrum—high functioning, between the ages of 17 and 24 years who are living at home and working in the community

   a. Discuss these examples with your instructor, other students, or colleagues. Organize the information provided for each of these examples into the following categories:

   Population:

   _____

   _____

   _____

   _____

   Conditions:

   _____

   _____

   _____

   _____

   Context:

   _____

   _____

   _____

   _____

   b. Identifying population, conditions, and context for the service profile you will develop, provide as much information as you have right now. With the help of your student group or colleagues, delineate the following categories as you did in the previous examples:

   Population:

   _____

   _____

   _____

   _____

   Conditions:

   _____

   _____

   _____

   _____

   Context:

   _____

   _____

   _____

   _____

When you have completed this exercise, you will have the anticipated service profile for the population you have selected. With this profile, you are now ready to research your textbooks, library, and Internet resources to learn as much as you can about the population, the conditions expressed and experienced by this population, and the context within which you will find this population and within which services will likely be conducted. You will have generated enough information with this recent research and the preliminary community profile to begin a program development file for this specific program. You can index the file in the same way the chapters of this text are organized, or you can develop your own system. By the end of the process, you will have collected a substantial amount of information and resources from which you will develop your formal program proposal and, perhaps, a funding application. When you have completed the research to further develop the anticipated service profile, you will be ready to develop the formal "on the ground" needs assessment. The results of the needs assessment will help you identify areas where you may wish to do further research to enhance the accuracy of what will become your specific service profile and to complete the data collection for the comprehensive community profile.

Researching the Literature and Finding Evidence

What Is Evidence-Based Planning and Practice?

The movement to encourage evidence-based and more scientific medical practices has evolved over many decades. According to Drake (2005) and Guyatt and Rennie (2002), the term *evidence-based medicine* was first introduced in 1990 to refer to a systematic approach to helping practitioners apply scientific evidence to decision making relative to a specific consumer. According to Relman (2007), the concept "evidence-based" developed when medical practitioners were charged with greater responsibility for monitoring their practice standards, initiating what would be described as the "age of accountability" (p. 95). Over time, the need for accountability broadened to include other health care practitioners. The term *evidence-based medicine* evolved into the more inclusive term *evidence-based practice*. Occupational therapy practitioners cannot avoid using evidence to support their practices and thus to produce evidence-based decision making. Insurance companies are using evidence-based practice (EBP) guidelines to determine standards of care, including the nature of services they will routinely fund. Hospital and rehabilitation facility administrators support evidence-based measures by advocating for data (evidence) to document client/patient outcomes, and Kellegrew (2005) notes that the inclusion of educational systems in this impetus for accountability likely began with the No Child Left Behind Act, which called for evidence-based education in classrooms.

Scaffa and Brownson (2014) tell us that **evidence** can be defined as data that inform decision making (p. 77). Program planning begins with the best evidence available to the planner. **Evidence-based planning** for health includes the best information available from clinical, epidemiological, administrative, demographic, and other relevant sources to clearly describe current and desired outcomes for an identified population (Ardal, Butler, Edwards, & Lawrie, 2006, p. 1). Epidemiological and demographic data comprise information about a population usually derived from a census or survey. Accessing these kinds of data was mentioned earlier in our discussion of profiles. Such data are almost always included in our program proposals.

According to the Institute of Medicine (2001), "effectiveness refers to care that is based on the use of systematically acquired evidence to determine whether an intervention, such as a preventive service, diagnostic test, or therapy, produces better outcomes than alternatives—including the alternative of doing nothing" (p. 46). In community programming development and practice, where we often rely on grant or foundation funding, we are held to the same standards for evidence to support our designs and programs as practitioners in institution-based practices. We must always ask ourselves the following question: Will this program produce the desired outcomes, and will it do so over other alternatives, including doing nothing? Generally, we would assume that "doing nothing" was not an alternative, but selecting another trajectory for action might be.

Drake (2005), writing from an occupational therapy mental health practice perspective, describes the "science-to-practice gap" in issues of prevention and wellness (p. 45). This gap is that between what we may know works and what we actually offer clients. We all recognize that this gap must be closed, and that efforts must be made to inform clinicians of the best and most efficient ways to first find evidence, which is then utilized in developing practices. Titler (2010), writing from a nursing perspective, also expresses concerns regarding the gap between evidence and actual practice. She tells us that evidence-based health care practices are available for a number of conditions, such as asthma, smoking cessation, heart failure, and the management of diabetes—areas in which many programmers are interested. However, these practices are not routinely implemented in care delivery, and variations in practices are broad. She suggests that to advance knowledge about promoting and sustaining the adoption of EBPs in health care, translation science needs more studies that test translating-research-into-practice interventions. She sees EBPs as innovations, and the adoption of any innovation is influenced by the nature of the innovation (e.g., the type and strength of evidence; the clinical topic), and the manner in which it is communicated (disseminated) to practitioners within a social system (organization, profession). Titler (2010) is describing **translation/implementation science**, the investigation of methods, interventions, and variables that influence the adoption of EBPs by individuals and organizations to improve clinical and operational decision making in health care.

It is not uncommon for health care consumers to research their diagnoses and accompanying treatment to advocate for their own effective and efficient services. It is likely that this trend toward self-advocacy in matters of illness and health will grow stronger over time. David Sackett, a Canadian physician, and his colleagues (1996) proposed early on that "evidence is high-quality current research or high-quality information that contributes to a decision about the care of a particular patient" (pp. 71-72). In the mix of factors that influence clinical decision making, the astute therapist knows that the consumer's values, preferences, and choices are of significant importance (Haynes, Devereaux, & Guyatt, 2002). These authors write from a mental health perspective, but, as occupational therapy practitioners, we are all very much proponents of client-centered approaches and the assurance of mechanisms for shared decision making between consumer/client, sometimes family and significant others, and therapist. In order to provide the best practice and to satisfy the consumer/advocate, the therapist must maintain a sophisticated understanding and translate the current research. The therapist, generally through his or her educational background, learns to review and critique research studies, and this leads to evidence that will inform our practices. How is this done? There are generally three parts to a thoughtful critique of relevant literature: (1) What are the study findings? (2) Is this study of sufficient rigor and quality? and (3) How can the results help me do what is best for my client/patient?

Before we continue this discussion, you may wonder, "What did we rely on before the push for practices supported by evidence of effectiveness became so prevalent?" Likely, most practitioners relied on theory, opinion, their education and experiences, and sometimes intuition. In adding EBP to the mix, these elements of clinical reasoning are not lost but simply expanded to include everything that is available to us that will provide evidence that we are on the right track. Kellegrew (2005) describes an evidence-based approach as a "style of thinking that incorporates research findings as one part of the **clinical decision-making** process (p. 12). EBP supports clinical experience, but does not replace it. The effective therapist combines multiple kinds of research alongside clinical experience in a reasoning process to shape his or her practice. Law (2002, 2005) is a strong proponent for the integration of individual knowledge and expertise with the best available external clinical evidence that can only be obtained from systematic research. We must also remember that there are qualitative/narrative measures to consider in our clinical reasoning process as well, and these studies are not as prevalent in the bank of evidence-based data as are quantitative approaches. This also prompts us to consider our role and responsibility, as therapists and programmers, in generating many kinds of data to construct evidence.

Finding "Evidence" to Support Need and to Guide Programming Goals, Objectives, and Interventions

Systematic Reviews and Clearinghouses

Evaluating research for application to practice takes some expertise as well as time—time that a therapist, particularly one engaged in program development, may not have. The **systematic review** is a way for therapists and students to utilize research findings without doing a full analysis of individual research studies, and it is often the most useful and efficient way to find and evaluate evidence to support their programming ideas. Reviews identify, assess, and synthesize research evidence from a number of individual research studies. There are a variety of sources of systematic reviews of research. The systematic review was initially introduced by the Cochrane Center, which is now referred to as the *Cochrane Collaboration* (www.cochrane.org). This organization aggregates multiple studies on many topics to determine the effectiveness of an intervention or practice. The studies selected are current and considered of high quality in their method. The Cochrane Collaboration is a clearinghouse for a wide array of practice specialists, pharmaceutical clinical trial data, and consumer information.

In support of the growing importance of EBP to the practitioners in the broad field of psychiatry and mental health (both of interest to community-based practices), the journal of the American Psychiatric Association, *Psychiatric Services*, dedicated 2001 to articles dealing with EBPs. Drake and Goldman offer most of these in their 2003 book, *Evidence-Based Practices in Mental Health*. The following topics of interest to occupational therapy practitioners and other providers for clients with severe and persistent mental illness are addressed among others:

- Strategies for disseminating EBP to frontline providers
- Ways to integrate EBP into the recovery model
- EBP in child and adolescent psychiatry
- EBP in services for family members of persons with psychiatric disorders

Other clearing houses and organizations that provide a research synthesis or critiques are ERIC Digests (www.eric.ed.gov.); the What Works Clearinghouse (www.whatworks.ed.gov); the Orlena Hawks Puckett Institute (www.puckett.org), dealing specifically with early childhood; and of similar concern with early childhood is the Center on the Social and Emotional Foundations for Early Learning (www.csefel.uiuc.edu). The latter two are representative of a research-to-practice orientation that not only includes a synthesis of relevant research, but also companion research-based consumer handouts. Other clearing houses of interest include Best Practice Initiative (www.osophs.dhhs.gov/ophs/BestPractice); Campbell Collaboration Library (www.campbellcol-laboration.org/library); Evidence-Based Mental Health (www.ebmh.bmj.com); and the National Guidelines Clearinghouse (www.guideline.gov).

General Guidelines and Databases for Practice Supported by Research

Practitioners can access EBP guidelines from national and international health care organizations. The National Guidelines Clearinghouse website (www.guideline.gov) documents the ways in which each guideline was developed, including the quality of the research evidence. Although these may be helpful, presently they are somewhat narrowly focused and one does not find standard practice guidelines that are tailored for occupational therapy implementation from any one group. However, the thoughtful practitioner will not select only one method to obtain evidence for effective practice, but many methods to provide the best care.

Also to be considered are databases. There are many that now support an EBP approach to include Medline and PubMed (www.ncbi.nlm.nih.gov/entrez/); the National Rehabilitation Information Center (NARIC) (www.naric.com), Agency for Healthcare Research and Quality (www.ahrq.gov); the National Institute of Mental Health (NIMH) (www.nimh.nih.gov/); and the Substance Abuse and Mental Health Services Administration (SAMHSA) (www.samhsa.gov). Currently, SAMHSA is funding an evaluation of EBPs through the Implementing Evidence-Based Practices Project. Of specific interest to occupational therapy practitioners in mental health and community practices, this includes, among other topics, the following:

- Assertive community treatment
- Integrated dual-disorder treatment
- Supported employment
- Illness management and recovery
- Family psychoeducation
- Medication management

Kellegrew (2005) recognizes that we must find better and more efficient ways to find evidence and utilize it in our work. She notes that the ability to use EBP requires some specialized skills and resources. She expands on this further with ideas for how to help the clinician to include Journal Clubs, developing a "favorites" list of evidence-based databases, using software such as *EndNote* to develop a customized database of one's most useful resources, updating critical appraisal skills at EBP workshops or in a college research methods course, and many other useful suggestions for the practitioner (Kellegrew, 2005, p. 15).

Evidence-Based Decision Making in Practice Supported by the Resources of the American Occupational Therapy Association

In response to what they describe as a reluctance by occupational therapists to let go of unsubstantiated traditions and a hesitancy to embrace scientific evidence, Fleming-Castaldy and Gillen (2013) challenge the profession to engage in a culture shift to a profession informed by evidence (p. 364). Evidence-based decision making and science-fostered innovation in practice are key objectives of the Centennial Vision (American Occupational Therapy Association [AOTA], 2007); however, the profession seems to be slow in moving forward to the use of evidence to support their practices. Many challenges are involved in integrating evidence into practice and, particularly, integrating evidence into community programming. What can happen if we do not place our programming on a foundation of evidence? Likely, these programs will not obtain expected outcomes, there will be a lack of or loss of funding, and lowered expectations by consumers of our ability to provide effective interventions to name a few potential repercussions. Many of our practice partners in the community are also lacking in their generation of evidence and/or their use of it to inform their work, although the disciplines associated with community development are making a strong claim for its importance.

EBP is based on the integration of critically appraised research results with the clinical expertise and the clients' preferences, beliefs, and values. The AOTA is committed to the generation of research to advance occupational therapy and to ensuring the viability of the profession. Resources toward this commitment include the EBP resource directory, evidence exchange, the journal club toolkit, the researcher database, and many research opportunities (http://www.aota.org/practice/researchers.aspx).

The Evidence Exchange was developed in 2011 as a central repository for high-quality, evidence-based literature reviews and related resources (www.aota.org/practice/researchers/evidence-exchange). The Evidence Exchange houses **critically appraised papers (CAPs)**, which are summaries of individual research articles selected for their value in providing evidence that can be easily implemented in practice. The CAPs posted on the Evidence Exchange go through a review process to make sure all information presented meets strict requirements. The CAPs reviewers represent all areas of occupational therapy practice and also professional expertise: clinicians, educators, and researchers (Arbesman, Goetz, & Lieberman, 2015, p. 21).

The profession also organizes and distributes practice guidelines. The newest EBP guidelines published by AOTA include *Occupational Therapy Practice Guidelines for Early Childhood: Birth Through 5 Years* (Frolek & Kingsley, 2013) and *Guidelines for Older Adults With Low Vision* (Kaldenberg & Smallfield, 2013). Occupational Therapy Practice Guidelines for Mental Health Promotion, Prevention and Intervention for Children and Youth (Bazyk & Arbesman, 2013) is an update of Occupational Therapy Practice Guidelines for Children with Behavioral and Psychosocial Needs (Jackson & Arbesman, 2005). Of course, practice guidelines provide clinicians, educators, and program planners with a concise summary of the existing evidence on a given topic. Practice guidelines are available at the AOTA online store (http://store.aota.org).

OT Search is a subscription service operated by the American Occupational Therapy Foundation (AOTF) through the Wilma West Library. OTSeeker (www.otseeker.com) is an occupational therapy database housed in Australia and is useful for the entire international occupational therapy community. Another subscription data base, OTD-BASE (http://www.otdbase.org), catalogues occupational therapy journals.

In October 2015, the AOTF sent a press release announcing their research priorities to work toward their vision of having a vibrant science that will support effective, evidence-based occupational therapy. In this press release, they announced new research initiatives to include health behaviors to prevent and manage chronic conditions, functional cognition, safety and injury prevention in home, clinical and community settings, technology and environmental supports in home and community, development and transitions for individuals and families, emotional and physiological influences on health, family and caregiver needs, and health care experience that includes access, care coordination, and utilization. Within these priorities we find many that are of interest to community programming planners, which may serve to remind us that we can also gather and provide data to contribute to these research priorities.

Organizing Your Literature Review to Support Your Profiles and Your Programming

Sometimes, it is a challenge to organize the literature you have found into a format that supports your ideas and helps you refine your programming interests. Generally, it is most helpful if you can organize your materials into themes or groupings of similar ideas. There are options for how to do this. The more primitive way is to make literature review notations on 3 × 5 cards, lay these cards out on a table, then move them around to represent ideas and developing themes. However, it is not likely that students today even know what a 3 × 5 card is, perhaps not even for its original usage of containing your grandmother's recipes. Today, there are more contemporary guidelines for both how to read a research paper and how to organize your reviews into themes. You may wish to choose a version of a CAPs approach to guide your reviews and organization of the articles you find. If you wish to organize your literature in this fashion, or are curious, visit the American Occupational Therapy Association (AOTA) website for more information and their guidelines for researchers and authors on how to proceed (www.aota.org/practice/researchers/evidence-exchange). Your proposal structures the research you are doing to support your programming ideas and, likely, you will include literature from several disciplines in addition to occupational therapy literature, so you may choose to organize your review summaries by discipline and/or by topic/population. The summaries of individual research articles provide evidence to strongly suggest your programming will be successful in one or more elements of your planning process.

Another method of organizing your review, favored by some granting organizations and planners, is a **synthesis matrix** (Parker-Karst & Walker, 2015). For the synthesis matrix your literature

How to create a synthesis matrix:

- Open your Microsoft Word document for Table Options
- Choose columns for the number of topics you expect to have
- Choose rows for the number of sources you plan to synthesize
- Begin to add information
- Adjust column width as needed
- Click Microsoft Word "Help" for more information on tables

Sample Synthesis Matrix

	Topic 1	Topic 2	Topic 3	Topic 4	Topic 5
Source 1					
Source 2					
Source 3					
Source 4					

Figure 7-3. Synthesis matrix with instructions for how to create the actual matrix format. (Adapted from Parker-Karst, K., & Walker, P. (2015). *Health sciences literature made easy: The matrix method*. Retrieved from https://www.youtube. com/watch?v=mPK6Lnbwrms.)

review may be organized in several ways. For one, it can be organized around ideas that emerge across several sources. Your topics/paragraphs will be based on themes or patterns. The synthesis matrix helps you to visualize the ways in which your sources/ideas are related to one another. Your matrix, then, will likely include your organizing thoughts as you select your early proposed need, possibly anticipated assets of this community/population, literature support for the profiles you are developing, and anticipated programming and effectiveness. A synthesis matrix is ongoing through your planning processes and often through implementation and evaluation. Figure 7-3 provides an example of what a synthesis matrix might look like, with topics/ideas at the top and sources along the side, along with instructions for creating the actual matrix box. Figure 7-4 provides a blank matrix example that is organized with sources at the top and the main ideas along the side. Try one to develop your own topic.

To begin to use the blank matrix, label the columns across the top of your matrix with the author's last name or with a few keywords from the title of the work. The sides are labeled with the main ideas that your sources discuss about your topic. As you read each of your sources, make notes in the appropriate column about the information discussed. You can also group the readings by subsidiary ideas. As you record in the matrix table, include page numbers and/or complete citations so you can return to the sources later. When you have completed the matrix, focus on the columns to compare the studies. Look for themes and update over time. Over the course of your education, you may have discovered another method that works well for you in reviewing and synthesizing literature; certainly do use whatever works best for you and whatever your instructor might recommend. A word about "searching the literature": in other course work, you may have learned about searching the literature to prepare to write a paper or perhaps for a project that required a more extensive synthesis. Therefore, only a very cursory summary is offered here for those who may need a refresher.

	Source 1	Source 2	Source 3	Source 4	Source 5
Main Idea 1					
Main Idea 2					
Main Idea 3					
Main Idea 4					
Main Idea 5					

Figure 7-4. Blank working matrix. (Adapted from NC State University Writing and Speaking Tutorial Service. *Writing a Literature Review and Using a Synthesis Matrix 2006.* Retrieved Sept 10, 2015 from http://www.ncsu.edu/tutorial_centr/ writespeak/download/Synthesis.pdf.)

These steps (adapted from Parker-Karst & Walker, 2015) comprise the following:

- Choose a topic (population/diagnosis/condition)
  - e.g., juvenile diabetes
- Refine the topic (who, what, when, where, how)
  - e.g., Mexican American children, Los Angeles, CA; at risk for diabetes
- Select key words
  - Juvenile diabetes
  - Mexican American children/health behaviors
  - Juvenile diabetes prevention
  - Interventions, programs
  - School, after-school programs
  - Nutrition/activity
  - Juvenile obesity
- Identify sources
  - Books
  - Reference books
  - Journal articles
  - Data
  - Guidelines
  - Systematic reviews
  - Conference proceedings
  - Reviews

Depending on what you are able to find, you may choose to enter your findings immediately into the suggested matrix, or you may wish to first organize using another method. Planners may choose from several tools to organize their references, such as RefWorks, EndNoteWeb, EndNote, Reference Manager, Zotero, MS Word 2007, and others.

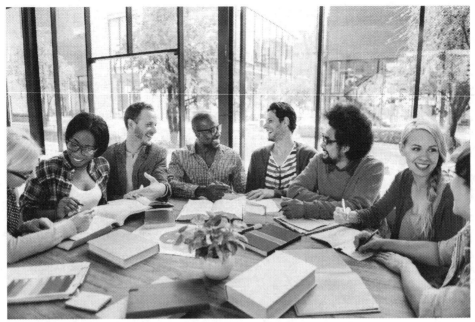

A student group works together to create themes from their literature reviews.

Expert Opinion to Support Profiles and Programming

We have mentioned that you will need to thoroughly examine the available research and practice literature to fully understand your population, the conditions, and the problems they are experiencing. We have also begun to investigate the context where you will find them and their communities. As you entertain program goals, objectives, and potential programming, there is another resource to explore. Finding an **expert** who knows your population or has done similar programming to what you are considering is a beneficial supplement to what you have already accomplished. If you are a student, this may be one of your instructors or perhaps an occupational therapy practitioner who has published his or her work in *OT Practice*, the *American Journal of Occupational Therapy*, and/or other relevant publications. It may be an author/researcher from one of the articles you have discovered in your literature reviews. You may also wish to speak with other practitioners who are not occupational therapists. Although not likely working from a perspective of "occupation," they may provide sound information to validate your present and projected work or offer suggestions. Visiting similar programs to the one you are proposing will help you see firsthand what works well and what may not. You can match your proposed population and context to the ones observed and discuss the differences with the programmer and personnel.

As an experienced programmer, you may be less in need of **expert opinion**, but you always want to remain apprised of the work being done by others with similar interests and experiences to your own. Forming networks of like-minded programmers, clinicians, and academicians leads to better outcomes for everyone involved. You will most certainly want to seek any available evidence that your early programming goals, objectives, and actual program/interventions will achieve the results you wish. Searching for accounts of practices that mirror or strongly reflect the work you wish to do and that demonstrate its effectiveness is a necessity in today's practice environment.

This subject-matter expert you will choose is someone who is knowledgeable regarding the population and health/need problem for which you will be planning your program. You may want to consider beginning your query with something like this either in person, telephone, or email:

"During our/my preliminary research regarding the needs/concerns (of whatever population you choose), we found (summarize the two or three main themes that you found). Are we on the

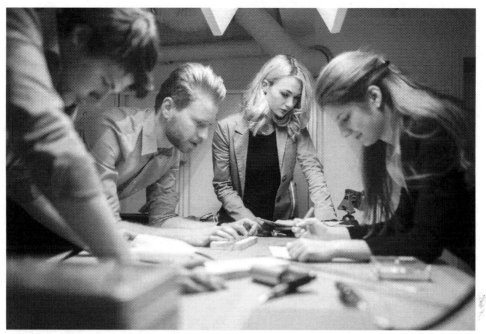

Identifying similar programming and experts to support programming ideas.

right track? Are there aspects of the population/need that we have not addressed? Of the themes that we have identified, are some more or less important than others? In our research of potential programming to meet the needs, we have identified (summarize your main findings). Do you have any recommendations for additional literature we should review? Do you have any other recommendations?"

You may also wish to ask if you can contact this person again later in your planning if need arises. If you intend to quote this expert in the body of your proposal, be sure to obtain a signed permission to do so that will be placed in the appendices. Certainly a formal thank you is merited. Remember that you are forming your professional networks throughout this process.

Ardal et al. (2006) tell us that consultation with experts can be a source of evidence. Such expert opinion is often sought to validate our thinking, helping us to formulate needs assessment and profile questions as well as to identify additional sources of information and evidence. It may also be useful as we interpret our findings later on.

The Case for Trusting the "Art" of Practice: Seeking Synergy Between Judgment, Experience, and Evidence

At this writing, EBP is all the buzz. Granted, accountability is a good thing, but the pendulum of trusting in evidence to support practice exclusively will likely need to swing back a bit. Polkinghorne (2004) makes a convincing case for what he describes as a **judgment-based practice of care**. Over recent decades, the practices of care (teaching, nursing, social work, psychotherapy, occupational therapy, and others) have become part of what Polkinghorne describes as a general cultural shift toward a technified worldview (p. 1). In his observations, practitioners have been challenged to "substitute a technologically guided approach for determining their practice in place of situationally informed judgments" (Polkinghorne, 2004, p. 1).

The human being is unique; perhaps the singular variable in the larger dynamic of practice that cannot be controlled or ever fully understood. When two of these unique individuals come together—the client and the practitioner face to face in an interaction focused on the reduction of injury, stress, illness, and emotional pain—can the outcome be anything less than limited in predictability? A practice model that will best prepare the practitioner will emphasize what Polkinghorne (2004) describes as the "situated judgment of practitioners" (p. 2). Certainly, every practitioner can benefit from scientifically validated knowledge (evidence) to support his or her practice. This knowledge provides the cushion of confidence for the practitioner; not controlling the nature of the interaction with the client, but permitting the practitioner to fully enter the therapeutic relationship with the freedom to explore and trust in his or her experiences, creative nature, empathetic foundation, and knowledge/skill base. In their discussions of clinical reasoning, Mattingly and Fleming (1994) suggest that it is this—what may be described as the "underground practice"—that most therapists employ in their actual work (p. 4).

What is the task of the practitioner—the provider of care? Is it not to work with the adult, the child, and the family to establish and accomplish goals that are situational and time-oriented? It is the practitioner who is the preliminary change agent, and it is his or her responsibility to rely on every resource available to orchestrate an effective intervention. Certainly tools, techniques, and evidence are important, but we must also put our trust in experience, knowledge, and the motivational impetus of "caring."

SUMMARY

In this chapter, we discussed the multiple layers of inquiry that must be conducted in order to design and develop a community-based occupation-centered program that meets the needs of our targeted population. Our first layer of inquiry resulted in the development of a community profile. We explored the demographics of our community and, later, we will match this information to our on-site observations. To our community profile, we added the profile of our targeted service population. This service profile represented the characteristics of our targeted population through our understanding of conditions and context.

Decisions about program goals, objectives, and interventions should be based on established best practice and research. Intervention effectiveness means that the intervention chosen has better results than the alternatives, including no intervention. This chapter has provided you with tools, information, and resources to help you prepare your review of the literature, which will include practice and programs that have offered evidence of their effectiveness. This is the evidence you will need. The chapter has also included a brief suggested dialogue to help you engage with an expert who is familiar with your population and your proposed programming. Suggestions for how to organize your literature review so that emerging themes can be identified have been offered to resolve the dilemma of how to utilize the literature to support what you wish to do. This chapter has been identified as the first part of the needs assessment—time with the computer before you enter the community itself. It is from the results of the work described in this chapter that you will enter the community with confidence.

There are numerous resources that can and will offer you working links to AOTA. Whether through this organization, your state and/or regional organization, or others of your choice, it is strongly recommended that you begin forming associations with other programmers, practitioners, and researchers who are doing work similar to yours. Talk to them about supporting their efforts through your own data gathering. We all share an obligation to contribute to the body of developing literature through our own publications, presentations, and posters. Last, you are encouraged to recognize that practice represents a synergy between judgment, experience, and evidence.

REFERENCES

American Occupational Therapy Association. (2007). AOTA's Centennial Vision and executive summary. *American Journal of Occupational* Therapy, *61*, 613-614.

Arbesman, M., & Lieberman, D. (2013). Highlighting newly published AOTA evidence-based practice guidelines. *OT Practice, 18*(15), 7-21.

Arbesman, M., Goetz, M., & Lieberman, D. (2015). Become a critically appraised paper (CAP) reviewer. *OT Practice, 20*(7), 21.

Arbesman, M., Lieberman, D., & Stutzback, M. (2014). Newly updated: AOTA's evidence-based practice website. *Evidence Perks, OT Practice, 19*(3), 20.

Archbishop of Canterbury's Commission on Urban Priority Areas. (1985). *Faith in the city: A call to action by church and nation.* London, UK: Church House Publishing. Retrieved from https://www.churchofengland.org/media/55076/faithinthecity.pdf

Ardal, S, Butler, J., Edwards, R., & Lawrie, L. (2006). Evidence-based planning: Module 3. In *The health planner's toolkit* (pp. 1-9). Ontario, Canada: Health System Intelligence Project.

Baldock, P. (1974). Community work and social work. In *Library of social work.* London, UK: Sage.

Bazyk, S., & Arbesman, M. (2013). *Occupational therapy practice guidelines for mental health promotion, prevention, and intervention for children and youth.* Bethesda, MD: AOTA Press.

DiLima, S., & Schust, C. (1997). *Community health education and promotion: A guide to program design and evaluation.* Gaithersburg, MD: The Aspen Reference Group.

Drake, R. E. (2005). The principles of evidence-based mental health treatment. In R. E. Drake, M. Merrens, & D. Lynde (Eds.), *Evidence-based mental health practice* (pp. 15-32). New York, NY: W. W. Norton and Co.

Drake, R. E., & Goldman, H. (2003). *Evidence-based practices in mental health care.* Washington, DC: American Psychiatric Association.

Fleming-Castaldy, R. P., & Gillen, G. (2013). Ensuring that education, certification, and practice are evidence-based. *American Journal of Occupational Therapy, 67,* 3.

Frolek, G., & Kingsley, K. (2013). *Occupational therapy practice guidelines for early childhood: Birth through 5 years.* Bethesda, MD: AOTA Press.

Guyatt, G., & Rennie, D. (2002). *User's guides to the medical literature: A manual for evidence-based clinical practice.* Chicago, IL: American Medical Association.

Haynes, D., Devereaux, R., & Guyatt, G. (2002). Clinical experience in the era of evidence-based medicine and patient choice. *American College of Physicians Journal Club, 136,* AN.

Henderson, P., & Thomas, D. (1987). *Skills in neighborhood work* (2nd ed.). London, UK: Unwin Hyman LTD.

Institute of Medicine. (2001). *Crossing the quality chasm: A new health system for the 21st century.* Washington, DC: National Academy Press.

Jackson, L. L., & Arbesman, M. (2005). *Occupational therapy practice guidelines for children with behavioral and psychosocial needs.* Bethesda, MD: AOTA Press.

Kaldenberg, J., & Smallfield, S. (2013). *Occupational therapy guidelines for older adults with low vision.* Bethesda. MD: AOTA Press.

Kellegrew, D. (2005). The evolution of evidence-based practice: Strategies and resources for busy practitioners. *OT Practice, 10*(12), 11-15.

Law, M. (2002). *Evidence-based rehabilitation: A guide to practice.* Thorofare, NJ: SLACK Incorporated.

Law, M. (2005). Evidence-based practice: What can it mean for me? *Occupational Therapy Association of California Newsletter, 9*(30), 15-16.

Mattingly, C., & Fleming, M. (1994). *Clinical reasoning: Forms of inquiry in a therapeutic practice.* Philadelphia, PA: FA Davis.

Ohmer, M., & DeMasi, K. (2009). *Consensus organizing.* Los Angeles, CA: Sage.

Parker-Karst, K., & Walker, P. (2015). *Health sciences literature made easy: The matrix method.* Retrieved from https://www.youtube.com/watch?v=mPK6Lnbwrms

Polkinghorne, D. (2004). *Practice and the human sciences: The case for a judgment-based practice of care.* Albany, NY: State University of New York Press.

Relman, A. (2007). *A second opinion: Rescuing America's health care.* New York, NY: Perseus Books.

Sackett, D., Rosenberg, W., Gray, J., Haynes, R., & Richardson, W. (1996). Evidence-based medicine: What it is and what it isn't. *British Medical Journal, 312,* 71-72.

Scaffa, M., & Brownson, C. (2014). Program planning and needs assessment. In M. Scaffa, & S. Reitz, *Occupational therapy in community-based practice settings* (2nd ed., pp. 61-79). Philadelphia, PA: F. A. Davis.

Titler, M. (2010). Translation science and context. *Research and Theory for Nursing Practice: An International Journal, 24*(1), 35-55.

Internet Sites Related to Evidence-Based Practice

ACP Journal Club of the American College of Physicians: www.acpjc.org

American Occupational Therapy Association's Evidence-Based Practice (EBP) Resource Directory: OT Search: www.aota.org

Center on the Social and Emotional Foundations for Early Learning: www.csefel.uiuc.edu

CINAHL: www.cinahl.com (fee)

Cochrane Collaboration: www.cochrane.org

ERIC Digests: www.eric.ed.gov

Evidence-Based Medicine Web Tutorial: http://www.usc.edu/hsc/nm/lis/tutorials/ebm.html

Evidence-Based Practice Centers: http://www.ahcpr.gov/clinic/epc/

National Guideline Clearinghouse website: www.guideline.gov

National Institute of Mental Health (NIMH): www.nimh.nih.gov/

National Rehabilitation Information Center (NARIC): www.naric.com

Orelena Hawks Puckett Institute: www.puckett.org

OT Seeker (free online database that contains systematic reviews and randomized controlled trials relevant to occupational therapy): www.otseeker.com

OTD-BASE (20 occupational therapy journals): http://www.otdbase.org

PubMed (free public access to the MEDLINE database): www.ncbi.nlm.nih.gov/entrez/

RehabData Collection of the Agency for Healthcare Research and Quality: www.ahrq.gov

Substance Abuse and Mental Health Services Administration (SAMHSA): www.samhsa.gov

TRIP (Turning Research Into Practice): www.tripdatabase.com

What Works Clearinghouse: www.whatworks.ed.gov/

8

Continuing the Needs Assessment in the Community

Fazio, L. S. *Developing Occupation-Centered Programs
With the Community, Third Edition* (pp 119-133).
© 2017 Taylor & Francis Group.

What Is . . .

(CURRENT STATE, SITUATION, PROBLEM, OR CONDITION)

What Should Be . . .

(DESIRED OR PREFERRED STATE, CONDITION, RESOLUTION

OF PROBLEM OR SITUATION)

Figure 8-1. Identifying need. (Adapted from Altschuld, J. & Kumar, D. (2010). *Needs assessment: An overview.* Los Angeles, CA: Sage.)

OBTAINING THE NEEDS OF A COMMUNITY

This chapter and the previous one formally introduce the term *need*. Some background information for how need is used in discussions of community programming is appropriate. Leagans (1964) has suggested that a need is the difference, or gap, between "what is" and "what should be" (or, what is reasonably possible) (p. 4). Altschild and Kumar would concur (2010, p. 3) (Figure 8-1).

The gap between what is and what should be must be measurable; thus, the two conditions (what is, what should be) must be measurable as well. If they are not, we cannot really know if there is a need and we cannot easily determine whether we can satisfy it. We can "believe" we know what the need is, based on what we have read, but it is only with the **on-the-ground needs assessment** that we can determine whether the need is truly valid (for our specific population and the communities they claim). A **needs assessment** or **assessment of needs** represents a systematic set of procedures and methods designed for specific purposes that are used to determine needs, examine their nature and causes, and set priorities for future action (Watkins & Meiers, 2012).

Between different needs, there are going to be different levels of risk or consequence for not meeting them. The weight of the consequence will help you determine which needs should be satisfied first. As we have indicated, the needs assessment actually begins with our literature reviews, our research, and the completion of the profiles. We want to gather as much information on the topics as we possibly can. By initiating our visit to the community, we have begun to add new information and bring together what we have learned with what we have yet to discover. The on-the-ground needs assessment is really a verification of a match or fit between all that we now know of the actual community and the nuances specific to this community. Altschuld and Kumar (2010) refer to the full needs assessment process in terms of preassessment (what is already known, has been compiled, or has been written by others), assessment (gathering new data about the need), and postassessment (design and implementation of solutions).

Needs assessment is a comprehensive process; however, for the purposes of this text, we are separating the process into two phases. The first phase, or early stage, contains all of the research we have done, and are continuing to do, to develop our profiles and learn as much as we can about the population and the community. This portion of the needs assessment is used to identify the results of the literature review, expert opinion interview, and the development of profiles. The second phase of the needs assessment is referred to as *on-the-ground* and includes the walking and/or windshield surveys; visit to a partnering agency or facility; and the interviews and surveys that are used for agency administration/personnel, stakeholders, and the targeted population themselves. Although not an assessment of need, we would now add an assessment of resources/assets that may overlap both phase I and phase II of information gathering.

As with all models, this is a recommended structure to facilitate your understanding of a phenomenon (the assessments of needs and assets/resources to facilitate community program design and development). Your process may vary somewhat from this model but still be entirely thorough. Blurring of the phases is inevitable and sometimes desired (as in continuing the literature review based on the need for additional information that is prompted by the on-the-ground findings or a visit to the community if a partnering agency/facility has been identified early on).

As mentioned in the previous chapter, several layers of inquiry are necessary to determine what programming services are needed by a population. We initiate the investigation of these layers of inquiry first at our desks, and then we are ready to continue in the community itself. From your research into the literature, you now have the information needed to know the community where you will provide services, and you may know the assets of the community, or at least some of them. You know a good deal about the targeted population that will receive services, and you know your own potential for providing them. We still have a few more layers of inquiry to investigate: (1) who will be our partnering agency/facility, (2) what does the agency/facility administration want for the clients/patients, (3) who are our stakeholders, (4) what do the stakeholders want for the population, and (5) what do the clients/patients want for themselves. You may have some of this information already, such as the agency/facility that you anticipate will be your partner. You also may know some of your stakeholders, who are likely included in the previously mentioned groups, but there may be others. If any of these areas are neglected in the early stages of planning, it is likely that you will not be as successful as you could be.

Now that you have learned all you can from other sources and have well-developed profiles, it is time for a visit in order to match what you have learned with what you can observe. This is sometimes done en route to your first on-site appointment with an agency, but you can also explore the area before you schedule the appointment to begin the process of determining programming needs. Either way, this first visit will permit you to make some useful observations and to ask yourself some questions pertinent to your program design and development. Ohmer and DeMasi (2009) refer to this method of on-site data gathering as a **walking or windshield survey**. A walking survey involves first identifying your neighborhood of interest and walking through the area during the daylight hours (returning at night if relevant to your programming). Walking in a neighborhood provides a feel for the community, and you will meet people along the way. You may want to start by visiting business establishments and have lunch at a local café. The people you meet can help you make connections to partners and stakeholders. An important word of advice is to be safe. Before you go, contact the local police and find out when it is safe to visit. Visiting a library, public space, and/or a business is far wiser than attempting to obtain data in an alley at 2 a.m.!

A windshield survey involves driving through a community/neighborhood to get a visual picture of what the area is about. You are obtaining an on-site view (to add to what your research has contributed) of the physical conditions, including the condition of the housing, public amenities (e.g., parks and community centers), institutions, and businesses. Remember your census data may be a few years old. Things change and demographics shift. Gentrification may be occurring. As you begin to explore the community, you might ask yourself the following questions:

- What is the standard mode of housing?

- Are there playgrounds, parks, and recreation facilities?

- Are there adults and children on the streets? If so, what are they doing?

- Are police visible?

- Are there as many churches and schools as liquor and convenience stores?

- Are there graffiti, including gang signs?

- What are the languages displayed on signs, billboards, and advertisements?

- Do these observations match the statistical/demographic information already gathered?

When you are ready to visit the potential partnering facility for your first appointment with the administrator or another professional, you will already have gleaned substantial information from your demographic research and these early observations. You will have established the foundation for any questions you will wish to ask in order to center your targeted population in the community. Again, it is important to remember that sometimes the population to be served by a program may live in a completely different community or many different communities. This is an important question to ask, and the answer might prompt you to extend your community profile to other communities in addition to the one where services will be located.

Your observations might also prompt the need for community information beyond what you have collected previously. In addition to census bureau data, you might wish to examine national and local marketing and survey data; government documents, reports, and statistics; or data from other agencies. Your collected information may include ranges of income, the incidence of single-parent families, employment, education, religion, ethnicity, crime and police statistics, and other information of specific interest to you as you develop your ideas for programming. Many times, the facility/agency can provide you with some of this information since it is often used to justify funding for programs and, in fact, might justify the funding for the one you are proposing. You might also want to consider community newspapers, newsletters, or posted materials describing local interests and events. Items posted on a town hall or grocery store bulletin board can tell you a great deal about the community.

THE NEEDS ASSESSMENT: AGENCY/FACILITY AND STAKEHOLDERS

The earlier preliminary work we have accomplished to develop our community profile and the profile of our anticipated services sets the foundation for what we are beginning to define as the needs of this particular population in this particular community. Up to now, we have been working with primarily demographic quantitative data collected by others and with some qualitative generalizations formed through our observations. Perhaps we also have had brief conversations during an early, informal community visit. For example, from our preliminary research into the demographics of the community, we might know that there are a certain number of adolescent girls with infants living in their single mother's households, and we might know that these girls did not finish high school. We might also know that pregnancy prevention, parenting classes, or other services for these girls are nonexistent (or they exist but appear to be ineffective). Perhaps we have also talked informally with those who may be stakeholders: a school counselor, a minister, or a teacher who could confirm some of these data. In our preliminary research efforts to develop the profiles, we may have identified existing programs for similar populations. These programs may offer evidence to support their effectiveness, and we will return to these when we develop specific programming.

At this point in our inquiries, we have not formally asked other professionals in the community what kinds of services are needed for these girls and their families, and we have not asked the girls or their families what kinds of services they need (as for education, skill building, prevention, remediation, and so on).

In short, we still must formally or specifically assess or define the needs of our community population. In other words, we now must conduct the formal on-the-ground needs assessment. We can say that there are two **phases of the needs assessment process**. The early phase consisted primarily of literature review and research, identification of an expert, and perhaps a very cursory visit to the community. The second phase is "on the ground," and there are at least two parts to determine formal assessment of the needs of the targeted population—first, from those who may be involved with them at some level, and second, the perceived needs of those to be served. The first assessment might include input from other health care professionals, teachers, counselors, police, parents, spouses, and caregivers. It may be that the proposed population is already being seen by an occupational therapist, perhaps in the school system, and you want to extend services to a camp program or after-school enrichment program. If we are working with an agency, the first part of the needs assessment is initiated with the professionals at the site (the facility, institution, or agency). For the example in question, this may be the principal or the counselor at the school. On the other hand, if we know that there is a community agency already providing services to meet the needs of this population, we may go directly to the agency. We have indicated that it is advisable to be as familiar as possible with the demographics of the community and with the proposed population before going on site. From this information, you will develop the structure of this first visit and interview with the agency representatives.

The Interview

Face-to-face **interviews** are often considered the most thorough way to collect information, but they can be difficult to schedule. They do permit the possible addition of an interpreter, which is sometimes helpful. A telephone or email interview can be conducted if distance is a problem, and both are good for detailed answers, though telephone is perhaps better. In general, this visit begins with your self-introduction (or the introduction of your group). This interview also includes the purpose of your visit and sometimes an explanation of the parameters of your assignment (if you are a student) and explanations of occupation-centered practice. Much of this will depend on how your instructor elects to structure the experience. Although this chapter focuses on *need* as the starting place for program development, it is worth mentioning that our assessment of need is often complicated by *want*. It is important to clearly distinguish between the two. We certainly do wish to help the agency/facility achieve its needs; however, at the level of the clients/patients, we wish to address not only their needs, but also their wants. It is through our ability to meet needs and wants that we are able to offer programs that our target population will find meaningful. If programming is not meaningful to our clients/patients, there cannot be successful goal development or positive outcomes. We are now ready to conduct our interview with a potential partnering organization or perhaps a stakeholder or stakeholders. Adler and Elmhorst (2010) offer some recommendations for information-gathering interviews (pp. 172-175):

- Plan your interview: What is your goal?
- Collect background information (prepare topics and questions..open and/or closed)
- Choose the right interviewee and know about him or her before you go
- Choose the best interview structure for your purpose
- If you can, arrange the setting to meet your needs and anticipated goals
- Be cognizant of time

You will want to begin by fully explaining who you are and what you are interested in; you may have already done this with an introductory communication. You might also want to include why you selected this agency for your first interview.

Our initial needs assessment interview with a facility or stakeholders is semi-structured; often, it begins in an appropriately conversational manner. Your questions may vary depending on what you already know from your research; however, the interview generally consists of a discussion centered on the following core set of questions (**the interview questionnaire**) that you have developed:

- How would you describe your purpose (i.e., the mission and philosophy) of your organization?
- What group of individuals (i.e., your targeted population and others served by this organization) do you serve?
- What are some of the characteristics (i.e., their ages, abilities, and so on) of this population?
- What kinds of programming (i.e., treatment, prevention, group, individuals, and so on) do you offer?

- What are your funding sources? Are you a for-profit organization, or is your organization not for profit?

- Do our ideas for programming seem realistic to you? Would they add value to your services? Are there other, unmet programming needs (from the perspective of the interviewee) that you, as an occupation-centered practitioner, might be able to consider? Be careful with this; you may open a "can of worms." Sometimes, it is best not to ask unless you are really looking for more.

We describe this interview format as conversational because we will find that the interviewee's responses to our core questions will often prompt other questions. This is also your opportunity to introduce information you have collected from your earlier work developing the foundational community and service profiles. The interviewee can validate and perhaps dispute your information and may direct you elsewhere for more research. It is very appropriate to note the responses under each question. In these interviews, it is expected that you will be taking notes so that you will not be likely to miss important information.

When you have completed this interview, you can use the answers to your interview questionnaire to check the accuracy and scope of your preliminary community and service profiles. Based on the information you have received, you might find that you do not need all of the information you have collected to form a comprehensive picture of the population identified by the agency. To this end, you might want to synthesize, from the earlier work, information specific to the group where needs have been identified by the representatives of the agency/facility. Even if it is not immediately needed, retain all of the demographic and observational information you have collected for future options, such as the extension of services or alterations in the way services are provided. It is important to be very open with this interview; sometimes, actually conducting the proposed programming is not feasible within the time constraints of your educational agenda. If this is the case, be clear that you are conducting the interview to gather needed information on the basis of which to develop the programming proposal, but that you will not be able to conduct the actual programming. In these cases, you may wish to present and give the completed proposal to the agency for them to utilize as they wish in order to initiate the programming themselves.

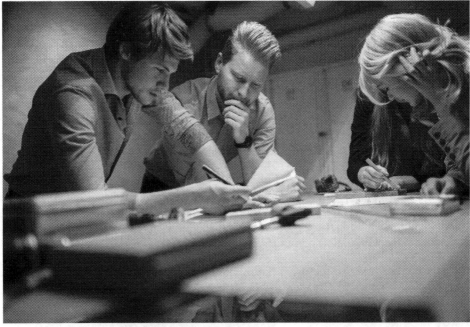

Developing good interview questions takes collaboration.

THE NEEDS ASSESSMENT: THE TARGETED POPULATION

There are several methods that can be used to assess the need for services; we have already mentioned one of these—the interview—in our earlier discussion and also when we talked about the interview of an expert. When this method is used in conducting formal research to obtain quantitative data, the interview instrument (the interview questionnaire) establishes a prescribed, structured set of questions that is given to each participant. There are no open-ended questions. The interview format we have described for use with the agency/facility or other community service providers is not entirely true to this definition. We are using a structured set of questions we want interviewees to answer, but we are also hoping to generate more questions. We can appropriately call this approach a semi-structured interview, which is more characteristic of qualitative research methods where in-depth interviews are conducted via probing and open-ended questions. This would seem to fit our more conversational, open-ended exchange. Our interest in having a core set of questions answered and perhaps generating more questions makes this method very appropriate for the facility/stakeholder portion of our needs assessment.

If we decide to again use an interview questionnaire when we prepare our second set of questions targeting the specific needs of the population for whom we wish to develop programming, it is likely that it will not be as open-ended as the first one prepared for the agency or other care providers. We use the results of the first interview to prepare the second interview questionnaire, which is more focused and contains fewer, if any, open-ended questions.

The Focus Group

Also very appropriate to assessing the need for community-based programs is a **focus group.** Such a group may be used in all portions of our needs assessment. Although a focus group is typically fairly small (usually six to ten members), it can comprise up to as many as 30 members when several planners are conducting the group. With several planners, one or more may take notes or one of the group members might be asked to record the proceedings on a flipchart. If the group agrees, audiotaping is a good way to capture all of the discussion. Members do not usually know each other but probably share some common characteristics that relate to the focus of the group. For successful outcomes, Dumka and Michaels (1998) recommend careful consideration to seemingly simple things such as a convenient and comfortable location and a convenient time. The group focuses on a set of questions provided by the facilitator (planner). Like an open-ended interview, the intent is not only to get questions answered, but also to generate questions. When a focus group is used with the stakeholder assessment, the planner guides a group of interested community members (such as professionals, service providers, and potential collaborators) through increasingly focused issues related to the core set of questions or concerns and may utilize the same process with potential clients/patients/members. When used with potential clients/targeted population, the questions prepared for the focus group will likely have been generated from the results of previous interviews; in some cases, the process of formalized needs assessment may begin with this group. Generally, the focus group generates diverse ideas and allows members to influence each other by listening and responding to the ideas presented in the discussion. A successful focus group experience can result in a developing network of support for the program. In addition, a focus group can be an opportunity to establish/improve community stakeholder relations (Morgan, 1993).

DiLima and Schust (1997) recommend the use of a focus group when one wishes to find answers to the complicated issues of health beliefs and behaviors, barriers to health care, and cultural influences on care. These issues often make the difference in the success or failure of a community program. Using members of such a focus group for a continuing advisory council or board or developing new focus groups during programming can assist in finding answers to programming questions in an efficient and effective manner.

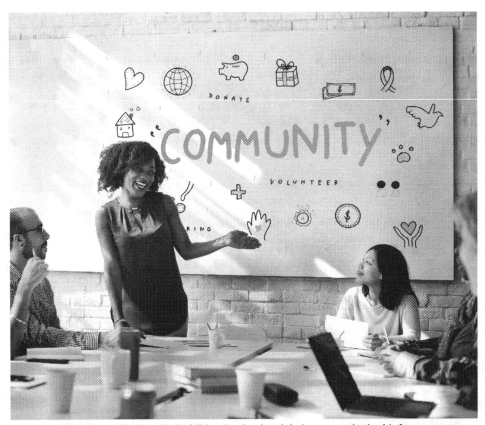

Parent–stakeholders talk about their children's school and their community in this focus group.

Analyzing the Results of Your Focus Group

Krueger and Casey (2000) recommend a careful analysis of your focus group results with the following considerations:

- Begin your analysis while still with the group by listening, and resolving if you can, inconsistent comments.

- Offer a summary of key questions when preparing to end the group.

- Make your notes as soon after the group closes as you can.

- Consider organizing your results under individual questions asked.

- You can use bullet points and/or narrative. Add quotes to illustrate strong comments (p. 32).

Surveys

In some cases, when the use of interviews or focus groups is not practical (e.g., the population may be quite large or is not readily accessible, or respondent anonymity is desired), a **survey** may be the preferred instrument. A survey is most often conducted via a questionnaire that is distributed on site, via email, or by surface mail. Its intent, of course, is to collect information from a sample of the population.

In our case, we wish to collect information with regard to the community programming services people may need and want. As in the other methods described, our sample, or those we wish to survey, will be selected from our initial target population.

Our survey questions are developed around the initial identification of need provided by the facility, but they are now developed toward the specific sampling of our proposed population. In considering a web-based survey, SurveyMonkey (http://www.surveymonkey.com) and Qualtrics are two to consider. These are web-based online survey tools packed with industry-leading features designed and tested by noted market researchers. A good survey is very difficult to develop, so you might wish to visit the SurveyMonkey site for recommendations and tips on how to put together a good, focused set of questions. For a paper survey, you can hand out the survey when your target population is already convened; this facilitates the return rate. One week after the initial survey has been delivered, you may also want to consider reminding people at last once to respond. For those wishing to know more about the survey sampling method, Fink and Kosecoff (1985) and Fowler (1993) offer in-depth explorations of survey design and development. In general, these are guiding questions for you to consider in developing your survey instrument:

- What is the goal of this survey?
- Why are you creating this survey?
- What do you hope to accomplish with this survey?
- How will you use the data you are collecting?
- What decisions do you hope to affect with the results of this survey?

In summary, methods that can be utilized in assessing the need for community-centered services include the following:

- Structured or semistructured interviews (face-to-face, by email, or by telephone)
- Focus groups
- Surveys (electronic, mailed, or in-person handouts)

All of the aforementioned methods are appropriate for the student programmer as well as the experienced therapist. Depending on the characteristics of the population and the nature of service provision, there are additional mechanisms for obtaining data related to needs.

For example, never neglect information that has already been collected, assuming permission to review can be obtained. We have already discussed ways to access demographic data, but there are other existing data banks that may provide programmers with useful information. Medical charts, institutional survey results, quality-assurance studies, end-of-year reports, and other such institutional information are all examples of existing data banks that may be useful to support the need for occupation-centered services. Local and regional regulatory agencies collect and maintain information on items such as indicators of health status, which may also be useful to preliminary programming work. Collection of data may vary from one region to another, but reviewing what is available in your area is well worth the time.

Remember that the questions designed to structure the needs assessment are prepared within the parameters of the therapist's expertise or that of previously considered resources (i.e., other persons, instructional aids, or further training within a realistic time frame). In many cases, one round of needs assessment following the first interview with the agency/facility or others may be all that is necessary; however, the on-the-ground needs assessment most often is a process involving several formats, each one more specific and more targeted. For example, following the review of survey results, the planner may wish to conduct focus groups or interviews. It is not uncommon that need may continue to be assessed while the programming is being conducted. For example, ongoing information regarding needs and wants may be gleaned from the care provider, patient, parent, child, social service worker, house manager, vocational counselor, and perhaps others who are in contact with the population for whom you are providing services. This continuing assessment of need is often included in program evaluation if the programmer asks the clients/patients/members and perhaps others questions regarding satisfaction with services and what additional services they might need.

You will use the results of the needs assessment to guide the establishment of goals and objectives for programming. It is important to remember that the needs assessment guides the services that will be provided but does not establish them. The establishment of programming will require substantial negotiation between everyone involved in the process. For example, the needs identified in your interviews with the stakeholders and those identified by the targeted population may be in disagreement, or the needs as they are identified may be outside the purview of the programmer. It is the task of the programmer to ensure that once negotiations end, he or she has crafted a program that represents the needs of all of those concerned.

In summary, the following are steps to identifying the needs of your targeted population:

- Develop the community profile
- Develop the service profile
- Conduct the first part of the needs assessment (interview the agency/facility director and the stakeholders and others involved with the target population; select methodology in addition to interview if needed)
- Conduct the second part of the needs assessment (select a methodology and obtain the needs as identified by your target population)

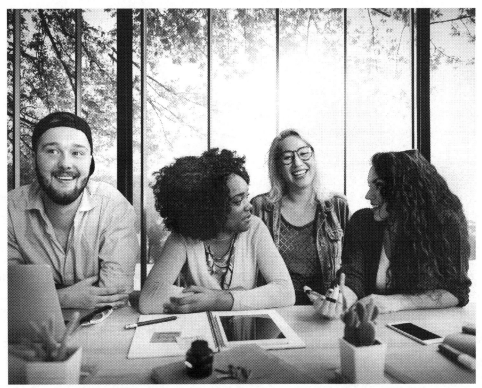

A group of teachers and case workers share information and energy in this focus group.

Synthesizing the Data From the Needs Assessment

Depending on your methods of data collection, there are several ways to synthesize your information. You may choose quantitative and/or qualitative methods. A combination of both is usually required. Put the data into a form that is useful for making decisions. Keep it organized, short, and simple. Determine how the data will be used (i.e., for decision making regarding goals, objectives, programming, evaluation, etc.) and let this help you organize the results.

Exercise 8-1

Developing the Needs Assessment: Assessing Need From a Partnering Agency

Develop the specific questions you will ask in your initial interview according to the parameters recommended earlier and according to what you already know: What is the purpose of your organization (mission and philosophy)? Whom do you serve? What are the characteristics of your service population? What services do you currently offer? Are there any unmet needs? Tailor the questions to your specific circumstances.

1. Based on what you have learned while developing your community and service profiles, write the questions you will ask when you have your first interview with the representatives of the facility/agency where you expect to develop your program.

   Your questions will provide a structure so that you do not forget anything you wish to know, but they may be altered as you move through the interview.

> Drawing from our previous example, the work accomplished in developing the community and service profiles for the homeless adolescents in Denver might prompt the following question to the director of a sanctuary:
>
> I see from your mission statement (hanging on the wall when you entered the building) that you provide free meals, a shower, and a bed in a safe environment for adolescents who are homeless. Are there other services you provide as well?
>
> The answer will satisfy several of your questions and will likely prompt the director to think about other things he or she does or wishes to do at the sanctuary.

Draft the questions you will ask here:

_____

_____

_____

_____

_____

2. Are there others you would like to interview for this initial assessment of need? Note here who they might be and what questions you would like to ask them:

_____

_____

_____

_____

_____

3. Following your first interview, are there persons you would like to add to the earlier list? Any you wish to delete? Will you need to alter your questions? If so, note the changes here:

_____

_____

_____

_____

_____

4. Following your first interview, review the answers to the questions you listed previously. Are there any areas you will need to research further before developing the assessment for the targeted population? If so, note them here:

_____

_____

_____

_____

_____

5. What did the director or others at the facility identify as an unmet need or needs?

_____

_____

_____

_____

_____

The mission of the sanctuary for homeless adolescents identifies the purpose of the sanctuary to be the satisfaction of what Maslow (1970) would describe as basic biological needs—physiological needs and safety. In keeping with this purpose and the characteristics of the population (adolescents), the director might identify an unmet need of programming for "safe sex."

Note here any unmet needs that were identified during your interview with the facility and/ or stakeholders:

_____

_____

_____

_____

_____

6. Review all of the information you have to date, including the results of any additional research or interviews you may have conducted. Discuss the unmet needs that have been identified during your assessment process. Ask the following questions:

a. Are the identified unmet need(s) appropriate for occupation-centered programming? Why or why not? If you said no, you might need to return to your definitions of *occupation*; they may be too limiting. Note your responses here:

_____

_____

_____

_____

_____

"Safe sex" was identified earlier as an unmet need for our community of adolescents. Is the expression of sexuality occupation, and is it, therefore, appropriate to our interests as occupation-centered programmers? To help answer this question, we might turn to
(continued)

occupational science. The activities and behaviors associated with sexual expression lend themselves to the three major research orientations of occupational science as described by Larson, Wood, and Clark (2003) and Clark, Wood, and Larson (1998). These activities and behaviors exhibit directly observable aspects of occupation (form); collectively, they serve adaptation (function), and they provide significance within the context of the adolescent's life and in the culture (meaning).

If we use the parameters established by occupational science of form, function, and meaning to understand the occupational patterns of developing sexuality in our population, and if we further use them to consider the multiple expressions of sexuality as adaptive responses to the potentially dangerous context of homelessness, we have the scaffold on which to build a significantly meaningful program. If we add to this developing theoretical construct what we know of the adolescent's developmental "window" for cognition, emotion, and morality, we further strengthen the potential for a successful program (Austin, 1995; Cronk, 1992; Garsee & Schuster, 1992; Schuster, Cronk, & Reno, 1992). For the creative occupation-centered programmer, meeting the need for "safe sex" is more than displaying a basket of condoms and a few pamphlets. This seemingly simple need might open a door to multiple programming objectives. It is not likely that we could have arrived at these conclusions without substantial investigation of the relevant research literature. A good programmer is an avid consumer of research.

Exercise 8-2

Assessing Need From the Targeted Population

1. Review the recommended methods for assessing the needs expressed by your targeted population. Match these methods to what you know about the population. Discuss the pros and cons of structured or semi-structured interviews, focus groups, or surveys. You might wish to review the references at the end of this chapter or other sources for additional information.

   Select the method you wish to use, and begin to develop the instrument. Remember that you begin with the needs that were identified by the partnering facility, or stakeholders and perhaps were also informed by your research into evidence-based practice and other sources (assuming that these were acceptable to you and that you have the knowledge and skills to provide programming to meet them). Also, remember that during all phases of assessment, you can negotiate.

In our "safe sex" example, a focus group might be successful with our population of adolescents, particularly if it could be organized at the time of a meal served by the sanctuary. Group process might diffuse some of the suspiciousness that individual interviews would likely prompt. A survey could be tried to supplement the focus group, but it is not likely that this population would fill out even a brief survey unless a substantial reward were offered for doing so. Occasionally, rewards (such as food, movie tickets, or concert tickets) are given to solicit cooperation in the types of programs we are suggesting, but if true need is defined, this should not be necessary. In general, homeless adolescents are not anxious to be identified. Most are running away from life circumstances that they found to be compromising and/or dangerous. They do not wish to be found by a parent, stepparent, foster parent, or care provider. They are more likely to cooperate with programming if their anonymity can be protected.

(continued)

The first question or questions for our focus group would be designed to determine if the group supported the facility identified need for safe sex. As the answers to this question or questions emerged, we would then develop further questions to identify what sexual behaviors are being practiced and what this population means by safe sex. If new needs are introduced in the discussion and we feel we could design programming to meet those needs as well, we would take note of them and bring them back to those first interviewed to see if there was consensus. This process is what we described as *negotiation*. In many ways, you are the arbitrator/negotiator between the agency, stakeholders, and your targeted population. The needs of both must be met in order to elicit the cooperation and support that will be needed to offer the program.

a. Note here the method you will use to conduct the needs assessment with the targeted population:

_____

_____

_____

_____

_____

b. Draft the questions you would like answered to support the identified earlier needs. The nature of your questions will likely be different depending on whether you wish to use an interview questionnaire, a focus group, or a survey. You might also wish to offer some programming options based on the early expressed needs, particularly if you use a survey instrument.

_____

_____

_____

_____

_____

When you have your draft of questions completed, develop your final instrument.

c. When you have field-tested your instrument, discuss the responses with your instructor, group, or colleagues. Do you have the answers you need to finalize one or two goals for your program and related objectives? Do you need to draft another instrument or try a different methodology? It is often the case that you will have to assess your population again for more focused questions. If you have what you need to continue the design of the program, you can always return later with more rounds of focused questions (such as where and when would you like the programming to be conducted).

SUMMARY

This chapter focused on what we are calling the on-the-ground needs assessment, when we enter the community to verify what we already know from our research and to ask the questions that remain. This first needs assessment was conducted through a semi-structured interview with a representative of the agency/facility where we would access our targeted population. Through this interview and perhaps others, we would determine what services the agency/facility already provided and what the agency/facility considered to be needs still unmet for our targeted population. We then would evaluate the expressed need for appropriateness with occupation-centered programming, and we would evaluate our skills and expertise to determine whether we could realistically meet the need as expressed. We would also determine the accuracy of our earlier work and what areas we might need to further research. At this juncture, we may also choose to obtain more formal information from our stakeholders.

Using all of this information, we then determine the questions and methodology we wish to use to assess the needs as expressed by the targeted population. An instrument format appropriate to the methodology is selected, and questions are developed to determine whether the targeted population supports the needs expressed by the earlier respondents. Depending on the responses of the targeted population, we may then return to those we questioned earlier and begin the process of negotiation between the two groups. We may find it necessary to return to the targeted population with more specific questions with regard to how the program will be implemented, and we likely will continue our processes of assessing unmet need throughout the program via our program evaluation procedures. When we are comfortable that we have identified the needs for which we will develop programming, we are ready to finalize our goals and objectives.

REFERENCES

Adler, R., & Elmhorst, J. (2010). *Communicating at work*. New York, NY: McGraw Hill.

Altschuld, J. & Kumar, D. (2010). *Needs assessment: An overview*. Los Angeles, CA: Sage.

Austin, E. W. (1995). Reaching young audiences: Developmental considerations in designing health messages. In R. Parrott, & E. Maibach (Eds.), *Designing health messages: Approaches from communication theory and public health practice* (pp. 114-143). Thousand Oaks, CA: Sage.

Clark, F., Wood, W., & Larson, E. (1998). Occupational science: Occupational therapy's legacy for the 21st century. In M. Neistadt & E. Crepeau (Eds.), *Willard and Spackman's occupational therapy* (pp. 13-21). Philadelphia, PA: Lippincott-Raven.

Cronk, R. (1992). Cognitive development during adolescence. In C. Schuster & S. Ashburn (Eds.), *The process of human development: A holistic life-span approach* (pp. 513-531). Philadelphia, PA: Lippincott.

DiLima, S., & Schust, C. (Eds.). (1997). *Community health education and promotion: A guide to program design and evaluation*. Gaithersburg, MD: The Aspen Reference Group.

Dumka, L., & Michaels, M. (1998). Marketing prevention services in a community context. Workshop conducted at the American Association for Marriage and Family Therapy, Annual Conference, July 12-15, 1998, Dallas, TX.

Fink, A., & Kosecoff, J. (1985). *How to conduct surveys: A step-by-step guide*. Newbury Park, CA: Sage.

Fowler, F. (1993). *Survey research methods*. Newbury Park, CA: Sage.

Garsee, J., & Schuster, C. (1992). Moral development. In C. Schuster & S. Ashburn (Eds.), *The process of human development: A holistic life-span approach* (pp. 330-350). Philadelphia, PA: Lippincott.

Krueger, R. A., & Casey, M. A. (2000). *Focus groups: A practical guide for applied research* (3rd ed.) Newbury Park, CA: Sage.

Larson, E., Wood, W., & Clark, F. (2003). Occupational science: Building the science and practice of occupation through an academic discipline. In E. Crepeau, E. Cohn, & B. Schell (Eds.), *Willard and Spackman's occupational therapy* (pp. 15-26). Philadelphia, PA: Lippincott-Raven.

Leagans, P. J. (1964). A concept of needs. *Journal of Extension, 2*(2), 89-96.

Maslow, A. (1970). *Motivation and personality* (2nd ed.). New York, NY: Harper and Row.

Morgan, D. (1993). *Successful focus groups: Advancing the state of the art*. Newbury Park, CA: Sage.

Ohmer, M., & DeMasi, K. (2009). *Consensus organizing*. Los Angeles, CA: Sage.

Schuster, C., Cronk, R., & Reno, W. (1992). Psychosocial development during adolescence. In C. Schuster & S. Ashburn (Eds.), *The process of human development: A holistic life-span approach* (pp. 532-543). Philadelphia, PA: Lippincott.

Watkins, R., & Meiers, M. W. (2012). *A guide to assessing needs: Essential tools for collecting information, making decisions, and achieving development results* (p. 15). Washington, DC: The World Bank.

9

Identifying and Building Assets, Developing Community Capacity, Knowing Your Stakeholders, and Sustaining Programming

LEARNING OBJECTIVES

1. To define *sustainability* as it relates to community programming

2. To articulate the multiple dimensions of sustainability

3. To explain the *natural step* approach to sustainability and relate its objectives to occupation-centered, community-based programming

4. To identify the elements of a sustainability plan

5. To demonstrate an understanding of community development, capacity, asset identification, and building

6. To understand how human and social capital can support sustainability in community programming

7. To identify potential stakeholders in community programming

Fazio, L. S. *Developing Occupation-Centered Programs
With the Community, Third Edition* (pp 135-147).
© 2017 Taylor & Francis Group.

KEY TERMS

1. Sustainability
2. The Natural Step (TNS)
3. Community development
4. Capacity building/asset building
5. Community assets
6. Community capital: social capital and human capital
7. Communities of place/communities of interest
8. Stakeholders
9. Coalitions
10. Consensus organizing

WHAT IS COMMUNITY SUSTAINABILITY?

The title of this chapter identifies five closely linked features (factors) that are all about sustaining your program. Green and Haines (2016) tell us that one of the many goals of community development is to sustain places and people, using all forms of community capital to do it (p. 57).

There are many definitions of **sustainability.** According to *The International Webster New Encyclopedic Dictionary*, to sustain means "to keep in existence, to maintain and endure" (1975, p. 988). The Sustainable Community Roundtable Report (2006) offers this definition: "a healthy and diverse economy that adapts to change, provides long-term security to residents, and recognizes social and ecological limits." Sustainability is about preserving the health of the planet and the people who live on it.

"The practice of sustainability is about creating new ways to live and prosper while ensuring an equitable, healthy future for all people and the planet" (The Natural Step, 2006). Sustainability can be viewed as a concept, a method, or even a way of life. There has been recent emphasis all over the globe on the conservation of resources and attention to "wasteless" lifestyles. Some of our student programming has been directly connected with recycling and the conservation of resources. Our alliance with such international organizations as Roots and Shoots is one example (see Chapter 19). Communities of the homeless are perhaps one of the best examples of communities who make recycling of bottles and cans a priority, and central to their economy. Other programming may appear less obviously connected to sustainability, but anytime we help a group of people develop their knowledge and skills, we are building a sustainable life.

Dimensions of Sustainability

We would like to contribute to sustainable communities proactively, but much of what is going on today is reactive. In the United States alone, the loss of farmland and open space and problems in management of solid waste, crime, homelessness, and widening income disparities are pushing sustainability discussions and actions. Green and Haines (2016) have sifted through many definitions of sustainability; they propose three common themes among the definitions: (1) a focus on current behavior to benefit the future, (2) the link between economy and ecology, and (3) a general dissatisfaction with current human lifestyles and behaviors (p. 58). They go on to suggest that there are three important dimensions of sustainability, referred to in the literature as the *three Es*. These dimensions that underlie sustainability are: economics, environment, and equity (or social justice) (Green & Haines, 2016, p. 59). Each of these needs to be in balance with the others for sustainability to be achieved. However, and likely to no surprise to you, there are inevitable conflicts of interest represented by a potential conflict between social equity and environmental protection (development conflict); tension between current use and long-term demand for natural resources (resource confict); and potential conflict between private interest and the public good (property conflict) (Berke & Kartez, 1995; Campbell, 1996; Green & Haines, 2016). All we need do is look around our own cities and neighborhoods to see a demonstration of one or all of these conflicts. Many of you are working individually and in small grass-roots groups to address them, but why are communities, local governments, and community-based organizations adopting community sustainability approaches? Why are "we" writing community programming proposals with sustainability as part of our planning?

Why Sustainability?

There are trends driving our actions and the actions of our communities. One trend that is undeniable is seemingly uncontrolled human population growth. Human populations have increased from 2.52 billion people in 1950 to 7.2 billion in 2013. By 2050, the United Nations (2013) estimates that the human population will have increased to 9.6 billion. James, Power, and Forrest (2000) add the repercussions of climate change and suburban sprawl to the list of trends. The spillover from urban sprawl is interesting and includes segregation/unequal opportunity, traffic congestion and smog, and disproportionate exposure to environmental hazards.

In 2001, some 1.1 billion people survived on less than $1 per day of income, with roughly 70% in rural areas where they are highly dependent on shrinking and endangered agriculture, grazing, and hunting for subsistence. Even though we have increased the world's per capita food production in the last four decades, an estimated 852 million people were undernourished in 2000–2002, up 37 million from the period 1997–1999. Some 1.1 billion still lack access to an improved water supply. Water scarcity affects roughly 1 to 2 billion people worldwide (Millennium Ecosystem Assessment, 2005; United Nations, 2013).

What Can "We" Do?

In our work with communities (large and small), there are a number of approaches to sustainability that may be used to inform our thinking. One internationally favored approach is **The Natural Step (TNS)**, a systems-based approach. Begun in Sweden, it has now spread internationally. There are four scientific principles that, if followed, would allow both organizations and communities to move toward a sustainable world (James & Lahti, 2004). In Sweden, about 70 municipalities follow TNS principles and, in the United States, cities that have used the framework include Pittsburgh, PA; Madison, WI; and Santa Monica, CA. Companies using the TNS framework include Nike, Interface, Electrolux, Ikea, and others. The four principles of the Natural Step System are represented in the box next.

THE NATURAL STEP SYSTEM: CONDITIONS AND PRACTICES

Guiding Objective	Examples of Practices
1. Eliminate our community's contribution to fossil fuel dependence and to wasteful use of scarce metals and minerals.	Transit and pedestrian-oriented development; renewable and alternative energy; incentives for organic agriculture
2. Eliminate our community's contribution to dependence on synthetic substances.	Healthy building design and construction that doesn't rely on toxic building materials; landscape design and park maintenance that uses alternatives to chemical pesticides and herbicides
3. Eliminate our community's contribution to encroachment on nature (e.g., land, water, wildlife, forest, soil, ecosystems)	Redevelop existing sites and buildings before building new ones; conservation and preservation; recycling of water and resources
4. Meet human needs fairly and efficiently.	Affordable housing; locally based business and food production; use of waste as a resource; participatory community planning, and decision making

Adapted from James, S., & Lahti, T. (2004). *The natural step for communities: How cities and towns can change to sustainable practices.* Gabriola Island, British Columbia, Canada: New Society Publishers.

Exercise 9-1

You may notice that several aspects of this plan are appropriate to occupation-centered programming, and you may think of other programming agendas where your impact will meet one or more of Natural Step objectives or other objectives leading to sustainability. Take a moment to write your thoughts here; and discuss these with your planning group:

_____

_____

_____

_____

_____

Sustainability and Occupation-Centered Community Programming

We initiated our discussion of sustainability with broad definitions that will help us to seat our programming within the larger picture and ensure that we are contributing to the larger agenda of creating a sustainable world. We now turn our discussion to some of the literature, focusing more specifically on what may become occupation-centered programming agendas. Much of what we hear about sustainability from granting agencies consists of reminders to build in a plan for how programming will be sustained once the grant funding ends. However, you are probably becoming aware that simply having funding to continue a program is not all there is to sustainability. We must go beyond program implementation to connect with the community and build their capacity to include the programming, and to make it their own (Akerlund, 2000; Edberg, 2007).

Our assessment of needs may begin with attention to a population, and sometimes appears to end there if our population represents a community of interest/shared concerns and problems, but in most of our programming, we must go beyond to include the needs of the larger community and should extend to an assessment of the social, economic, and environmental conditions that affect the community and the program. This positions the program to be responsive as community needs and desires change. Sustainability and programming flexibility are intertwined.

What Does a Sustainability Plan Look Like?

The sustainability plan encompasses an overall strategy for program maintenance that includes specific goals for sustainability along with an action plan to address those goals (Doll, 2014; Pluye, Potwin, & Denis, 2004; U.S. Department of Justice, 2005). The sustainability plan will have goals and objectives for what you will do and a date for accomplishment. This is already what you are doing to ensure that the program will happen—your implementation plan; only now you are ensuring that it will continue to happen! The development of this plan includes the community, the volunteers and team members, and the stakeholders. This group can help identify challenges to sustainability so that planning is proactive.

ELEMENTS OF A SUSTAINABILITY PLAN

1. Methods and plan for collection of data to demonstrate program effectiveness. Very important for newer programs

2. How will activities and infrastructure be sustained once initial funding ends? Also very important for newer programs

3. Will the target population be enlarged? Particularly for experienced programs

4. Will you transfer "best practices" to other programs? Particularly for experienced programs

5. Will you build new relationships with other agencies?

6. How will you build more efficient mechanisms for funding (such as repurposing of existing resources through improved alignment, and coordination of complementary activities and resources)?

7. Will you collect additional data that demonstrate program efficiencies and effectiveness, community advocacy, funding diversification, and collaborative partnerships that can maximize resources?

8. What are your plans for developing community assets through staff/volunteer training and programming?

9. Do you have other plans for developing community assets?

Adapted from Doll, J. D. (2014). Program design implementation. In Scaffa, M. & Reitz, S. M. (Eds). *Occupational therapy in community-based practice settings* (2nd ed., pp. 80-95). Philadelphia, PA: F. A. Davis; Pluye, P., Potwin, L., & Denis, J. L. (2004). Making public health programs last: Conceptualizing sustainability. *Evaluation and Program Planning*, (27), 121-133; and University of Kansas Work Group for Community Health and Development. (n.d.). *Community Tool Box*. Lawrence, KS: University of Kansas. http://ctb.Ku.edu/en/tablecontents/chapter 1046 htm.

Developing Communities

When we discuss communities as a core component of our planning efforts, we need to familiarize ourselves with the people who make this discipline their primary emphasis in research and study. Generally, we will find this body of work in academic departments of community and environmental sociology, colleges of natural resources, and urban and regional planning. While our work in occupation-centered programming is generally much smaller in scope, we nevertheless are benefitting from the foundations these groups of researchers and scholars are constructing as well as validating and adding to their investigations through our own publications. We must always be careful not to work in a bubble of isolation.

Community development has always had a diverse set of objectives: solving local problems (e.g., unemployment and poverty), addressing inequalities of wealth and power, promoting democracy, and building a sense of community (Rubin & Rubin, 1992). Green and Haines (2016) define *community development* as "a planned effort to build assets that increase the capacity of residents to improve their quality of life" (p. xiii). Is this not what we expect to do with our programming and for our populations? Rubin and Rubin (1992) go on to distinguish between development and growth. *Growth* refers to increased quantities of specific phenomena, such as jobs, population, or income. The word could also be used to refer to changes in quality, such as "better" jobs. *Development*, on the other hand, involves structural changes, especially in how resources are used, the functioning of institutions, and the distribution of resources in the community (Green & Haines, 2016, p. 5). It also implies that there is an effort to balance economic growth with social justice and environmental protection.

A fundamental tenet of community development is that the ultimate goal is to help communities learn to help themselves. **Capacity building** can broadly be defined as the ability to become active agents (rather than objects) of change (Green & Haines, 2016, p. 8). Typically, there are four key components of capacity building: (1) a sense of community, (2) a level of commitment, (3) the ability to solve problems, and (4) access to resources (Green & Haines, 2016, p. 9). These authors go on to further discuss **community assets** in terms of several forms of **community capital**. Assets may be understood and grouped in terms of community capital to include physical, human, social, financial, environmental, political, and cultural (Green & Haines, 2016).

Human and Social Capital

Certainly, our programming could target looking for assets (think of it as a treasure hunt) and building assets in any of these domains, but it would seem most likely that occupation-centered interests and the interests of occupational therapy practitioners would fall into the realms of human and social capital. We briefly described Putnam's work regarding **social capital** in Chapter 1. Anyone working in the community would recognize the importance of social relationships in organizing and mobilizing community residents. These social relationships and ties are a form of exchange or capital that facilitates collective action in communities (Green & Haines, 2016; Ohmer & DeMasi, 2009; Putnam, 2000). Social capital can be considered an asset that contributes to the development of other forms of social capital—human, financial, physical, political, cultural, and environmental (Green & Haines, 2016). As an asset, we must recognize it as it occurs in our populations and communities of choice; we must learn to build on it and to increase it. Social capital as it occurs in **communities of place** (social relationships in a particular locality) as contrasted with **communities of interest** (social relationships based on a common set of interests or concerns) is not as strong as it once was, although most people still interact with a few neighbors and families, and these relationships are often based on expectations of mutual support. In our programming, we often work with populations representing "communities of interest/shared concerns" rather than "place." Incarcerated populations and homeless populations represent a shared problem or problems and may be found in transient or fluid communities, spilling in and out of more stable communities (locale or place). Asset identification may target the population more than a community, but reciprocity and social capital is always important.

Many of our occupation-centered programs encourage the building of social capital through communities of interest such as neighborhood arts programs, club structures, and others highlighted in this text. This building of social capital between "participants and members" is then used

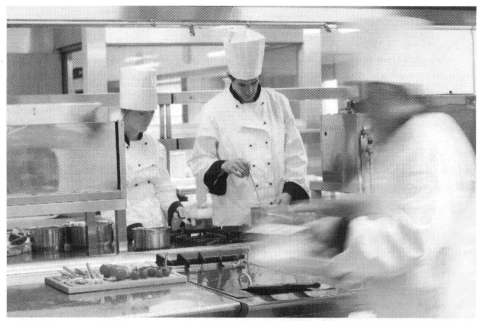

Apprentice chefs, from a life of dependency to an important position in the community: building social capital.

to leverage developing relationships with the larger neighborhood/community. Opportunities for social connections, networks, and mutual support are among the most significant assets we can offer in the building and strengthening of sustainable communities.

Human capital is the other essential community asset of primary interest to occupational therapy programmers. It can include general education background, work/labor market experience, artistic development and appreciation, health, and other skills and knowledge (Green & Haines, 2016). All of our programs focus on people. In most cases, we emphasize individuals but do so in collectives/communities so that assets are built between human and social capital arenas. Several authors caution community developers who wish to educate and train (provide knowledge and skills) individuals toward work that they do so while taking into consideration local labor market conditions (Chaskin, Brown, Benkatesh, & Vidal, 2001; Green & Haines, 2016; Ohmer & DeMasi, 2009). Asset building, then, focuses on the individual (the person) and the needs of the local employers. This bridging between our program participants (often our community of interest) and our community of place (building assets in both) more closely assures that our programs will be successful and sustainable.

A program idea need not be complicated to demonstrate the encouragement of human and social capital as well as sustainability within a community. In 2009, a journalist started an environmental initiative to reduce waste in Holland. He started a *Repair Café* where fix-it volunteers do repairs or show how to do it yourself—everything from toasters to clothing. This group sponsors free events that bring volunteers who like to fix things together with people who have broken items that need fixing! With the assistance of grants from the Dutch government, foundations, and individual donations, there are now 40 repair cafes in that country. The Repair Café Foundation is now helping to start similar programs all over the world. To date, you can find one or more Repair Cafes in Toronto, Melbourne, and Southampton; in the United States, they may be found in Portland, OR; Oak Park, IL; the Hudson Valley; and Palo Alto and Santa Cruz in California. Visit their website for more information: repaircafe.org.

Stakeholders

This may be a good place to talk about our program and community stakeholders. Scaffa, Reitz, and Pizzi define **stakeholders** as "persons who may or may not benefit directly by being involved in the potential program, but who may have a stake in the program's outcome and often the ability to influence that outcome" (2010, p. 204). Bryson, Patton, and Bowman (2011) speak to the importance of stakeholders to the programmer's evaluation process. They identify stakeholders as "individuals, groups or organizations that can affect or be affected by an evaluation process and/ or its findings" (2011, p. 1). In their discussion of the development of a program evaluation plan, they place the identification of stakeholders at the top of the list. Their list of possible stakeholders includes the following: (1) persons having authority over the program, such as funders and advisory boards; (2) persons having responsibility or oversight for the operations of the programs, such as program managers and administrators; (3) persons who benefit from the program, including program participants and their families; (4) persons who may be disadvantaged by the program in some way; and (5) members of the general public who may have a direct or indirect interest in the outcomes of evaluation (Bryson et al., 2011, p. 1). Stakeholders who will be the primary users of the evaluation findings are always included in the evaluation process.

Scott (2014) speaks of the importance of stakeholders to the actions of advocacy; in particular, for accessibility and community integration. In her discussion, stakeholders may be individuals, family members, business owners, employers, advocates, or government entities or officials. They have an interest in the cause and/or a self-interest based on personal need (Scott, 2014, p. 328). This last reference to personal need is an important one; family and friends should probably be placed high on the stakeholder list. These people come from many walks of life, and often these groups of stakeholders are the best advocates, fundraisers, and friends a programmer can have.

Before we leave this discussion of stakeholders, we should mention **coalitions** and other collaborative linkages. Coalitions, partnerships, alliances, consortia, and other collaborative linkages are some of the structural forms that result when stakeholders, interested parties, members of the targeted audience, and professionals with expertise agree to work together toward the common goals of community (and health) improvements for common constituents. The term *coalition* is used as the umbrella term for such agreements (Issel, 2014; W. K. Kellogg Foundation, n.d.). Coalitions in whatever form can be viewed as potentially having power and being power brokers. There is growing evidence that collaboration among stakeholders is key to ensuring effective community involvement and to decreasing health disparities (Braithwaite, Taylor, & Austen, 2000). Both the W. K. Kellogg Foundation (http://wkkfoundation.org) and the Robert Wood Johnson Foundation (http://rwjfoundation.org) as well as several federal agencies have funding priorities related to health disparities that require programs to engage in coalition development, often in the form of community engagement.

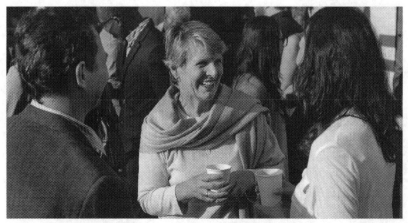

A community event to identify and organize stakeholders.

Identifying and Building Community Capacity

When we review the four components of capacity building presented by Green and Haines (2016), they seem to be very straightforward. Our community will experience a sense of belonging to "a community"; they will be committed and will know how (have the necessary tools) to solve their own problems. They will also have access to resources to make change happen. We know that program sustainability relies on these capacity-building components. How do we encourage the necessary individual assets that will contribute to a community's capacity to develop, change, and sustain? Community programmers and developers tend to rely on four broad strategies, even though their approaches to these may be quite different.

The first is leadership development. In every community, there is a need to identify and expand the pool of leaders to improve public participation and the quality of leaders in the community. We know something about leadership because we have been expanding our own leadership potential through the addition of knowledge and skill building; we can now use those skills to help our stakeholders and community members. There are many full leadership programs available from which we can draw more information should we wish to do so. The Blandin Community Leadership Program (http://bclp.blandinfoundation.org/program/) and Leadership Wisconsin (http://leadershipwisconsin.org/) are examples. In our own occupation-centered community programming, we can offer leadership skill training and opportunities to assume mentored leadership roles toward personal empowerment.

A second strategy is organizational development. Sometimes, this is about strengthening existing organizations by improving board management, member recruitment, and resource allocation. Sometimes, it requires establishing new organizations that address community needs. The establishment of a nonprofit organization might be an example.

Community organizing is a third strategy toward capacity building. In this strategy, we might help community residents become more aware of their common interests to work together. **Consensus organizing** is one way this can occur. It is one approach to community organizing. Consensus organizing uses a technique called *parallel organizing*, in which community organizers mobilize and bring together the interests within the community as well as the political, economic, and social power structure from outside of the community (Chaskin, Brown, Venkatesh, & Vidal, 2001; Eichler, 2007). The goal is the development of deep, authentic relationships and partnerships among and between community residents and stakeholders and members of the external power structure to facilitate positive and tangible community change. If you wish to know more about consensus organizing, please refer to Ohmer and DeMasi (2009) *Consensus Organizing: A Community Development Workbook*.

The fourth strategy is organizational networks. One of the important keys to success in community development is the ability of local organizations to access resources and information outside of the immediate community. Capacity building, therefore, involves the establishment of mechanisms for interorganizational connections. Regional organizations as well as building social ties with key leaders outside of local communities can lead to the building of power and a mass-based social movement to promote social change. Within our occupational therapy profession and other health professions, you can see how networks have evolved to gain strength in overcoming health care access issues and inequities. We can do much in all four of these aforementioned strategies for capacity building before, during, and following programming.

Recognizing and Building Assets in the Community and the Recognition of Needs

Kretzmann and McKnight (1993) defined assets as "the gifts, skills and capacities of individuals, associations and institutions within a community" (p. 25). Oliver (2001), the former vice president of the Ford Foundation, has further elaborated on asset building:

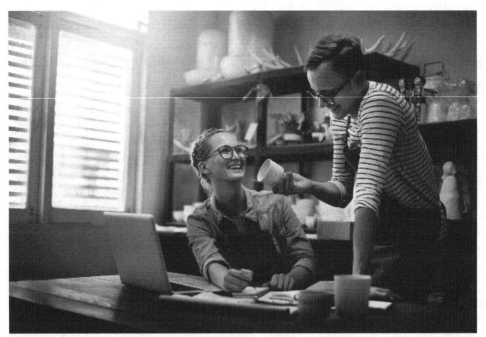

Collaborating with a local business to market handmade pottery sustains a community of craftsmen.

An "asset" in this paradigm is a special kind of resource that an individual, organization, or entire community can use to reduce or prevent poverty and injustice. An asset is usually a stock that can be drawn upon, built upon, or developed as well as a resource that can be shared or transferred across generations. As the poor gain access to assets, they are more likely to take control of important aspects of their lives, to plan for the future and deal with economic uncertainty, to support their children's educational achievements, and to work to ensure that the lives of the next generations are better than their own. (p. xii)

Remembering that assets can take many forms—including financial, physical, natural, institutional, human, cultural, political, and social assets—the focus on community assets rather than needs represents a significant shift in how community programmers and developers have approached their work over the past couple of decades. We have most often begun our programming efforts with a needs assessment that has examined problems and most often focused on a population and/or community's weaknesses. There is an advantage to a needs assessment in that problem identification can help mobilize communities to address local issues and it can help retain a focus on energy and resource allocation. The tendency, though, is for participants to look to others outside of the community, especially to professionals, for help. By relying on professionals and other forms of external assistance, communities become more dependent on outside resources and often lose any control or need they may have had to care for themselves.

In response to these tendencies, Kretzmann and McKnight (1993) emphasize the importance of looking to community assets as a way to identify strengths and resources that can contribute to a planning process. Helping our communities gain skills and knowledge to solve their problems and supporting them through this process is empowering. The distinction between needs and assets does not mean that practitioners have to make a decision to use one approach or another. In many cases, it makes more sense to begin by identifying a community's or population's assets and then examine its needs. Every community/population can benefit from an identification of goals and strengths; from this perspective, problem-solving "needs" are easier to deal with.

In our occupation-centered program planning processes, we create profiles. This is our opportunity to identify assets. We can identify the capacities of our population, and we can identify community organizations and institutions that may be of interest. If we find assets that are underutilized, we can examine why and help provide bridges to better utilization. We can identify and map both formal and informal organizations and services. Sometimes, the informal ones are most useful, such as block clubs, neighborhood watches, and garden clubs. Community institutions purchase goods and services that can contribute to the local economy. They have facilities that may be used for events and classes. They employ workers. Farm-to-school programs have developed in recent years. These programs improve markets for local farmers and improve the quality of food in the school diets of children. Schools can also provide meeting spaces since they are seldom utilized in the evenings and on weekends. Youth groups can use recreational and sports facilities when school children are not using them. School grounds are being increasingly used for community gardens. Schools have kitchens that can be used to provide equipment and facilities to entrepreneurial programs for budding caterers, chefs, and bakers. Classrooms can provide space for classes of adults in the evening and on weekends, offering courses in English as a second language or various skill and knowledge-building curricula. Many of our occupation-centered programs have been offered in a class format for adults and families. When we identify assets in the community, we can often use our negotiation and communication skills to encourage reciprocal relationships. Assets can be found in our populations and in our communities; we just need to learn to identify them.

Adding Assets to Our Community and Population Profiles

It has always been the practice of this text to include assets in our development of the profiles (See Chapters 7 and 8), although it has not been explicit in labeling them as *capacity* and *assets* or linking them to sustainability. That will be our intent here. So, what is it exactly that we are looking for in assets and capacity? We have already identified some things within the broader areas of financial assets, physical assets, natural assets/resources, institutional assets, human assets, cultural assets, social assets, and political resources/assets. What and who is there in this community to help our program find a niche and be successful? We can locate a substantial amount of this information on the Internet; however, the W. K. Kellogg Foundation, in their learning module *Developing Community Capacity: Sustaining Community-Based Initiatives*, remind us that we are likely to get much of it from asking people, just as we do when we conduct our on-site, on-the-ground assessments of need. Among other methods, they recommend community meetings, focus groups, and citizen surveys; we would add to these interviews of stakeholders. Conducting group meetings is always good because you can provide information while you are also collecting it.

If you would like to expand your knowledge of identifying and developing community capacity and assets as well as the additional roles of building capacity and assets, please take advantage of the numerous resources at the close of this chapter—in particular Green and Haines (2016), Ohmer and DeMasi (2009), and the W. K. Kellogg website.

Exercise 9-2

Revisit the profiles you developed in Chapters 7 and 8. After reading this chapter, how will you include a review of assets and capacities in your community? Consider what you already know. How will you determine assets and capacities in your target population (members of this community by place or representative of a community of interest, problems, or concerns)? Remember that where there are needs, there are also assets. Discuss and write your thoughts here:

_____

_____

_____

_____

SUMMARY

In this chapter, the reader is introduced to language, definitions, and concepts from the world of community development. Program sustainability has fairly recently come to our attention as we have designed and conducted occupation-centered community programming. With "sustainability" have come a host of questions. What is it? Is it only about paying for our programs? Do we only have to consider it if we want to apply for a programming grant? By itself, the word can be confusing, but with appropriate background and foundation and the tools and knowledge provided by the multiple disciplines engaged in community development, we can more readily see how the work we've been doing can easily encompass the wider agendas of capacity and asset building and how our programming can be sustained.

Determining the capacity of a community to help itself and the work that can be done to assist them may require additional assessments by the programmer; however, much of this kind of assessment can simply be added to our profiles. We just need to remember that we are looking for strengths and resources, not only problems and needs (although we want to identify these as well). Your curriculum and the time you have to develop a program and implement it will determine whether you have the additional time to conduct further assessments into the community or whether you just need to broaden and/or reframe what you are already doing. Whatever portions of program design, development, and implementation you are able to accomplish will be worthwhile and of great help to you in your practices and in your future ventures into community programming. There is no doubt, though, that the words from the title of this chapter will become familiar language should you decide to make community programming a part of your present and future. Please refer to the references for more in-depth information.

REFERENCES

Akerlund, K. M. (2000). Prevention program sustainability: The state's perspective. *Journal of Community Psychology, 28*(3), 353-362.

Berke, P. R., & Kartez, J. (1995). *Sustainable development as a guide to community land use.* Cambridge, MA: Lincoln Institute of Land Policy.

Braithwaite, R. L., Taylor, S. E., & Austin, J. N. (2000). *Building health coalitions in the black community.* Thousand Oaks, CA: Sage.

Bryson, J. M., Patton, M. Q., & Bowman, R. A. (2011). Working with evaluation stakeholders: A rationale, step-wise approach and tool kit. *Evaluation and Program Planning, 34*(1), 1-12.

Campbell, S. (1996). Green cities, growing cities, just cities? *Journal of the American Planning Association, 62,* 296-312.

Chaskin, R. J., Brown, P., Venkatesh, S., & Vidal, A. (2001). *Building community capacity.* New York, NY: Aldine DeGruyter.

Doll, J. D. (2014). Program design implementation. In M. Scaffa & S. M. Reitz (Eds.), *Occupational therapy in community-based practice settings* (2nd ed., pp. 80-95). Philadelphia, PA: F. A. Davis.

Edberg, M. (2007). *Essentials of Health Behavior: Social and behavior health in public health.* Boston, MA: Jones and Bartlett.

Eichler, M. (2007). *Consensus organizing: Building communities of mutual self-interest.* Thousand Oaks, CA: Sage.

Green, G., & Haines, A. (2016). *Asset building and community development.* Los Angeles, CA: Sage.

Issel, L. M. (2014). *Health program planning and evaluation.* Burlington, MA: Jones and Bartlett.

James, S., & Lahti, T. (2004). *The natural step for communities: How cities and towns can change to sustainable practices.* Gabriola Island, British Columbia, Canada: New Society Publishers.

James, S., Power, J., & Forrest, C. (2000). *APA policy guide on planning for sustainability.* www.planning.org/govt/sustdvpg.htm

Kretzmann, J., & McKnight, J. (1993). *Building communities from the inside out: A path toward finding and mobilizing a community's assets.* Evanston, IL: Center for Urban Affairs and Policy Research, Northwestern University.

Millennium Ecosystem Assessment. (2005). *Ecosystems and human well-being: Synthesis.* Washington, DC: Island Press.

Ohmer, M., & DeMasi, K. (2009). *Consensus organizing: A community development workbook.* Thousand Oaks, CA: Sage.

Oliver, M. (2001). Foreword. In T. M. Shapiro & E. N. Wolff (Eds.), *Assets for the poor: The benefits of spreading asset ownership* (pp. xi-xiv). New York, NY: Russell Sage Foundation.

Pluye, P., Potwin, L., & Denis, J. L. (2004). Making public health programs last: Conceptualizing sustainability. *Evaluation and Program Planning,* (27), 121-133.

Putnam, R. D. (2000). *Bowling alone: The collapse and revival of American community.* New York, NY: Simon and Schuster.

Rubin, H. J., & Rubin, I. S. (1992). *Community organizing and development* (2nd ed.). Boston, MA: Allyn and Bacon.

Scaffa, M. E., Reitz, S. M., & Pizzi, M.A. (2010). *Occupational therapy in the promotion of health and wellness.* Philadelphia. PA: F. A. Davis.

Scott, J. (2014). Rehabilitation and participation. In M. Scaffa & S. M. Reitz, *Occupational therapy in community-based practice settings* (2nd ed., pp. 321-331). Philadelphia, PA: F. A. Davis.

Sustainable Community Roundtable Report. (2006). *About the roundtable.* Retrieved from http://www.sustainable-southsound.org/about-us/

The International Webster New Encyclopedic Dictionary. (1975). Chicago, IL: The English Language Institute of America, Inc.

The Natural Step. (2006). *What is sustainability?* Retrieved from http://www.thenaturalstep.org/our-approach/

United Nations, Department of Economic and Social Affairs, Population Division. (2013). *World population prospects: The 2012 revision, key findings and advance tables* (Working Paper No. ESA/P/WP.227). New York, NY: Author.

University of Kansas Work Group for Community Health and Development. (n.d.). *Community Tool Box.* Lawrence, KS: University of Kansas. http://ctb.Ku.edu/en/tablecontents/chapter 1046 htm

U.S. Department of Justice. (2005). *Developing a sustainability plan for weed and seed sites.* http://ojp.usdoj.gov/ccdo/pub/pdf/ncj 210462.pdf

W. K. Kellogg Foundation. (n.d.). *Sustaining community-based initiatives, Module 1: Developing community capacity.* www.kellogg.org.

10

Developing and Finalizing the Projected Impact and Outcomes for Your Population, Developing Program-Specific Goals and Objectives, and Choosing a Guiding Theory

LEARNING OBJECTIVES

1. To review steps to accomplish in preparation for writing goals and objectives for programming

2. To appreciate the process of clinical reasoning as it may be used to describe the complex course of first establishing programming goals and then helping patients/clients/members reach those goals

3. To learn to recognize and develop empowering goals for occupation-centered, community-based programs

4. To learn to develop measurable objectives to support a program goal

5. To appreciate the complexity in developing a program goal and accompanying objectives to meet multilevel missions

6. To understand the relationship between the program goal, related objectives, and the design of programming

7. To understand the relationship between theories, theoretical frames and models used to guide practice, and intervention strategies and the program evaluation purpose and methodology

8. To identify specific theories both in occupational therapy and in health education, public health, and health psychology that may be used to guide occupation-centered programs

9. To explore the relationships between your program goal/the accompanying objectives and your selected theory, theoretical frame, model, or approach and intervention strategies for practice

Fazio, L. S. *Developing Occupation-Centered Programs With the Community, Third Edition* (pp 149-170). © 2017 Taylor & Francis Group.

KEY TERMS

1. Goal
2. Objective
3. Outcomes/impact
4. Mission
5. Theory/theoretical orientation/theoretical frames and models
6. Occupational science
7. *Occupational Therapy Practice Framework: Domain and Process* (OTPF)
8. *International Classification of Functioning, Disability and Health* (ICF)
9. The Model of Human Occupation (MOHO)
10. Ecology of Human Performance (EHP) model
11. Person-Environment-Occupation (PEO) model
12. Person-Environment-Occupational Performance (PEOP) model
13. Kawa (River) model
14. Health belief model
15. Social learning-cognitive theory (SCT)
16. Self-determination theory (SDT)
17. Transtheoretical Model of Health Behavior Change
18. PRECEDE-PROCEED planning model

Using imagination and creativity, occupational therapy practitioners and occupational therapy students develop inventive ways to engage their patients/clients in meaningful occupations. Because they have many ideas and know how to access resources, they seldom have problems in developing programs. However, developing realistic, needs-based, measurable goals and objectives for community-based programming can be challenging.

Let us consider what we have accomplished. First, we explored our own knowledge, skills, and experience in preparation for program development. We then identified the population with which we would work and, in some cases, the agency/facility or site where we would develop programming and the community that agency served. We researched the literature to learn as much as we could about our selected population and the programming that had been done for them. We also found one or more "experts" who knew our population and our anticipated programming. Next, we developed some ideas for occupation-centered programs that we thought might be appropriate for our population. This was followed by brainstorming practice in matching these ideas to tentative goals and program outcomes. Next, we selected our facility/site and specific population and we developed our community profile and our service profile. In this phase of program development, we also looked at the assets and capacities our population and our community demonstrates. A visit to our facility (or programming site) helped us to obtain more information about the facility's mission and goals (in addition to a review of their website), to learn something more about the population, and to gain some sense of the unmet need for services and the community's assets and capacities. We will now go to the targeted population and conduct an on-the-ground needs assessment. We will identify potential collaborators, partners, and stakeholders if we have not already done so, and we will continue to explore the research and practice literature to learn more about our population and our programming context. Based on the results of all of this, we will be able to initiate a firm plan for a sustainable occupation-centered community program. The next step is to firm up a goal or goals and objectives for the specific community program we are developing and select a theory or model to guide our programming and help us with the selection of program evaluation language and method.

To summarize, the steps to accomplish in preparation for writing goals and objectives for programming are as follows:

- Investigate what you can bring to programming—your knowledge, skills, and experience.

- Investigate trends and explore ideas for occupation-centered programs.

- Select your population and identify what you believe will be the purpose of the program (considering tentative goals and outcomes).

- Develop the profiles of the community and the service population where you wish to conduct your program.

- Conduct the needs assessment as well as the assessment of community assets.

- Compare the results of your needs assessment and your literature reviews with what you have accomplished thus far.

- Select a theory or model to guide programming and evaluation.

This is the time to ask yourself the following: Do I need more information? For the community? For the service population? Will my skills and knowledge base permit me to meet the expressed need? Do my earlier ideas regarding the tentative purposes and outcomes of the program still fit? Do I have a developing sense of what my outcomes will be and the results I hope to achieve?

LEARNING TO WRITE GOALS FOR OCCUPATION-CENTERED COMMUNITY PROGRAMS

Occupational therapy practitioners and students have spent considerable amounts of time drafting goals. Practitioners familiar with Medicare and other insurers have learned that the key to reimbursement for services is a goal that is functional, measurable, and objective. In the language of patient care, the term *goal* is used to describe what happens following evaluation by the therapist. A **goal** is what you aim to have happen, or your target. In general, a treatment plan developed by a practitioner will establish long-term goals (what will be accomplished at the end of the treatment process) and short-term goals (what will happen along the way to the accomplishment of the long-term goal).

For example, a long-term goal for a head-injured patient might be, *Patient will be able to shop independently for necessary grocery items.*

The accompanying short-term goal would be, *The patient will be able to generate a shopping list with minimal assistance.*

You might have considerable experience writing goals using this sort of structure; even if you do not, you likely have used goals to structure your personal growth and progress. Over time, many of us have set ourselves the goal of losing or gaining something. For example, we might aspire to lose weight or gain friends. Goals often define what we vow to do in the passion of some fairly intense emotion. If these are left as general goals, nothing much happens, but if we attach a short-term goal—an **objective** that we can measure—results are likely to follow.

In our developing language for describing the processes of occupation-centered program development for the community, our use of the term goal will generally be reflective of the needs of the community of clients/patients/members, and the use of the term objective may take into account the profiles of individual participants. This will also be the case if we choose to develop goals and objectives with our community volunteers and/or staff. When our goals and objectives are tightly connected and our objectives are measurable, we can determine the first measure of program effectiveness. Of course, our interest is that the goals of the program should benefit all of our clients/patients/members; however, unlike individual goal setting, if all participants do not meet their personal objectives, this does not mean that the program is a failure. This distinction between goals developed for ourselves or for individual patients and the goals we will develop for occupation-centered community programs and, most particularly, our expectations for outcome will take some practice. This is quite a different orientation from what we may have become accustomed to in more traditional occupational therapy treatment environments. In writing goals for a community as opposed to an individual, we must consider the needs of the community and write goals for the community (of individuals). By assessing the need from both those who are observing what they believe to be the needs of the service population and those who are directly receiving services, we have a good idea of goals that will be meaningful for everyone involved.

Our shared knowledge base and our understanding of occupation permit us to translate the expressed needs into goals that are meaningful for occupation-centered intervention. In our earlier community gardening example, the city officials who responded to the early phase of the needs assessment expressed the need to find a place other than the street and the city parks for the homeless population, including those who were homeless with severe and persistent mental illness. In addition, something was needed to keep them busy/occupied. In the parent-child program example, the children's teachers wanted parents to become involved in their children's education, and the administrators of the Sea Grant Program specifically wanted to encourage the children's interest in science and science-based careers.

In discussions of the needs related to these programs, an attempt was made to synthesize and distill the expressed needs into what was considered to be motivating and inspirational language. It was believed that the needs expressed by the city officials could be satisfied and that the population would benefit from the creation of an occupation-centered community. In the second example, the response to teachers and administrators was to create a parent-child program around the development of teams and team building to focus on the academic progress of the child and, again, to go beyond to benefit the parent-child relationship in many other ways. Before conducting additional needs assessments, the concept of community was researched and translated into occupation-centered language. What is meant by teams and team-building and what this might have to do with parenting was also explored.

The broad goal of the gardening program, then, might be to build community, and the broad goal of the parent-child program might be to build teams. The broad goal of the homeless adolescent program discussed earlier might be to encourage self-efficacy and/or develop self-determination. You will recall that the early need for the population of adolescents who are homeless was simply for "safe sex." Based on our community profile and our service profile, we believed that we could meet the expressed need to explore safe sex with this population, but our discussions prompted us to consider what safety might mean to these adolescents in the practice of their daily occupations. The issue seemed much larger than the early expressed need; the issue seemed to be about self-efficacy and the components of what Ryan and Deci (2000) describe as self-determination (confidence, relatedness, and autonomy) . Thus, our broad goal for this program was to encourage the development of self-efficacy and self-determination for the adolescents who participated.

In all of these examples, we are careful not to negate the earlier assessed need. In the discussions of that need, we develop a language for the following assessment that offers more definition and perhaps not only explores the needs already identified but also might offer a few additional options. Our later focus group might include not only questions for discussion around what the adolescents themselves identify as sexual concerns (such as safety), but also other daily/weekly occupations where safety might be an issue (such as drugs, solicitation for prostitution, and so on). The questioning could include consideration of the factors involved in self-protection (for example, issues of confidence, information, and skills that affect self-esteem and self-efficacy). We can then develop objectives for occupation-centered programming that are closely aligned with all phases of the needs assessment results and, in this way, continue to invite the support and cooperation of both groups. With this support, the program becomes a part of the community.

These goals and others like them are empowering; they virtually invite investment and interaction of the participants. They excite not only us, but also those who may wish to fund our programs. However, as they stand now, they tell us very little. Trying to evaluate the goals of building community, or teams, or encouraging efficacy in such a way that one can measure effectiveness is not possible. Goals are not measurable as they are expressed; thus, we must couple these lofty, idealistic statements with clear, sound objectives that are measurable.

Outcomes and Impact

Before you go further to develop measurable objectives for your programming goals, let us revisit your "working" logic model. Remember that our model consisted of inputs and outputs that would lead us to programming **outcomes**, and these outcomes would ultimately carry a larger **impact**. The University of Wisconsin Extension (2008) logic model example considers progress toward outcomes and impact to be measured in terms of short-term results, medium-term results, and ultimate impact. They consider short-term results to be about learning (knowledge, attitude, skills, etc.); medium-term results are action (behavior, decision making, social action, etc.), and impact is about change in conditions (social, economic, civic, environmental). We can think of short-term results as our objectives and their measurement (knowledge, skills, attitudes, etc.). Medium-term results are more ambiguous and need our accompanying objectives to obtain a measure. We can think of these as our associated goals. When we have accomplished our objective measures and satisfied our objectives, we can assume that we have, at least in part, satisfied our goals and that our outcomes and impact should be viable. As you review your model, make note of updates in your information. It should be making sense as you use an if-then narrative. "If" we do this, as we intend, "then" we can expect the desired outcome and anticipate a specific impact.

Exercise 10-1

Review the previous examples from the parent-child Sea Grant program and the community gardening program or the program for homeless adolescents. In small groups, discuss the goals and objectives of these programs. Can you identify outcomes and the long-range impact that might be expected for these programs?

_____

_____

_____

_____

_____

WRITING MEASURABLE OBJECTIVES TO ACCOMPANY PROGRAMMING GOAL

From our research and our dialogues, we develop one or perhaps two goals for occupation-centered community-based programs. Our goals are sufficiently global and comprehensive that we will not need many to address the expressed needs for programming. Settling on appropriate goals takes some work, and in the process, we must offer definitions and tease out meaning. In considering the previous examples, what does *community* mean? What about *team building, self-efficacy,* or *self-determination*? As we grapple with the many ways in which we can translate the expressed needs into goals, we generate terms and phrases that will become our objectives.

DiLima and Schust (1997) provide us with a list of characteristics for community programming objectives. They recommend that objectives must be performance-, behavior-, or action-oriented. They must be clear and must state the level, condition, or standard of performance that is expected. They must be results-oriented and must include stated outcomes that are directly observable. They must have a specific time for completion and, perhaps most importantly, they must be measurable (DiLima & Schust, 1997, p. 209).

To summarize, the objectives for community programs must do the following:

- Be performance-, behavior-, or action-oriented
- Be expressed in clear language
- State the level, condition, or standard of performance that is expected
- Be results-oriented
- Have stated outcomes that are directly observable
- Be oriented to time
- Be measurable

When we write objectives, we select from an assortment of verbs. Some examples include to learn, explore, promote, discuss, evaluate, identify, understand, determine, illustrate, recite, write, construct, define, demonstrate, challenge, accept, and support. Certainly, there are many more from which to choose. With whatever we select, however, we must be able to determine when the action has occurred and to measure the outcomes. Our choice of verbs indicates the action that will be performed. We will then follow the verb with a noun that will identify the expected outcome. We finish with the level or condition we expect and when we expect it to occur. Note the following example:

The members will *demonstrate* their *commitment to the community* by *working in the community garden 6 hours each week* for the *12 weeks of the program.*

You may have only one goal, but several objectives may be required for the participants of your program to be able to satisfy the goal. Your objectives offer the structure for your program. Keep them as simple and uncomplicated as possible because you will have only a certain amount of time to accomplish them, and everyone involved in the program—therapist, client, volunteer, and student—must be able to observe and recognize when the objectives have been accomplished.

For example, your goal for a day camp may be *to encourage movement and socialization through play.* You may enroll six children (or perhaps as many as 12) for four 5-hour days each week (or perhaps four 2-hour days each week) for a period of 2 weeks; then you will have another group of children. Regardless of the number of children you decide to accommodate or the specific daily schedule, the objectives to meet the goal of encouraging movement and socialization through play must be accomplished in 2 weeks. Consider the following example of a measurable objective to meet this goal in the time specified:

The children (or each child) will participate in *one group game each day* that will require *movement through a flexible crawl tube.*

Anyone working in the program described can observe and note when the objective has been satisfied; however, it would be virtually impossible for observers to consistently note the encouragement of movement and socialization through play. These four terms—*encourage, movement, socialization,* and *play*—are all open to broad, subjective interpretation; none is measurable without a specific objective. You might wish to practice defining these four terms for yourself; in the process, you will have begun to generate objectives for such a program. You may look at the goals of this program and the objectives. "If" the objectives are accomplished, we should expect to see increased movement and higher measures of socialization; this can be measured by different instruments over time, and we can group our measures to determine outcomes. The literature would indicate that movement is important for a young child and that there is a connection to the development of social skills. Ultimately, it will likely be "socialization" and connected measures (success in school, well-being/happiness) where we will look for impact over time.

THE INFLUENCE OF "MISSION" ON GOALS, OBJECTIVES, AND PROGRAM DESIGN

We cannot draft goals and objectives for programming without first having sufficient knowledge of the umbrella organization or organizations (i.e., that organization that sponsors or supports the selected facility/agency) and the **mission** and purpose of that organization. Sometimes, our programs may be free-standing, but most often there will be a partnering group. Our Denver sanctuary, for example, might be sponsored by Catholic Charities; a similar program might be provided under the auspices of the Red Cross. The after-school delinquency-prevention program we will be describing in Chapter 19 is provided under the multiple umbrellas of the Community Development Commission of the City Housing Authority, the University Extension Urban 4-H Club, and the City Parks and Recreation Department. There are many stakeholders, as well, represented within these groups, along with parents, neighbors, and others from the associated community.

As noted earlier, the mission of the sanctuary example was to provide free meals, showers, and beds in a safe environment. The need expressed by agency/facility administrators or other professionals working in that environment will reflect the mission and the purpose of the sponsoring organization; that must be our first consideration in the design of programming. It may be an obvious oversimplification, but we would not expect to design a for-profit program to provide services for the homeless adolescent population frequenting the sanctuary. We also would not develop a "wellness" focus for a community-based program to serve the needs of a hospital whose mission it is to serve the acutely ill. However, the latter might be appropriate if the hospital's mission also included concern and protection for the health and welfare of the community being served. This could also be an example of a program intended to satisfy a gap in services, which is often a motivation for program development.

When you review the programming narratives described in Part V, you will see that almost all of the examples work from an early identification of the mission of the institution, agency, or organization. This is of significance when you are developing programming to support a particular community mission. Of course, if you are developing a free-standing program, perhaps a nonprofit, you will establish a mission of your own from which your programs will develop. Missions describe a purpose.

The following example will demonstrate how the multiple missions of several umbrella organizations and their combined needs can be translated and melded to form an occupation-centered program; it also demonstrates how collaboration and partnering may develop:

1. *The Community Development Commission/Housing Authority expressed an original need to occupy the children who resided in housing authority projects during after-school hours until their parents returned home from work. Although not explicitly expressed, this need may have been prompted by recurring problems associated with graffiti, property damage, and gang violence.*

2. *Most of the children living in housing authority buildings attended a nearby public school. The teachers of the school supported the need for such a program and responded to this need with a structured way to encourage the children's after-school interest in education that would be engaging and fun. A science teacher at the school had heard a recent talk by primatologist Jane Goodall and wanted to sponsor a Roots and Shoots program for students.*

3. *The City Parks and Recreation Department sponsored the activities of a facility adjacent to the projects. They were interested in having the neighborhood children frequent their facility, particularly to encourage attendance at their weekend programming, but were understaffed in the afternoons when the housing authority needed programming. With the support of the school and the University Cooperative Extension, they had initiated an urban 4-H Club chapter earlier in the year, and most of the chapter's activities were conducted on Saturdays.*

Granted, this is an extremely complex example, but it is likely that you will have a number of missions to consider when you identify an opportunity to design a program; as well as multiple stakeholders and partners. In the preceding example, the missions did not appear to be competing with each other; they seemed, in fact, to be mutually supportive, and the needs assessment confirmed these observations. There are recurring themes of community throughout these missions. The missions of the school and the Community Development Commission of the City Housing Authority were directed toward the education, protection, and development of children. The school's specific mission was to provide education to children in grades two through five. The Housing Authority not only provided housing to low-income families, but it also financially supported programming for the children in the community through the Community Development Commission. The city Parks and Recreation Department encouraged the health and fitness of children and adults through selected activity.

Two additional organizations were embedded in this mix. Through the sponsorship of the University Cooperative Extension, the 4-H Club's mission is "to enable youth to make wise choices and positive contributions to society throughout their lives." The club's mission is articulated through its motto: to "pledge my HEAD to clearer thinking, my HEART to greater loyalty, my HANDS to larger service and my HEALTH to better living" (4-H Clubs of America: http://www.4h-usa.org/). The science teacher brought another mission to the forefront through his interest in sponsoring programming developed around Jane Goodall's Roots and Shoots projects for children around the world. Encompassed by the mission were the three major directives for this organization: demonstration of care and concern for the community, the environment, and for animals (Herold, 1983). This programming is described in more detail in Chapter 19.

The combination of these missions provided an excellent opportunity to combine the interests and support of several organizations in the development of after-school occupation-centered programming for inner-city children. Skillful program design would be responsive to the sociocultural development of the children through a structure of clubs rather than gangs. Goals and objectives would support community building, education, and perhaps a future orientation. As occupation-centered practitioners, there are very few missions we encounter to which we are unable to relate. The previous example offers multiple opportunities for engagement in community-building while providing personal growth for each child involved in the program. The following is an example of a suggested goal for a program that will meet the anticipated needs and the combined missions.

Combined Missions: To *build* community

Proposed Goal: *To demonstrate* care and concern for the community through club projects that encourage *thinking, caring*, and *helping*

A suggested objective to help us meet this goal might be:

The children will cooperate to plan and carry out one neighborhood activity in the celebration of Earth Day.

Exercise 10-2

In this example, we have used caring and concern as indicators of investment in shared community, and cooperation has been defined as one measure of what we mean by community. Can you think of other ways to define community? Consider the foregoing example. As it is expressed, does the goal capture all of the interests of those involved in providing mission statements? Does it capture all of the needs expressed in our brief description of the early phase assessment results? Does it generate excitement, interest, and spirit? These multiple organizations also provide good examples of community assets and capacity. Identify what you think are some of the assets and capacities expressed by these organizations/this community:

_____

_____

_____

_____

_____

Exercise 10-3

Writing Goals and Objectives to Meet Multilevel Missions and Early-Phase Needs

1. Write a goal for the "combined missions" example:

_____

_____

_____

_____

_____

Discuss your goal with classmates or colleagues. You might wish to reread the example, highlighting those portions that describe the collective missions and the needs.

2. Review the objective provided in the example. As the objective is written, you might suggest that it cannot be measured. How will you measure "to cooperate?" What might be a more measurable way to indicate cooperation? Rewrite the objective so that it is more measurable:

_____

_____

_____

_____

_____

3. Now write a measurable objective (or more than one) for the goal you wrote in step 1 of this exercise:

_____

_____

_____

_____

_____

Exercise 10-4

Writing Goals and Objectives for Your Program

Review all of the information you have collected as you have moved through the exercises to prepare for this step. Consider the data gathered to develop your community and service profiles. If you have a sponsoring organization, review its mission and purpose. Re-examine the results of your assessments of need. Discuss how you will respond to the needs. What do you want to accomplish for your targeted population? Will you provide prevention by offering programming to reduce the risks of illness, disability, or criminality? Will you provide remediation for the effects of illness and disability? Will you provide promotion and maintenance of health and wellness? Will you provide a combination of all of these things? What difference do you want to make, what impact? You will want to revisit your early tentative ideas for goals and you might wish to return to some of the examples offered in this chapter. Write here your ideas for a program goal.

1. Ideas for a program goal:

_____

_____

_____

_____

_____

Review the goal you wrote in the previous step. What does the goal mean to you? How will you define it for your community?

2. Develop several objectives that will permit your population to achieve the goal you have established. Write these objectives here:

_____

_____

_____

_____

_____

Review your objectives according to the criteria listed earlier in this chapter. Are your objectives written clearly? Are they measurable? Do you include the action that will occur, the outcome, the condition, and the time? Does each objective directly relate to the program goal? If an objective does not contribute to the satisfaction of the goal, then it must be rewritten or deleted. Make sure that you do not have more objectives than you can realistically measure. If more practice is needed, continue to work on these exercises until you have achieved the tight linking and clarity you will need to further develop the program. The quality of your goal statement and the accompanying objectives will establish the success of your program. There is sometimes a tendency to want to fold into your objective your rationale for selection of the objective (why and how) you will accomplish or meet the objective (your actual programming). The following is an example:

The students will learn to identify stress signals and to create a plan of action in order to decrease stress (thereby decreasing any guilt they may have felt when engaging in leisure).

We can understand what the programmers are trying to say, but the objective is confusing and difficult to measure in this format. If you find yourself writing such comprehensive and confusing objectives, consider practicing the following approach:

Objective: *The students will learn to identify stress signals (in 2 weeks of programming).*

Rationale: *This will be done in order to decrease stress that may be prompted by guilt over engagement in leisure.*

Programming: *helping the students to create an action plan to balance engagement in occupations.*

It is now time to outline what sort of programming you will provide, on what kind of schedule, and for how long. Your goal and the accompanying objectives will provide the structure for this process. Your goal describes what you feel is most important to accomplish. It is the link to outcome and impact. Your objectives define, refine, and delimit the qualities that characterize your goal. The objectives describe not only what your population will do, but also when they will do it. Now your task is to develop the programming that will enable your population to meet the objectives that will satisfy the goal. It is a detailed and methodical process, and the links between actions and outcomes are equally as intricate.

WHAT PROGRAMMING WILL YOU PROVIDE?

As you have accomplished the planning tasks in preparation for the work in this chapter, you have been developing the program you will ultimately provide. Many planners begin with the idea for a program and then seek to position and justify it through the steps of program development; this is often the course for students and new programmers. The excitement generated by the idea springboards the work necessary to bring it to fruition. Those who consult and are responsive to community requests are generally first driven by need, although programming to meet that need can be equally as creative and exciting.

We have all of our traditional options and more for how to practice in the community. Earlier, we discussed the several roles—including prevention, restoration, maintenance, and promotion—that we might choose to develop a structure for our programs. Certainly, these roles are not mutually exclusive; one program might, in fact, provide a goal and objectives to meet several of these directives. Regardless of the directive we select, there are some assumptions surrounding community-based practices. Practice in the community suggests that we become a part of our practice site—the community. Whether we reside there or not, we understand it and share in its problems and victories. There is an implicit expectation that we are responsive to the needs of the community, just as we are responsive to the needs of our client/patient/member. We understand that our client/patient/member is not only a member of the larger community, but of many other communities as well, and it is our task to encourage and enrich this person's contributions to all of these communities. We are aware of and responsive to what we might describe as the greater good. Although community-based programs need not always be charitable in structure, there is an expectation of charity in spirit. Occupation-centered, community-based practitioners share in common a pervasive altruism.

In summary, the shared assumptions of community-based practitioners, then, include the following:

- We become part of our practice community.
- We are responsive to the needs of our community.
- We encourage and enrich the contributions to their many communities by our clients/patients/members.
- We share with other occupation-centered, community-based practitioners a pervasive altruism and a belief in the greater good.

These assumptions are directed toward strengthening community and, in the process, strengthening its members. Alongside those who receive our services, we are its members. The assumptions listed in the previous paragraph could be described in the same way we have discussed goals; they are empowering, and they help us feel connected to a greater purpose. However, just as we have acknowledged with regard to goals, these assumptions do not structure what we will do; they only make us want to do! Where do we go from here?

THEORETICALLY FRAMING YOUR COMMUNITY-BASED PROGRAM

Goals, objectives, programming, and evaluation are derived from the theory that is selected to guide programming. The supporting theory or theories explicates the connection between what is done and the intended effects and outcomes. Practitioners develop organized ways of thinking about what they see, what they do, and how these things are inter-related. Reed (1998) describes this as **theory.** She suggests that occupational therapy theory is concerned with occupational endeavor translated through four major concepts: the person, the environment, health, and occupation (Reed, 1998, p. 521). From our discussions of occupation-centered community-based practice, it would seem that we are certainly relying on occupational therapy theory to not only frame our discussions of this phenomenon, but also to guide our program design and development. In trying to understand and articulate the placement of occupation-centered intervention in the community, the author draws heavily on the theoretical orientation of **occupational science** (Clark, 1993; Clark et al., 1991; Clark, Wood, & Larson, 1998; Yerxa et al., 1990). Larson, Wood, and Clark (2003) remind us that occupational science is an academic discipline. The formulating ideas for this discipline are extremely helpful as we think about the development of community-based programming, but we do not currently find the structure that is implicit in a fully developed formal practice model such as the Model of Human Occupation (MOHO). Crepeau and Schell (2003, p. 204) distinguish between professional models (e.g., the AOTA *Occupational Therapy Practice Framework* [OTPF], 2014); formal theory (e.g., MOHO, ecology of human performance [EHP], occupational adaptation, and person-environment occupation model), and a frame of reference (e.g., sensory integration). Reitz, Scaffa, and Merryman (2014) offer a discussion of concepts, principles and models, theory, paradigm, and conceptual models of practice offered in ascending order of complexity from basic building blocks of theory and then higher levels of conceptualization. A *conceptual model of practice* is perhaps a more favored term today than a *frame of reference.* Kielhofner (2009) has identified conceptual models used in occupational therapy as the biomechanical model, cognitive model, functional group model, intentional relationship model, MOHO, motor control model, and sensory integration model. Many of these offer substantial guidance in our community-based practices. Theories and models may also inform intervention strategies or approaches. Two examples used a bit later in this discussion are neurodevelopmental theory and learning theory. Both of these provide fairly detailed guidelines for the application of these theories to practice or intervention strategies and approaches. In addressing the questions stimulated by the interweaving of community, occupation, and intervention, we are searching for meaningful ways to integrate these concepts into a practice discipline appropriate for today and the future. In this process, we may rely on all of the previous examples.

Practitioners generally bring to the community one or more theoretical approaches that offer structure for the way he or she provides comprehensive services to patients/clients/participants. How do we select a theory or model that is the right one and the most comfortable one for us to employ in our practices? Selection of a theory or model (or more than one) for practice is first based on one's belief system; that is, it is based on what we believe about the world and what we believe about the people who occupy it. If we believe people define their own purposes in life and act on the world with intention, then we would seek an approach that offered respect for that belief and not one that might be antagonistic to it.

Occupational therapy practitioners commonly use the term *occupation* to describe how people act on or react to the world. The language of occupation is widely used today; however, there is still considerable variability in how this language is translated through the various theories and models. Perhaps this is how it should be; occupation unites us, but our choices of theories and models set us apart. This eclecticism will permit us to meet the wide variability of community-based need in many creative ways while remaining true to our foundations.

As mentioned in Chapter 2, we will also adopt larger, more comprehensive theories and models to umbrella our interventions that are most descriptive of the interactive community systems where our populations are served. Community models and occupation will provide the foundation for structures that will encapsulate other strategies to guide individual intervention in the form of goal structures, objectives, and programming.

Professional Models to Guide Our Program Development Processes

Although first based on our philosophical orientations, the next step in the selection of a specific theory or model for practice may be quite pragmatic. There are two documents, specifically, that provide a comprehensive structure to assist the practitioner in developing a foundation for first understanding, and then implementing practice. These documents are (1) the official document of the American Occupational Therapy Association (AOTA), **Occupational Therapy Practice Framework: Domain and Process** (OTPF; 2014), and (2) the World Health Organization's (WHO) international classifications, including the **International Classification of Functioning, Disability and Health** (ICF) (2001). They are discussed briefly at http://www.who.int/classifications/icd/en/ and http://www.who.int/classifications/icf/en. These documents may be described as professional models helping to define the purview of our practices and, in the case of the AOTA OTPF, the scope of practice. Both provide us with a way of thinking and understanding particularly suited to community practices. Such considerations as participation, health, and contextual factors are of utmost interest as we design community programs suited to adults and children. It is from a thorough understanding of these that practice theories may evolve to guide the practitioner.

The *Occupational Therapy Practice Framework: Domain and Process* and the *International Classification of Functioning, Disability and Health*

Practice in the community can be facilitated through exploration of a common foundation and language for all occupational therapy practitioners as well as others with whom we may wish to collaborate. The previously mentioned OTPF and the ICF offer such a foundation and descriptive language. In all of our community-based work we wish to improve occupational performance, health, participation, and quality of life. These are outcomes consistent with those of occupational therapy, as detailed in the OTPF. The profession, through the volunteer sector of the AOTA—specifically the Commission on Practice—provides us with guidelines and structures to assist our thinking, planning and accomplishment of best practices in occupational therapy. One of the most recent of these is the *Occupational Therapy Practice Framework: Domain and Process, Third Edition* (AOTA, 2014). This document continues to hone the language of occupation and the accompanying concerns of activity. It describes engagement in occupation to support participation in life. Words wisely chosen to reflect the even more global interest in establishing a common language for all health care practitioners is outlined in the *International Classification of Functioning, Disability and Health* (WHO, 2000, 2001). The overall aim of this document is "to provide a unified and standard language and framework for the description of health states" (2000, p. 2). As in the OTPF, the ICF uses the language of participation, activity, and context. The focus is on health as it is demonstrated (activities and participation) and as it is influenced by environmental and personal factors. The OTPF outlines performance in areas of occupation (what historically we termed *work, rest,* and *play*) to separate activities of daily living (ADLs) from instrumental activities of daily living (IADLs). IADLs are thought to be descriptive of those activities oriented toward interacting with the environment and, by nature, more complex (AOTA, 2014, p. S19). Because of the complexity found in the practice context of "the community," we may find that those ADLs described as instrumental are significant markers as we prepare to assist our community members to interface successfully with their environments. The OTPF describes engagement as realized through performance skills and performance patterns. The individual acts (performance) on his or her environment (performance skills and patterns) through chosen or prescribed areas of occupation. Such performance is influenced by the context, the demands of the activity necessary for performance, and the specific factors (body structures and functions) demonstrated by the individual/client. The combination of these two documents—the OTPF and the ICF—provides the practitioner with an appropriate and useful foundation to begin work in the multicontextual environment of the community with a focus on health, ability, and access.

Bringing Together Professional Models in the Selection of Theories and Frames of Reference to Inform Programming

Consider the following example using the two documents to inform our thinking as we continue the development of our programming ideas.

Our service population consists of children between the chronological ages of 5 to 7 years who have developmental ages of 2 to 4 years. The children are experiencing problems performing in their primary areas of occupation that may include toilet hygiene, dressing, feeding and eating, functional mobility, socialization or social participation, and functional communication (AOTA, 2014). Their problems may lie in what the OTPF defines as the performance skills of motor, process, and communication/interaction. Their immediate community consists of family and other children in the service environment. Context, then, is likely rich with cultural, physical, social, personal, and temporal parameters (AOTA, 2014). The ICF would describe these as environmental and personal contexts. Given this information, and more is available to us as we examine all of these documents, we might consider investigating two practice approaches—the sensory integration model (Baloueff, 2003; Mailloux & Burke, 1997; Parham & Mailloux, 2001) and the neurodevelopmental intervention approach (White, 2003)—that draw from developmental and neurological perspectives and theory to structure and guide our practice with these children. We might also wish to combine these with some aspects of a behavioral approach to intervention (Giles, 2003) drawn from learning theory or others that might be appropriate to meet the remediation, maintenance, and prevention needs of this service population and to ensure that they are fully engaged in the occupations of choice and need.

This example might also describe the ways in which we could structure our day camp program, mentioned earlier. The goal of that program was to encourage movement and socialization through play. We could broaden the objectives for that program to address not only functional mobility and socialization, but also functional communication, feeding, dressing, and toileting. We could attend to all of these "problem areas" through the medium of play guided by the theoretical frame of sensory integration, or we could combine sensory integration and neurodevelopmental theory and perhaps add others.

Whether your occupation-centered intervention is intended to help your population reduce risk and thus prevent illness, disability, or criminality; to intervene and remediate during the illness or disability process; or to maintain and encourage wellness and normal development, working from the structure and language of the OTPF or the ICF and selecting one or more theories, models, and/or intervention strategies will provide the programming parameters needed to ensure successful outcomes.

Occupational Therapy Theoretical Models to Guide Community Practice

There are some specific occupational therapy models that are comprehensive and offer language and foundation for translating occupation into community programming, and you will find several of them referred to in the programming examples. The MOHO and the ecological models are provided as examples.

The **Model of Human Occupation (MOHO)** was developed by Kielhofner and Burke in 1980. Of particular interest to community-based practice, it is a systems model describing a heterarchical system where each of the subsystems works together to perform occupational behavior, or purposeful interaction with the environment (Kielhofner, 1997). Communities can be very complex with many interactive systems, so this model is useful to us as we begin to determine how these systems contribute to our concerns for relevant programming and for the interpretation of outcomes. There is an excellent discussion tracing the history of changes in the model in Reitz et al. (2014, pp. 42-44). Of course, there are Kielhofner's original works (Kielhofner, 1980, 1985, 1995, 1997, 2002, 2004, 2009; Kielhofner & Burke, 1980, 1985).

In the 1990s, three groups of occupational therapists working independently created separate models to help practitioners understand the factors that influenced engagement in occupation. Brown (2014) refers to these as ecological models, and they include the **Ecology of Human Performance (EHP)**, developed by Dunn, Brown, and McGuigan at the University of Kansas (1994); the **Person-Environment-Occupation model (PEO)** (Law et al., 1996); and the **Person-Environment-Occupational-Performance model (PEOP)**, developed by Christiansen and Baum (1997). These three models consider occupational (task) performance as the primary outcome. In addition, all of these models indicate that occupational performance is determined by the person, environment (context), and occupation (task). One of the strengths of these models is the potential application across multiple settings, with intervention occurring at the level of person, program, or systems (Baum, Bass-Haugen, & Christiansen, 2005). Of particular interest to all of these developers was the construct of environment. In this text, we are using population, condition, and context to help frame our service profiles; therefore, all of these models are well worth our investigation. McIntyre (2008) discusses the PEO model as it has been used to structure community-based research using participatory action methods, which are of significant interest to community programming planners and evaluators.

The **Kawa (River) model** of occupational therapy was developed by a group of Japanese occupational therapists as a response to the challenge to find a culturally safe and relevant model of practice that accorded with the day-to-day realities of their clients (Iwama, 2005). The model arises from the Japanese social context and uses concepts drawn from the Japanese lexicon aligned in a structure that diverges from familiar scientific and rational form. Iwama describes the use of a common metaphor of nature in the model that allows a focus on harmony between the subject, be it person, group, community, or organization, and the context, and fits well with the East Asian worldview. If you are looking for a framework that will inform and guide your community program, and one that affirms and brings forward the importance of the client's world of meaning and emphasizes the importance of recognizing and responding to cultural differences, then it is recommended that you examine this model in more detail.

Theories From Other Disciplines of Particular Interest to Community-Based Practice

The fields of health education, public health, and health psychology have always been concerned with why people do or do not engage in health behaviors, and they offer extremely useful models to inform and guide community programming for occupational therapy practitioners. The interest in why people choose to engage in positive health behaviors has formed the work of those involved in these fields of study for well over 50 years. Some of the theories that have been developed to inform health behavior change include the health belief model, social learning-cognitive theory, self-determination theory, transtheoretical model of health behavior change, and the PRECEDE-PROCEED planning model.

The **Health Belief model** describes the relationships between what a person believes about health and his or her behaviors related to health (Rosenstock, 1974). According to the model, the beliefs that mediate health behavior are perceived susceptibility to the illness or problem, severity of the problem, benefits of the proposed intervention, and barriers to the change. The model is a planning framework comprising eight phases. These phases provide guidance for ethical health promotion interventions at the community or population level (Green & Kreuter, 2005). The health belief model has been used with a variety of health-related topics including diabetes self management (Bereolos, 2007); and general health habits of college students (Deshpande, Basil, & Basil, 2009).

Social learning-cognitive theory (SCT) as applied to health behaviors was described in 2004 by Bandura and included the core determinants of health behaviors, the mechanisms through which these core determinants work, and the application of social (learning) cognitive theory to prevention and health promotion practices. These core determinants include knowledge of the health risks and benefits of various associated/related behaviors, perceived self-efficacy, expectation of outcome, self-determined health goals and strategies, and perceived facilitators and impediments to health behavior change (Bandura, 1977, 2004,).

Self-determination theory (SDT) is the work of Ryan and Deci (2000) and is primarily concerned with psychological health and well-being. Although this work is not suggested as a structure upon which one would build an entire program, anyone who works with people hoping to make behavioral changes in their general health would be advised to become familiar with this body of research. These researchers pose that human beings can be proactive and engaged or, alternatively, passive and alienated, largely as a function of the social conditions in which they develop and function (Ryan & Deci, 2000). Through examination of factors that enhance versus undermine intrinsic motivation, self-regulation, and well-being, they postulate three innate psychological needs that, when satisfied, yield enhanced self-motivation and mental health. These three innate psychological needs are the need for competence, the need for autonomy, and the need for relatedness (Reis, Sheldon, Gable, Roscoe, & Ryan (2000). The need for competence is fulfilled by the experience that one can effectively bring about desired effects and outcomes; the need for autonomy involves perceiving that one's activities are endorsed by or congruent with the self; and the need for relatedness pertains to feeling that one is close and connected to significant others. If we take into consideration the satisfaction of these needs in our programming and build a context that will support and nurture them, we would probably find that they provide a foundation for more sustainable results in our outcomes.

The **Transtheoretical Model of Health Behavior Change** (also referred to as the *stages-of-change model*) was developed by Prochaska, Norcross, and DiClemente (1994). The model includes six stages of the change process: precontemplation, contemplation, preparation, action, maintenance, and relapse/recycling. There are processes associated with each of the change levels where actions may be instrumental in helping one to move forward through the stages. Processes may include consciousness-raising, self–re-evaluation, environmental control, and helping relationships. One particular unique feature of the model is the inclusion of relapse in the stages. This is of particular use when working with addictions where relapse may frequently occur, but there is a reinitiation of change following. As in SDT, this model is helpful to the programmer in better understanding and anticipating client responses to programming.

The **PRECEDE-PROCEED planning model** was developed by Green, Kreuter, Deeds, and Partridge (1980). Designed as a planning model for health education, it is based on principles from epidemiology, education, administration, and the social/behavioral sciences. In the PRECEDE-PROCEED framework, the acronym PRECEDE represents predisposing, reinforcing, and enabling causes in educational diagnosis and evaluation. A set of steps called PROCEED—standing for policy, regulatory, and organizational constructs in educational and environmental development—were later added to the original PRECEDE model (Green & Kreuter, 1991). The PRECEDE portion of the framework is in wide use across a variety of settings and is used to provide structure and organization to health education program planning and evaluation. The approach is considered unique in that it begins with the desired final outcome and works backward, taking into account factors that must precede a certain result. This attention to "final outcome first" is an approach to program planning and design that complements our use of the Kellogg model as a planning tool. The PRECEDE-PROCEED model is discussed in depth, including the illustrated framework in Green and Kreuter (2005, p. 17).

The models and approaches briefly introduced here have been used to guide similar programming to what you may be considering for your program. The descriptions are in no way intended to be exhaustive; however, there is enough information for you to determine whether you wish to pursue the references further. You will also find more descriptive use of theories and models as they inform programming in other chapters of this text. There are several theoretical orientations informing intervention strategies that are described in Part V of this text, including the MOHO, occupational adaptation, EHP, occupational science, social learning-cognitive theory, and SDT. Following Exercise 10-5 is an account of how theories and models may be connected to goals and proposed programming. If you would like to supplement your existing knowledge with regard to theoretical orientations and models used in occupational therapy intervention, review the extensive list of references at the close of this chapter.

Before we continue, we must revisit one more factor that was mentioned earlier in this chapter and one that contributes to the process of moving your patient/client/member from need to goal. This factor is clinical reasoning, or what Schell (1998) refers to as "the basis of practice" (p. 90). In many ways, clinical reasoning defines an occupational therapy practitioner's "way of being." Clinical reasoning describes the multifaceted process that encompasses all of the ways we utilize the information we have collected about a patient or client and the community (i.e., through our theoretical orientations, our practice knowledge, and our experience). It also captures what has been described as more covert practice enmeshed in the "stories" that we and our patient/client utilize to develop and meet our goals (Mattingly & Fleming, 1994).

Exercise 10-5

Selecting Theories, Models, and Intervention Approaches to Guide Your Developing Program

1. Review the goal and the related objectives developed in Exercise 10-4. Discuss with your group and/or colleagues some potential theories, frames of reference, and/or intervention approaches and strategies that will support the concepts of occupation for the program you are developing.

   If you are currently practicing, perhaps you are already using one or more theories or intervention strategies to guide your work. Are they appropriate to structure the program you are proposing to meet the objectives and to satisfy your goal?

Note here one or more of your choices that are compatible with and supportive of your program goal and the accompanying objectives:

_____

_____

_____

_____

_____

2. Are you comfortable with your selections? Is there agreement between these choices and your philosophical orientation? Your beliefs about people? Your beliefs about occupation? Is there sufficient breadth and guidance to provide the structure for any assessment you might wish to do? A guiding theory also guides evaluation. Is there a good fit with your purpose of remediation, maintenance, or promotion and/or prevention? Make any notes with regard to these questions here; consider further investigation and research that might be useful:

_____

_____

_____

_____

_____

The MOHO was selected to guide several of the programs described in this text. Because the model addresses the motivation for engagement in occupation, how one elects to pattern engagement in occupation, the relationship between skills and performance, and the influence of context/environment on occupation, it is sufficiently broad to meet the needs of a wide range of program participants. It is also appropriate to structure programs targeting prevention and wellness as well as those targeting remediation/intervention (Kielhofner, 1995; Kielhofner & Barrett, 1998).

The homeless adolescent sanctuary program mentioned earlier had as its goal "the development of self-efficacy." Objectives were developed to address the components of self-efficacy to include confidence, information, and skills. A review of the MOHO provides us with language (such as volition, personal causation, values, interests, habits, and roles) to structure our program. An investigation into SDT and the facilitation of intrinsic motivation, social development, and well-being further enhanced our understanding of self-efficacy.

In addition, the attention to the influence of environment on our population—within the context of urban homelessness—must be understood in the design of effective programming. This includes attention to what Dunn and colleagues (1998) describe as ecology, or "the interaction between a person and the context" with resultant effects on behavior and task performance (p. 531). In our homeless adolescent sanctuary example, we noted the multiple expressions of sexuality as adaptive responses to the potentially dangerous context of homelessness; therefore, the theoretical construct of adaptation is significant to understanding our population's response to the community and to our programming; it follows that we might also find it useful to include Schkade's and Schultz's (1998) work on occupational adaptation.

Clearly stated objectives guided by the selected theories, theoretical models, and intervention strategies provide the framework for the design and development of programming that will enable our population to satisfy needs and to meet the goal of services. The following boxed example summarizes this relationship.

OBJECTIVES + THEORIES, THEORETICAL MODELS AND INTERVENTION STRATEGIES = PROGRAMMING = GOAL

Objective: Adolescents participating in the program will be provided with *developmentally appropriate information and skills*, which they can use to make informed choices about practiced sexual behaviors.

Theories/Theoretical Models/Intervention Strategies: these might include the model of human occupation influenced by the theoretical underpinnings of the ecology of human performance and occupational adaptation.

Programming: Modules might be developed to include the acquisition of information and the development of skills structured around the subsystems of volition, habituation, and mind/body performance.

GOAL: To advocate for oneself by effecting positive change in one's relationship with the environment (efficacy).

Finally, to complete our equation, we must add clinical reasoning:

OBJECTIVES + THEORIES, THEORETICAL MODELS AND INTERVENTION STRATEGIES + CLINICAL REASONING = PROGRAMMING = GOAL

Exercise 10-6

Designing Programming

1. Following your goal, your objectives, the tenets of your selection of theories and models, and intervention strategies, what are your ideas for programming? (Refer to your textbooks and to Part V of this text for examples of programs if you need help.) Note your ideas here:

_____

_____

_____

_____

_____

Will your programming enable your service population to meet the established goal?

The mechanics of what materials we will select or develop to provide programming and exactly how we will structure it (i.e., weekly, daily, or monthly) will evolve as we continue to develop the program. For the beginner, developing programming in a step-by-step process is the best way to learn. For the experienced therapist, the process is less linear and problems are more easily anticipated and controlled during the planning process, but even experienced practitioners are often surprised and challenged by community practice environments and populations. Often, it might appear to be more akin to subtle chaos than order. There is always an element of trial and error in the best of planning.

Summary

The results of our earlier work in profiling our community/service population and in gathering the responses to the assessment of needs has resulted in a goal for our program, which includes what we wish to accomplish for and with our service population. Our tentative goal and initial ideas for programming have been matched to evidence for successful similar practices and may have been scrutinized by "experts" practicing with a similar population within like contexts.

Goals give us and our population an attractive and empowering incentive that keeps us engaged in the process of moving forward. However, without objectives to help us define and then measure these goals, they are useless in helping us to design programs for the community. It is from these objectives that our day-to-day programming and our evaluation measures evolve.

In community practice, we approach the individual's need through the combined need of the population; however, we maintain our responsibility to the individual by adopting a way of thinking, or a theoretical approach, theoretical frame(s) and models, and/or intervention strategies to guide our understanding and our choices of intervention. Our selected theories and intervention strategies can be compared to a pair of eyeglasses. When we put them on, we see the individual as an occupational being, but how we utilize occupation will be influenced by the theoretical orientation to practice that we have selected. Our selections provide us with ways to consider and to utilize occupation-centered thinking. How the program will actually look (the day-to-day activities) is a result of the goal, the objectives, and the theoretical orientation.

When you feel comfortable with your goal, objectives, theories, or frames/models and/or your intervention strategies, and when you have some ideas for programming that will move your population toward the expected outcomes, you are ready to go onto the next step of establishing specific programming, including planning for staffing, space, equipment, and supplies. Who will do it? Where will it be done? What will you need to accomplish the programming and outcomes?

References

American Occupational Therapy Association. (2014). *Occupational therapy practice framework: Domain and process.* (3rd ed.). Bethesda, MD: AOTA Press.

Baloueff, O. (2003). Sensory integration. In E. Crepeau, E. Cohn, & B. Schell (Eds.), *Willard and Spackman's occupational therapy* (10th ed., pp. 247-251). Philadelphia, PA: Lippincott, Williams, and Wilkins.

Bandura, A. (1977). *Social learning theory.* Upper Saddle River, NJ: Prentice Hall.

Bandura, A. (2004). Health promotion by social cognitive means. *Health Education and Behavior, 31*(2), 143-164.

Baum, C., Bass-Haugen, J., & Christiansen, C. (2005). Person-environment-occupation-performance: A model for planning interventions for individuals and organizations. In C. H. Christiansen, C. M. Baum, & J. Bass-Haugen (Eds.), *Occupational therapy: Performance, participation, and well-being* (3rd ed., pp. 373-385). Thorofare, NJ: SLACK Incorporated.

Bereolos, N. M. (2007). *The role of acculturation in the health belief model for Mexican-Americans with type II diabetes* (abstract). Denton, TX: University of North Texas. Retrieved from http://digital.library.unt.edu/ark:/67531/metadc4001/

Brown, C. (2014). Ecological models in occupational therapy. In B. Schell, G. Gillen, & M. Scaffa (Eds.), *Willard and Spackman's occupational therapy* (12th ed., pp. 494-504). Baltimore, MD: Lippincott, Williams and Wilkins.

Christiansen, C., & Baum, C. (Eds.). (1997). *Occupational therapy: Enabling function and well-being* (2nd ed.). Thorofare, NJ: SLACK Incorporated.

Clark, F. (1993). Occupation embedded in a real life: Interweaving occupational science and occupational therapy. *American Journal of Occupational Therapy, 47,* 1067-1078.

Clark, F., Parham, D., Carlson, M., Frank, G., Jackson, J., Pierce, D., ... Zemke, R. (1991). Occupational science: Academic innovation in the service of occupational therapy's future. *American Journal of Occupational Therapy, 45,* 300–310.

Clark, F., Wood, W., & Larson, E. (1998). Occupational science: Occupational therapy's legacy for the 21st century. In M. Neistadt, & E. Crepeau (Eds.), *Willard and Spackman's occupational therapy* (9th ed., pp. 13-21). Philadelphia, PA: Lippincott, Williams and Wilkins.

Crepeau, E., & Schell, B. (2003). Theory and practice in occupational therapy. In E. Crepeau, E. Cohn, & B. Schell (Eds.), *Willard and Spackman's occupational therapy* (10th ed., pp. 203-207). Philadelphia PA: Lippincott, Williams and Wilkins.

Deshpande, S., Basil, M. D., & Basil, D. Z. (2009). Factors influencing healthy eating habits among college students: An application of the health belief model. *Health Marketing Quarterly,26* (2), 145-164.

DiLima, S. N., & Schust, C. (1997). *Community health education and promotion: A guide to program design and evaluation* (p. 209). Gaithersburg, MD: The Aspen Reference Group.

Dunn, W., Brown, C., & McGuigan, A. (1994). The ecology of human performance: A framework for considering the effect of context. *American Journal of Occupational Therapy, 48*, 595-607.

Dunn, W., McClain, L. H., Brown, C., & Youngstrom, M. J. (1998). The ecology of human performance. In M. Neistadt, & E. Crepeau (Eds.), *Willard and Spackman's occupational therapy* (9th ed., pp. 531–534). Philadelphia, PA: Lippincott, Williams and Wilkins.

Fleming, M. H. (1994). Conditional reasoning: Creating meaningful experiences. In C. Mattingly, & M. H. Fleming (Eds.), *Clinical reasoning: Forms of inquiry in a therapeutic practice* (pp. 197-235). Philadelphia, PA: F. A. Davis.

Giles, G. (2003). Behaviorism. In E. Crepeau, E. Cohn, & B. Schell (Eds.), *Willard and Spackman's occupational therapy* (10th ed., pp. 257-259). Philadelphia, PA: Lippincott, Williams and Wilkins.

Green, L. W., & Kreuter, M.W. (1991). *Health promotion planning: An educational and environmental approach.* (2nd ed.). Mountainview, CA: Mayfield.

Green, L. W., & Kreuter, M. W. (2005). *Health promotion planning: An educational and ecocological aproach.* (4th ed.). New York, NY: McGraw-Hill.

Green, L. W., Kreuter, M. W., Deeds, S. A., & Partridge, K. B. (1980). *Health education planning and diagnostic approach.* Palo Alto, CA: Mayfield.

Herold, J. (1983). *The Jane Goodall Institute for Wildlife Research, Education and Conservation (1978). Roots and shoots fact sheet.* Ridgefield, CT.

Iwama, M. K. (2005). The Kawa (river) model: Nature, life flow, and the power of culturally relevant occupational therapy. In: F. Kronenberg, S. S. Algado, & N. Pollard (Eds.), *Occupational therapy without borders: Learning from the spirit of survivors* (pp. 213-227). London: Elsevier.

Kielhofner, G. (1980). A model of human occupation, part 3: Benign and vicious cycles. *American Journal of Occupational Therapy, 34*(11), 731-737.

Kielhofner, G. (Ed.). (1985). *A model of human occupation: Theory and application.* Baltimore, MD: Lippincott, Williams and Wilkins.

Kielhofner, G. (Ed.). (1995). *A model of human occupation: Theory and application* (2nd ed.). Baltimore, MD: Lippincott, Williams and Wilkins.

Kielhofner, G. (1997). *Conceptual foundations of occupational therapy* (2nd ed.). Philadelphia, PA: F. A. Davis.

Kielhofner, G. (2002). *A model of human occupation: Theory and application* (3rd ed.). Baltimore, MD: Lippincott, Williams and Wilkins.

Kielhofner, G. (2004). *Conceptual foundations of occupational therapy* (3rd ed.). Philadelphia, PA: F.A. Davis.

Kielhofner, G. (2009). *Conceptual foundations of occupational therapy* (4th ed). Philadelphia, PA: F. A. Davis.

Kielhofner, G., & Barrett, L. (1998). The model of human occupation. In M. Neistadt, & E. Crepeau (Eds.), *Willard and Spackman's occupational therapy* (9th ed., pp. 527–529). Philadelphia, PA: Lippincott, Williams and Wilkins.

Kielhofner, G., & Burke, J. (1980). A model of human occupation: Part 1. Conceptual framework and content. *American Journal of Occupational Therapy, 34*, 572-581.

Kielhofner, G., & Burke, J. (1985). Components and determinants of human occupation. In G. Kielhofner (Ed.), *A model of human occupation: Theory and application* (pp. 12-36). Baltimore, MD: Lippincott, Williams and Wilkins.

Larson, E., Wood, W., & Clark, F. (2003). Occupational science: Building the science and practice of Occupation through an academic discipline. In E. Crepeau, E. Cohn, & B. Schell (Eds.), *Willard and Spackman's occupational therapy* (10th ed., pp. 15-26). Philadelphia: Lippincott, Williams and Wilkins.

Law, M., Cooper, B., Stone, S. Stewart, D., Rigby, P., & Letts, L. (1996). The person-environment-occupation model: A transitive approach to occupational performance. *Canadian Journal of Occupational Therapy, 63*(1), 9-23.

Mailloux, Z., & Burke, J. (1997). Play and the sensory integrative approach. In L. D. Parham & L. Fazio (Eds.), *Play in occupational therapy for children* (pp. 112-125). St. Louis: Mosby.

Mattingly, C., & Fleming, M. (1994). *Clinical reasoning: Forms of inquiry in a therapeutic practice.* Philadelphia, PA: F.A. Davis.

McIntyre, A. (2008). *Participatory action research.* Thousand Oaks, CA: Sage.

Parham, D. L., & Mailloux, Z. (2001). Sensory integration. In J. Case-Smith (Ed.), *Occupational therapy for children.* (pp. 329-379). St. Louis: Mosby.

Prochaska, J. O., Norcross, J. C., & DiClemente, C. C. (1994). *Changing for good: A revolutionary six-stage program for overcoming bad habits and moving your life positively forward.* New York, NY: Avon.

Reed, K. (1998). Theory and frame of reference. In M. Neistadt & E. Crepeau (Eds.), *Willard and Spackman's occupational therapy* (9th ed., pp. 521-524). Philadelphia, PA: Lippincott, Williams and Wilkins.

Reis, H., Sheldon, K., Gable, S., Roscoe, J., & Ryan, R. M. (2000). Daily well-being: The role of autonomy, competence, and relatedness. *Society for Personality and Social Psychology, Inc., 26(4)*, 419-435.

Reitz, S. M., Scaffa, M., & Merryman, M. B. (2014). Theoretical frameworks for community-based practice. In M. Scaffa & S. M. Reitz (Eds.), *Occupational therapy in community-based practice settings* (pp. 31-50). Philadelphia, PA: F. A. Davis.

Rosenstock, L. (1974). Historical origins of the health belief model. In M. Becker (Ed.), *The health belief model and personal behavior.* Thorofare, NJ: SLACK Incorporated.

Ryan, R., & Deci, E. (2000). Self-determination theory and the facilitation of intrinsic motivation, social development, and well-being. *American Psychologist, 55(1),* 68-78

Schell, B. (1998). Clinical reasoning: The basis of practice. In Neistadt, M., & Crepeau, E. (Eds.), *Willard and Spackman's occupational therapy* (9th ed., pp. 90–100). Philadelphia PA: Lippincott, Williams and Wilkins.

Schkade, J. K., & Schultz, S. (1998). Occupational adaptation: An integrative frame of reference. In M. Neistadt & E. Crepeau (Eds.), *Willard and Spackman's occupational therapy* (9th ed., pp. 529–531). Philadelphia, PA: Lippincott, Williams and Wilkins.

University of Wisconsin Extension (2008). *Program development and evaluation.* Madison, WI: Author.

White, B. (2003). Neurodevelopmental theory. In E. Crepeau, E. Cohn, & B. Schell (Eds.), *Willard and Spackman's occupational therapy* (10th ed., pp. 245-247). Philadelphia, PA: Lippincott, Williams and Wilkins.

World Health Organization (2000, 2001). *International classification of functioning, disability and health (ICF).* Geneva, Switzerland: Author.

Yerxa, E., Clark, F., Frank, G., Jackson, J., Parham, D., Pierce, D., & Zemke, R. (1990). An introduction to occupational science: A foundation for occupational therapy in the 21st century. *Occupational Therapy in Health Care (6),* 1-17.

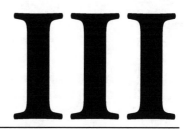

Developing the Program
Preparation and Implementation Phase

11

Supporting Your Programming
Staffing and Personnel

LEARNING OBJECTIVES

1. To learn to connect the program goal and related objectives to staffing needs
2. To consider direct and indirect services required to meet the needs of the service population
3. To understand the relationship between the nature of services offered and the selection of staff to meet the needs of the program
4. To understand the relationship between asset building, volunteerism, and community development
5. To become familiar with the many potential roles of occupational therapy practitioners
6. To become familiar with the guidelines for supervision of occupational therapy personnel
7. To develop the job description for the occupational therapy practitioners who will be hired for your program

---

Fazio, L. S. *Developing Occupation-Centered Programs With the Community, Third Edition* (pp 173-187).
© 2017 Taylor & Francis Group.

KEY TERMS

1. Personnel/staff/staffing pattern
2. Direct services
3. Indirect services
4. Occupational therapist
5. Occupational therapy assistant
6. Activity program coordinator
7. Credentialing/licensure
8. Accrediting agencies
9. Consultant
10. Entrepreneur/social entrepreneur
11. Supervision/supervisor
12. Asset building/human capital
13. Advisory board
14. Job description

As you make your way through this text, you may see (especially compared with the first and second editions) that we are beginning to shift toward programming that is about sustainability, asset and resource identification, and building; it is also much more about community members' involvement. In these programs, you will likely function as a consultant, helping a community's members to meet their own identified needs, to focus on their assets and strengths, and to gain the knowledge and skills needed to build and maintain their own programs. With your guidance, they may be making decisions about hiring personnel. You may stay on as a consultant once the program is in place or perhaps become a member of the board of advisors. In other cases, you may choose to develop a nonprofit yourself or a more traditional for-profit practice. You may or may not hire staff/personnel; however, this information is offered for those of you who choose to do so; it may be useful as well in many of your future professional roles. Although you do not necessarily need to address all of these questions now, they must be considered in your long-term planning. You might feel a bit overwhelmed with the demands of the initial planning process, but try to extend your thinking to first a 1-year plan, then a 2-year plan, and finally a 3-year plan. Make your plans for controlled growth or perhaps for stability. While growth seems to be the "American way," you should always ask yourself "why" before you decide to grow. Decide if there is a need and, most importantly, consider what will be necessary to maintain quality if growth is in your long-term planning. Chaos planning in response to emergencies is not the way to operate a program or to ensure balance in the life of the programmer.

MEETING THE NEEDS OF YOUR PATIENTS/CLIENTS/MEMBERS

The term *staffing* refers to the process of identifying, finding, and hiring those persons who will help to provide services to your population of choice. Braveman (2016) adds that staffing also describes the process of assuring that the right person is completing the right tasks within pre-determined work units, and that these persons have the necessary skills to do the job (p. 168). In some settings, these persons might be referred to as **personnel;** in others they might be referred to as **staff.** Often in the language of the community, they are referred to simply as *the people who work here.* In anticipating your staffing needs, there are several considerations. First, what are the occupation-centered services you wish to provide? To answer this question, return to your initial planning. What is your purpose, your goal, and your anticipated outcome? What are your daily and weekly objectives for the program? In anticipating your long-term outcomes—developing your goal and the accompanying objectives—you have carefully assessed the needs of the community and your population; you have identified their assets and strengths. Through this process and alongside your community, you have defined what services are needed.

However, you must also consider the number of clients/patients/members you can accommodate while offering quality services, and several things will affect that decision. Certainly, the funding for your program and the physical space where you will operate must be considered. It is possible that you will not have all of the answers to funding and space when you begin; rather, you might focus on designing a program that is somewhat conservative, but yet responsive to the need. You might then seek funding and space with a strong and well-planned program design. In seeking grant funding, the initial pilot program is often purposefully small so that it can be well controlled to ensure that outcomes are reached. An adequate funding amount can then be requested based on these early results. Training community members for programming roles may also be a part of programming needs, whether this will occur before meeting the needs of your targeted population or alongside.

We will want to know how services are offered to our population. We think of **direct services** as those services we provide that directly support the goal or goals of our clients/patients. In some of our programming, these services might consist of assessment and/or intervention offered by a therapist. The term *direct* is more important when used to determine the costs of billing for professional services. **Indirect services** likely are less costly and include those we provide through our programming that supports direct services. In the community programs described here, the distinguishing characteristics between these two kinds of services are not nearly as significant as they might be in a more traditional fee-for-service practice. Certainly, you will want to identify the nature of the services you wish to offer because this will significantly affect whom you hire and why. In considering staff to provide direct and indirect services, it will likely be the direct services that require specific and sometimes specialized knowledge and skills. Although more indirect services may be designed and coordinated by a practitioner with specialized skills and knowledge (perhaps as a consultant), the day-to-day program may be conducted by someone with more generalized skills, such as a member of the existing community. Green and Haines (2016) refer to our communities as *human capital* and see this as an essential community asset (p. 136). Empowering individuals in our communities to gain skills and knowledge is often as important or more so than the specific services we are providing to a target population within the community. As you make your decisions regarding the kinds of services needed to facilitate the goal achievement of your population, it may be helpful to review the most recent guide to occupational therapy practice provided by the American Occupational Therapy Association (AOTA; 2014).

In addition to knowing how our services will be offered, we will also want to know when our population is available to receive services. This information was likely obtained in the needs assessment process and must be considered now. The following example describes the reasoning that led to when this particular program was offered.

When parents in the parent-child program were surveyed during the needs assessment process, it became clear that all were working and would not attend a program that occurred immediately after school. Weekends were preferred for other things (such as shopping, laundry, and household chores). Early evening seemed the best time, although a potential conflict with dinner began to emerge. The solution was found through the simple inclusion of a shared meal as one aspect of the program that could then meet a number of the objectives as well as encourage attendance.

Finally, we must decide on the configuration of our service delivery; that is, will we provide direct and indirect services to individuals or to groups? If you choose a group model, the size of the groups will be determined by whether your population consists of children or adults and the nature of their needs (Cole, 2012; Howe & Schwartzberg, 2001; Malekoff, 1997).

For example, goal attainment for adolescents with behavior/conduct disorders requires the configuration of a smaller group size than might be successfully managed with a gardening group of individuals who are homeless. Likewise, a different level of staff expertise and supervision might be required for the two populations to meet their respective goals.

Direct group services to the adolescents in our example would likely require the education, skill, and experience of an intermediate or advanced practitioner (perhaps an entrepreneur). Although it would be designed and supervised by an intermediate or advanced practitioner/consultant, the gardening program could be conducted by an entry-level occupational therapist or by an intermediate occupational therapy assistant supervising occupational therapy aides, volunteers from the community, and both occupational therapy and occupational therapy assistant students. Supervision requirements vary by practice setting and the needs of the client and ultimately are guided by the agency of employment and the state practice requirements. Therefore, to anticipate staffing needs, you must determine the following:

- The needs and availability of the service population
- Will you train community members (volunteers), and what is their availability?
- Potential funding sources and estimated funds available to support the program
- Physical space where the program is likely to be provided
- The nature of services needed—direct or indirect
- Configurations of service delivery—individual or groups

When you have answered all of the relevant questions, you will be well on your way to identifying a **staffing pattern**, or the configuration of staff assigned to the varying responsibilities for maintaining programming, and for ensuring that the program will be sustainable.

OCCUPATIONAL THERAPY PRACTITIONERS

The Occupational Therapist

Our purpose is to design community-based programs that are occupation-centered, and at the center of all these programs will be one or more occupational therapy practitioners. Although they may not always be on site, they will always be responsible for maintaining occupation as the central organizing theme of the program. We are reminded that the focus of occupational therapy is to assist the client in "achieving health, well-being, and participation in life through engagement in occupation" (AOTA, 2014, p. 52). Other personnel may be involved to support the multiple functions of the program, but occupational therapy practitioners are the gatekeepers of occupation and the ones to ensure that programs remain occupation-centered.

Our next task will be to consider what practice skills are required to provide quality services to our population and, further, which occupational therapy practitioners can best provide these services. At some level, the program will require the skills and knowledge of one or more **occupational therapists**, perhaps to design and develop the program, to provide direct or indirect services, to train community members, or to supervise occupational therapy assistants or other personnel.

Generally, occupational therapists may be considered to be practicing along a continuum from entry level to intermediate level to advanced level based on their level of education, their experience, and their demonstrated practice skills. Whether your program will require the expertise of an entry-level, intermediate, or advanced practitioner will again depend on your anticipated outcomes, your goal and objectives, and the services you wish to provide. You will want to review the *Guidelines for Supervision, Roles, and Responsibilities During the Delivery of Occupational Therapy Services* (AOTA, 2014) and, of particular importance, your state's practice act as well as regulatory agency standards and rules to match the service needs of your population to the skills and experience of the practitioner you wish to employ. In all matters of responsibility, including the concerns of staffing, the occupational therapy practitioner is first guided by the *Occupational Therapy Code of Ethics* (AOTA, 2015). This document reminds us of our responsibilities to the client/patient and to the profession we serve. Refer to Chapter 12, Figure 12-2 on pp. 201-202 for a budgeting example that includes staff selection for a pediatric camp program.

To summarize, the program outcome, goal(s), and objectives, and planned services determine the following:

- The necessary level of education

- The level of experience

- The required skills and knowledge of the occupational therapy practitioner

The Occupational Therapy Assistant

The **occupational therapy assistant** may also demonstrate the three categories of ability—entry level, intermediate, and advanced—based on the same considerations that were applied to the occupational therapist. Requirements for supervision are provided in the *Guidelines for Supervision, Roles, and Responsibilities During the Delivery of Occupational Therapy Services* (AOTA, 2014). The specific frequency, methods, and content of supervision may vary and are dependent on several things, including the complexity of client needs, number and diversity of clients, type of practice setting, requirements of the practice setting, and the knowledge and skills of the occupational therapist and the occupational therapy assistant as well as other regulatory requirements (AOTA, 2014, p. 517). The guidelines do not constitute a standard of supervision in any particular locality or place. Practitioners are expected to be aware of and to comply with state and federal regulations and to maintain workplace policies. Both the occupational therapist and the occupational therapy assistant can serve as activity program coordinators. The **activity program coordinator** determines the activity needs and preferences of the clients and identifies specific activity plans to achieve the client's goals. Programs vary greatly but most often are preventative—that is, designed to maintain emotional, physical, cognitive, and social wellness. Adult day care programs and programs for the well elderly are examples of this type of programming, but increasingly more options are becoming available. These programming options are becoming ever more important as we plan and develop programming alongside present and future health care agendas to improve access to health care and maintain health and wellness.

Credentialing of Occupational Therapy Personnel

Credentialing is a process in which one receives written evidence of qualifications to practice. Occupational therapists are credentialed and **registered** under the auspices of the National Board for Certification in Occupational Therapy (NBCOT). In January 2007, all persons who sat for the national examination must have received a master's degree in occupational therapy and have completed the minimum of 24 weeks of full-time Level II fieldwork; these requirements remain current at this writing. When the candidate has successfuly passed the examination, he or she may use the designation **occupational therapist registered (OTR)** following his or her name. Credentialing by NBCOT is independent and separate from state regulation/**licensure**.

All states/jurisdictions—including the District of Columbia, Puerto Rico, and Guam—have some form of regulation of occupational therapy practitioners. Practitioners are encouraged to contact the appropriate state regulatory entity where they intend to practice. A most recent list of occupational therapy regulatory bodies can be accessed on the NBCOT website (http://www.nbcot.org).

Occupational therapy assistants are also credentialed and **certified** under NBCOT. Occupational therapy assistants must have completed a minimum of an associate in arts degree and 16 weeks of full-time Level II fieldwork to sit for the examination. When the candidate has successfully passed the examination, he or she may use the designation certified occupational therapy assistant (**COTA**) following his or her name, or simply OTA. In addition, as of 2015, occupational therapy assistants are regulated via licensure in all states, and the state office of employment should be contacted for any additional credentialing requirements.

Accrediting Agencies

Although indirectly associated with personnel, there may be additional credentialing required for your programming. If there is to be further credentialing/**accrediting** of your organization/program, you must become familiar with the agencies that provide this credentialing and must know their requirements as well (not only for staff but also for other aspects of your program). Some examples of **agencies** that set standards for operations of health care provision include the Commission on Accreditation of Rehabilitation Facilities (CARF; www.CARF.org) and the Joint Commission on Accreditation of Healthcare Organizations (JCAHO; www.jointcommission.org). Whether you will be required to meet the standards of these organizations or others will depend on the kinds of services you expect to provide and where they will be provided. You will need to explore this further when you initiate the early process of developing a program. If you are affiliating with another organization or agency, it can help you explore your role in any accreditation or credentialing procedures.

The Occupational Therapist as Consultant and Entrepreneur

Let us consider two other roles for the occupational therapy practitioner that are both very appropriate to many kinds of community-based programs in terms of both required expertise as well as the support of sustainable programming. In fact, it is proposed that these roles are and will continue to be the most significant to community programming. First, let us consider the role of the **consultant**. The consultant is one who provides consultation to individuals, groups, or organizations and does so within the systems related to practice, education, administration, or research. This role is not specific to occupational therapy nor is it restricted, within the profession, to occupational therapists. With consideration for state practice requirements and guidelines, the experienced occupational therapy assistant also may consult within his or her areas of expertise. Programming examples in this text span a broad arena of systems that a consultant with appropriate knowledge, experience, and expertise could first help a community design and develop a program and then consult through the continuing phases as more responsibility was shifted to the community itself. Epstein and Jaffe (2003) provide an insightful and comprehensive discussion of the various roles and responsibilities of the consultant, suggesting that the consultant would be significant in what we would see as "collaborative interventions for change."

The consultant has the opportunity—and, we presume, the ability—to see the "whole picture." Upon entering an agreement with an organization, the consultant is obligated to provide the best advice/plan possible to assist the organization to meet the needs of its service population and those of the organization as expressed through its mission and philosophy. The consultant is able to do this without becoming enmeshed in the day-to-day operations of the organization; therefore, his or her vision for the organization can remain unclouded. However, the programmer "who becomes" the consultant may not have this perspective.

The consultant's practice and programming experience permits him or her to provide the very best strategies and methods to accomplish the goals of the organization. In fact, the consultant, along with the members of the organization, may have assisted in establishing the goals. In our discussions of program development, it is possible that the consultant would be hired to do all aspects of development described in this text, including the recommendations for the personnel to operate the programs. The consultant might then stay on to consult at regular intervals. This role of consultant is not to be confused with the role of supervisor. In fact, the consultant might wish to supervise on-site professional personnel, but this would not be one of the expected roles of a consultant.

Hanft and Place (1996) mention "style" as one of the elements in their consulting model. They suggest that style, or how you present yourself and your information to the organization, may include the following choices: "tell, sell, teach/advise; and encourage or support" (p. 77). When you function as a program planner/consultant in the community, you must engage in all of these behaviors and more. The skills and information drawn from your intellect, education, and experience must be matched with strong qualities of leadership; you must have the ability to have a vision, to exude a sense of ethical responsibility (and as such, to merit trust), and to model a belief in the therapeutic and formative potential of engagement in occupation. Perhaps most importantly, you must be convincing in the belief that community is integral to our professional strength and must be encouraged and protected as an ideal.

The consultant may also be in a better position by nature of knowledge, skills, and experience to be comfortable with the additional roles of empowering communities to assume programming responsibilities for themselves. Public speaking, negotiation, and persuasive dialogue are described as important abilities for all program planners, but may be of particular importance to the consultant who specializes in program development and must begin most planning processes by gaining the participation of all community stakeholders, building partnerships, and coalitions.

The role of the occupational therapy **entrepreneur** is also very appropriate to our discussions and may simply be a companion term for what we have described as the programmer or planner. The entrepreneur is considered the practitioner who is most able to develop new and innovative models of service delivery. These new models may be in the form of a for-profit or nonprofit practice, or perhaps a hybrid venture. An entrepreneur can come from anywhere. His or her credentials vary substantially; however, by education and training, occupational therapists may be uniquely prepared to take on this role in community settings. We may already have many of the attributes of the entrepreneur. Bygrave (1997) noted decisiveness, determination, and a desire for control as commonly associated with entrepreneurship. Maybe, but it would seem that that is not all there is to it. As with any new endeavor, it is passion that spurs the energy and motivation and having the insight to acquire the necessary knowledge and skills to make changes. Present generations seem much more able to recognize the "wrongs" in the world. Previous generations may have had this ability as well, but today's generation wants to take action and right the wrongs. In many ways, this is the heart of the entrepreneur, most particularly, the social entrepreneur. As is often the case, it is one's character (ethics, moral commitment) and his or her communication skills that build trust in potential stakeholders, partners, and the community of interest. No entrepreneur works alone to achieve goals. Scaffa, Pizzi, and Holmes (2014) offer an interesting discussion specific to occupational therapy and entrepreneurship. Their discussion includes a qualitative analysis of interview content that produced general themes associated with the successful entrepreneur, such as the importance of trend identification, need to be visionary and future-oriented, and prepared to take advantage of opportunities; being an optimistic and persistent risk-taker rounded out the attributes for effectiveness as an entrepreneur. Of course, a recognition of research tracking, skill building, and planning were also important (Scaffa et al., 2014, pp. 119-120).

In recent years the term **social entrepreneur** has become a popular way to define those entrepreneurs who have the public good as their agenda, what Scofield (2011) refers to as "righting the unrightable wrong and finding your mission possible" (p. 1). Scofield (2011) goes on to tell us that there are now more than 3000 schools in the United States offering academic course work in entrepreneurship and some in social entrepreneurship (p. 255), although he suggests that most social entrepreneurs will continue to emerge from the ranks of those already employed. Many will come from the health care sector, from the ranks of the disenchanted, overworked, and undercompensated providers who are "rebelling against a totally broken, bankrupt system" (Scofield, 2011, p.

255). It seems feasible that many of these social entrepreneurs may come from the profession of occupational therapy, but why not early on in ones' career, in tandem with practice, and before disenchantment may occur? It is certainly my experience that many of my former students, having practiced for a few years, are now joining or starting nonprofits to pursue ideas that they had when they were students or new ideas that evolved from their practices.

The entrepreneur who is interested in righting social wrongs will likely have the necessary passion but may be lacking in capital. Possibilities for obtaining this capital are discussed in later chapters dealing with financing your program. We have suggested that social entrepreneurship has a specific agenda. Dees (2000) tells us that the social entrepreneur, similar to the business entrepreneur, wants to provide a superior product or service; the social entrepreneur, however, wants this product/service to result in social good.

SUPERVISING PERSONNEL

Collaborative **supervision** of numerous levels of personnel is the key to operating a successful occupation-centered program. Of course, the continuum of supervision depends on the experience and skills of the supervisee. As noted earlier, AOTA guidelines and state, federal, and workplace regulations establish the specific requirements for supervision. An aide, as in employed occupational therapy practice, is an individual who provides supportive services to the occupational therapist and the occupational therapy assistant. Depending on the setting in which service is provided, aides may be referred to as *rehabilitation* or *restorative aides, extenders,* and *paraprofessionals* as well as called by other names. In general, both the entry-level OTR and the entry-level COTA can supervise aides, technicians, care extenders, and volunteers; in addition, the entry-level occupational therapist may supervise all levels of occupational therapy assistants and Level 1 academic fieldwork students. Occupational therapists with 1 year of practice experience may supervise occupational therapy Level II fieldwork students; and occupational therapists or occupational therapy assistants with 1 year of practice experience may supervise occupational therapy assistant Level II fieldwork students. For more information, see Accreditation Council for Occupational Therapy Education (ACOTE; 2011).

Again, depending on your projected outcomes, goals, and objectives, your program may also benefit from the services of other professionals, including speech therapists, physical therapists, special education teachers, and others. Like occupational therapy personnel, if you wish to involve the services of other therapy specialists, you will need to carefully research their roles and requirements for supervision. The national and state organizations of other professions also publish documents describing service provision and supervisory requirements. If you plan to hire professional personnel in addition to occupational therapy practitioners, it would be necessary to contact these organizations.

Keep in mind, however, that the kind of programming that would require the consideration of multiple personnel at professional levels is more along the lines of a community-based, freestanding, or extended practice rather than much of the programming described in this text.

You will also need to become familiar with the credentialing of those personnel you intend to hire so that services are provided by properly credentialed and trained individuals. Academic standards for occupational therapy education are maintained by the Accreditation Council of the AOTA according to the guidelines provided by the *Standards for an Accredited Educational Program for the Occupational Therapist* (ACOTE, 2011) and a separate but similar document for occupational therapy assistants titled *Standards for an Accredited Educational Program for the Occupational Therapy Assistant* (ACOTE, 2011).

It is likely that you will want to staff your program with other personnel to assist in the provision of direct and/or indirect services or to offer other support to the program. Office staff may be necessary, particularly in a for-profit venture where billing and receipt of payment for services is an integral part of the success of the program. The multiple roles of reception will also be important to many settings. Clients/patients must be greeted, phones must be answered, messages must be received, records must be updated, and so on. The decision to either employ these persons or to employ an external service will need to be made based on your mission and your volume of services. If your service is offered in partnership with another agency or agencies, they may provide these services. As your program develops, or early on you will likely want to add opportunities for volunteers and or interning students. If you are designing and developing a community-based program as an experienced occupational therapy practitioner, you might want to contact the occupational therapy academic programs in your area to discuss their curricula and specific service learning/fieldwork/internship requirements. The costs of providing opportunities for students as opposed to the benefits has been a long-standing debate in the profession, particularly in recent "cost-crunching" times. However, in community-based programs, particularly those that are not for profit, students can learn while providing much needed services. This is also true for volunteers. Volunteers are a link to the community and often offer a wealth of assets, including skills, knowledge, and experiences, and are a valuable addition to a program. However, a program cannot expect to exist based on volunteer services or student services (volunteer, service learning, or interning) alone. There are two obvious reasons. First of all, both students and volunteers are time-limited. Since volunteers provide services because they want to and not because they have to, often they move on to other things, just as students will. Secondly, both groups are adjunctive intended to enhance professional services, and both groups must be supervised. Although this second reason of supervision is not prohibitive, it must be considered. Offering "volunteer to staff" training may be the answer for the program and for the community.

Asset and Capacity Building: Involvement of Volunteers/Staff From the Community

Green and Haines (2016), in their descriptions of **asset building** and community development, provide a focus on the important recognition of **human capital** as an essential community asset. In many of the communities where we recognize a need for programming, human capital is underused and likely underdeveloped; therefore, we have tended to design and develop programs *for* communities, not *with* them. Human capital may include such things as general education, experience in work/labor markets, artistic development and appreciation, general health care, and other knowledge and skills. These are areas that contribute not only to general subsistence, but to quality of life. Green and Haines (2016) are interested in asset building in part through community-based organizations that simultaneously improve the capacity of workers while meeting the demands of local employers. This approach builds on the experiences and interests of individuals and communities and matches them with the needs and opportunities in the region. Programs such as 'Home Boy" and "Home Girl" industries are examples (i.e., http://homeboyindustries.org; http://homegirlindustries.org). The program to provide asset building to victims of human trafficking is another such program (see Part VI, Chapter 24).

In many ways, these programs suggest a "train the trainer" model. There are many variations of this. One recent example, "Teach, Treat, Train," offers a collaborative model from mission work in Jamaica (Lehrer, 2015). This work is conducted by occupational therapists in brief visits, and you will see many of our interests in asset building and sustainability represented in the outcomes of this programming. Asset and capacity building may begin with our targeted population, but it may also be initiated alongside this programming by preparing other members of the community as volunteers and/or staff. Therefore, we would be offering knowledge and skill development on two levels—both important to the community now and in the future.

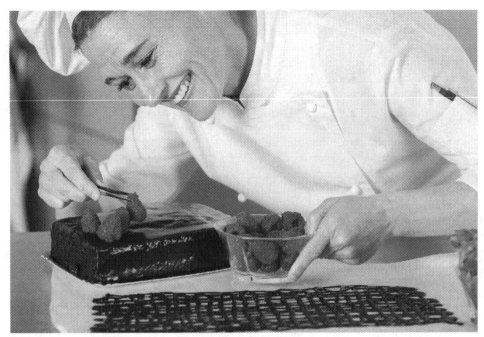

Learning a new "craft" feels good, and tastes good!

THE ADVISORY BOARD

The one other category of persons we should consider in the process of program development is the **advisory board.** Karsh and Fox (2003, 2014) describe the advisory board or committee as a "panel of representatives from all interested organizations and groups in the community who are concerned with a particular program and will help design, support, and oversee it" (2003, p. 287). They go on to describe how important a good advisory board is to the funding process. Today, advisory boards have become an important way of building collaborations and of strengthening relationships within and between communities. They should be selected with a great deal of strategic thinking and advisement from the communities of interest and should include representatives of all stakeholder groups. An astute programmer will recognize the advantages of appointing a group of persons from the surrounding community to assist in providing expertise and in offering links to those in the community who may be of assistance as we develop and market our program, including program participants, shareholders, and stakeholders. Members of this group may also provide mentoring to the programmer, which is particularly useful if the programmer does not share in the culture of the community.

Exercise 11-1

Developing Your Staffing Plan

In the previous chapter's exercises, you developed the anticipated outcomes of your programming, deciding on what impact you hoped to make; you then devised accompanying goals and objectives for your community-based service population. You may have selected a theoretical orientation or theoretical model to guide the selection and provision of services, and you began to develop your ideas for programming that would enable your population to meet the goals. Continue to develop your program by answering the following questions and noting your responses in the space provided.

1. What, if any, direct service(s) will your program provide?

_____

_____

_____

_____

_____

2. If you intend to provide direct services, what level of occupational therapy practitioner will you require?

_____

_____

_____

_____

_____

3. What, if any, indirect services will your program provide?

_____

_____

_____

_____

_____

4. If you are providing indirect services, who can best provide these?

_____

_____

_____

_____

_____

Although we will more carefully develop the volume of services and anticipated service configuration when we consider costs, these things will affect staffing in a number of ways; you might wish to consider them now. For example, offering services in less traditional time slots, such as evenings and weekends, might appeal to many patients/clients/members as well as staff who wish to work full-time during the days for another organization (perhaps another organization where benefits are paid). Such a schedule might also appeal to fieldwork students who seek part-time or nontraditional options. Weekend or evening time slots might also relieve concerns for space. When you survey your community, you may locate organizations that would make their facilities available after hours, since many occupational therapy clinics and facilities offer programming primarily in weekday formats. Leasing space for evening and weekend private practice might benefit everyone concerned.

If you intend to supplement your program with volunteers from the community, the day and time when services are offered will likely affect the age and experience of your volunteers. Retired adults may wish to volunteer during weekdays; students, on the other hand, might prefer to help after school and on weekends.

A combined volunteer model is recommended to supplement services for our earlier community gardening program example. In the gardening program described, retired gardeners preferred the early morning hours for working in the gardens, as did some of the members; other members, some retired volunteers, some working adult volunteers, and younger (working or in school) volunteers preferred the late afternoon and early evening. Still others were available on weekends. Service-learning students balanced out the options. On the surface, this might seem problematic, but with a continuous thread of direction and supervision (by occupational therapy practitioners and/or paid staff from the community), these options invite creativity and flexibility. They included tasks such as tilling, planting, weeding, and watering in the early mornings; picking, cleaning, preparing, and socializing under the trees in the afternoons; and viewing seed and equipment catalogues, researching options (such as a "taco" garden and an "early Native American" garden), building benches and ponds, and attending community meetings in the evenings or on the weekends.

The community garden was restricted by the fact that gardening space was at a premium. In order to involve as many members as possible, it was necessary to operate on a broad 7-day schedule. The garden also dictated this kind of attention. Thus, a wide array of personnel over a broad programming schedule was required. The two important requirements for the occupational therapy practitioners were (1) advanced supervisory skills and experience and (2) skills and experience in program management and coordination. There were other requirements, but the preceding were of most importance. For example, interest and experience in psychosocial/mental health practice and an interest in gardening were advantages but were not critical.

5. Considering the gardening example, what is your current planning with regard to how and when you will provide services? How will these plans dictate the paid and perhaps volunteer staff that you will require? If you are using community volunteers, as recommended, have you considered how you might want to build their knowledge and skills (asset building) to help sustain the program in the future?

_____

_____

_____

_____

_____

6. Consider what you will want your occupational therapy practitioners to do. Make a list of the tasks that will make up the job (separately if you anticipate hiring more than one).

Some examples for the occupational therapy manager of the community garden program include the following:

- Management of the gardening program to include staff, supplies, materials, equipment, scheduling, and budgeting
- Hiring, training, and supervision of staff
- Training and development of volunteers
- Supervision of students to include service learning, Level 1, and Level 2 fieldwork students

(continued)

- Monitoring program objectives and revising and updating as needed
- Monitoring all aspects of program evaluation
- Preparing statistics, documentation, and proposals for funding reapplication or new funding
- Maintaining collaborations with stakeholders within and between the communities of interest

Although in other kinds of programs, expertise and experience with a particular service population might be the most important factor, in this example, it was not.

List your tasks here:

_____

_____

_____

_____

_____

In the development of this list, you have created the **job description** for the occupational therapy practitioner or practitioners that will provide services for your program. If you are the one who will do this, can you do the job that is required? From the job description, you can identify the credentials and experience that will be required to perform the job and an advertisement can be written. You may wish to review examples of employment/ job listings in the AOTA's *OT Practice* (otpractice@aota.org). You may also wish to review newsletters and websites of your state organization.

7. Following your review of examples in professional sources, try writing a draft advertisement for the position you have described (the advertisement also markets your program, so you will want to describe it in the most accurate and positive way):

_____

_____

_____

_____

_____

You might choose to place your advertisement in national sources or local ones, or sometimes both. This choice is substantially influenced by cost and by what you believe to be the local/regional availability of qualified therapists. If you already anticipate funds to be limited, you might circulate a job description and advertisement in the form of a flyer to academic programs (for recently certified practitioners) or to State Association Chapter Newsletters for more experienced practitioners. A well-designed, strategically placed flyer is also an inexpensive and good way to attract volunteers. An even better way to inform the community or communities regarding opportunities for involvement and ownership is to make presentations in community meetings and/or in venues such as health fairs, farmer's markets, or other community events.

8. We have seen that there are all kinds of potential programs that we may choose to design and develop, all important and needed. If you feel a social obligation to build a community program that offers asset and capacity building to the members of the community

through volunteer development and/or through targeted population development, brainstorm some ideas for how this might be done and note them here:

_____

_____

_____

_____

_____

Will you use a "train the trainer" model? Maybe a mentoring model, such as is described in several of the programming example chapters? Do you have other ideas for how you will build a stronger "community" through your programming efforts?

Summary

Finding well-prepared, ethical, and creative staff may be one of the most complex challenges in the development of new programs. Once you have developed the outcomes, goals, objectives, and ideas for the program, it is usually not difficult to write a job description for the occupational therapy practitioners and other staff, volunteers, and community members. Sometimes, these positions are paid, and we advertise them in a conventional advertisement. Sometimes, they are not paid and our marketing is more informational, but these are "jobs," so a description of needed skills is important; although sometimes interest is enough. In considering the staffing of a new or extended conventional occupational therapy program, you must think about the match between the needs of the service population and the expertise and experience of the practitioner. If supervision of other personnel or students will be expected, the experience and practice credentials of the occupational therapy practitioner must be carefully considered. As with all developing programs today, the astute planner remembers that he or she is working "with" the community, not independent of it.

References

Accreditation Council for Occupational Therapy Education. (2011). *Accreditation standards for a master's degree level educational program for the occupational therapist; accreditation standards for an associate degree level educational program for the occupational therapy assistant.* Bethesda, MD: Author.

American Occupational Therapy Association. (2014). Guidelines for supervision, roles, and responsibilities during the delivery of occupational therapy services. *American Journal of Occupational Therapy, 68*(Suppl 3), S16-S22.

American Occupational Therapy Association. (2015). Occupational therapy code of ethics. *American Journal of Occupational Therapy, 69*(Suppl 3), 1-8.

Braveman, B. (2016). *Leading and managing occupational therapy services* (2nd ed.). Philadelphia, PA: F. A. Davis.

Bygrave, W. D. (1997). *The portable MBA in entrepreneurship.* Hoboken, NJ: John Wiley and Sons.

Cole, M. (2012). *Group dynamics in occupational therapy.* Thorofare, NJ: SLACK Incorporated.

Dees, J. G. (2009). Nonprofits. *Harvard Business Review,* (January– February), 55-67.

Epstein, C., & Jaffe, E. (2003). Consultation: Collaborative interventions for change. In G. McCormack, E. Jaffe, & M. Goodman-Lavey (Eds.), *The occupational therapy manager* (pp. 257-286). Bethesda, MD: AOTA Press.

Green, G., & Haines, A. (2016). *Asset building and community development.* Thousand Oaks, CA: Sage.

Hanft, B. E., & Place, P. A. (1996). *The consulting therapist: A guide for OTs and PTs in schools.* San Antonio, TX: Therapy Skill Builders.

Howe, M., & Schwartzberg, S. (2001). *A functional approach to group work in occupational therapy.* Philadelphia, PA: Lippincott, Williams and Wilkins.

Karsh, E., & Fox, A. (2003). *The only grant-writing book you'll ever need.* New York, NY: Carroll and Graf Publishers.

Karsh, E., & Fox, A. (2014). *The only grant-writing book you'll ever need* (2nd ed.). New York, NY: Carroll and Graf Publishers.

Lehrer, S. (2015). "Track, treat, train": Collaborative mission work in Jamaica. *OT Practice, 20*(17), 12-19.

Malekoff, A. (1997). *Group work with adolescents.* New York, NY: Guilford Press.

Scaffa, M., Pizzi, M., & Holmes, W. (2014). Entrepreneurship and innovation in occupational therapy. In M. Scaffa & S. M. Reitz (Eds.), *Occupational therapy in community-based practice settings* (2nd ed.). Philadelphia, PA: F. A. Davis.

Scofield, R. (2011). *The social entrepreneur's handbook: How to start, build, and run a business that improves the world.* New York, NY: McGraw-Hill.

Related Websites

Accreditation Council for Occupational Therapy Education: http://www.aota.org/students/standot.html

National Board for Certification in Occupational Therapy (NBCOT): http://www.nbcot.org

OT Practice: otpractice@aota.org

12

Supporting Your Programming
Space, Furnishings,
Equipment, and Supplies

Fazio, L. S. *Developing Occupation-Centered Programs With the Community, Third Edition* (pp 189-211).

KEY TERMS

1. Space/dedicated space
2. Environments
3. Negotiation
4. Context
5. Safety/ergonomics
6. Volume of services
7. Furnishings
8. Capital and noncapital equipment
9. Supplies (expendable and nonexpendable)
10. Cost projections
11. Overhead/direct and indirect costs

You now have taken your early idea and—either alone or with your classmates, colleagues, or partners—have developed a profile of the community or agency where you will partner and the population you will serve. You have assessed the need for services from those in the partnering agency/organization, the community, and from the population. You have reviewed developing trends and currently trending issues that may affect this program (issues of societal concern such as stress, violence, growing populations of homeless mothers and children, poor underserved elderly, and so on). From the results of this work, you have identified what you would like to accomplish, your outcomes, and ultimately the impact you hope to make, and you have selected a goal or goals and supporting objectives for the program.

Considering the ultimate change you hope to see for your population (outcomes/impacts) and the goals and objectives, you have identified specific directions for programming that will meet the needs of the organization and/or the community and service population. You have determined your staffing needs, including the levels of skill, knowledge, and expertise that will be required. You also know what levels of supervision will be needed. In some cases, you may have also designed a plan to train and educate members of your community or communities in addition to the programming for your service population. To review, you have accomplished the following:

- Profiled the partnering agency, community, and service population
- Assessed the need from the community and/or agency and the service population
- Reviewed trends and trending issues that might affect your program
- Selected an outcome/impact and a goal or goals for your program
- Selected objectives to support your goal or goals
- Designed programming to meet the objectives of your service population
- Identified the staff that will be needed to support the range, volume, and nature of programming required to satisfy the goals
- Outlined a plan to involve, train, and educate members of the community or communities

You are now ready to identify the remaining resources needed to conduct the program according to your design and plan.

PLANNING THE UTILIZATION OF EXISTING SPACE: ENVIRONMENTS AND CONTEXT

Let us consider space. Actually, that statement is a bit vague; what we are really doing is not just considering space but analyzing, designing, and engineering environments. **Space** happens to be where we complete these activities; it defines our parameters. Before you begin this process, think about **environments** and how they affect outcomes. Space denotes emptiness; think of it as a blank canvas on which you paint images. Just as you transform a blank canvas, you can transform the space designated for your program into a positive environment with color, light, and contours.

The same space can invite entirely different outcomes when the environment is created with the needs of the population in mind. For example, consider the choice of classical music and stimulating color for an older adult population or cartoon favorites and subdued color for a population of potentially hyperactive children (or perhaps the reverse depending on the theoretical orientation selected by the planner). In a recent American Occupational Therapy Association (AOTA) document, the profession of occupational therapy has given special attention to the importance of environments. They are particularly interested in the recognition of environments that either support or (limit) occupational performance and participation. Carving out an additional venue for the practices of occupational therapy in what may be limiting environments in the form of providing complex environmental modifications further causes us to be cognizant of environment as a significant concern for occupational therapists and occupational therapy assistants in all of our practices (Renda, Shamberg, & Young, 2015).

Now let us return to the tracing of our progress. If you have initiated planning at the invitation of an agency or organization to develop a partnership, it is likely that the agency or organization has identified some space it thinks would be suitable for the proposed programming. Although this offered space is often small and less than ideal, it is usually adequate to begin with. Remember that the space will, in part, structure the volume and design of the service being offered. Initially, you should be conservative until you have matched your objectives to outcomes, so a small space is not necessarily restrictive.

If space is offered by the agency or organization, it probably is not currently in priority use; for example, it might be a storeroom (to be emptied), a garage (to be cleaned out), a partially covered patio, or it might be a dining room or classroom to be shared. It may be an occupational therapy clinic space or another space that is available evenings and on weekends. If you will have **dedicated space** (used for your purposes exclusively), you will have much more flexibility in programming; if not, you will need to negotiate the sharing of space around other programming that may already exist. Occasionally, part of the **negotiation** process includes the need to revisit your objectives and the structure of your program as well as the volume of services you wish to provide. You might not be able to realistically meet the needs of the facility, community, or service population as they originally were assessed. If you are an inexperienced planner, this is an extremely challenging juncture because you want to meet all of the needs. This is a point when you will need to engage your stakeholders, your partners, and your community in order to choose the best path for everyone. You may wish to move forward with a pilot group. It is likely that if your program evaluation results indicate that you were successful with a smaller component of the population, you can negotiate for more (and maybe more desirable) space the next time. If your initial work was accurate, then your goal or goals do not change regardless of what negotiations you must make along the way.

Before you begin to actually identify and acquire space, revisit the work you have already accomplished, including your goals, your objectives, the nature of services you wish to provide, and the volume of services that you will provide to meet the identified needs. You cannot negotiate until you know what you want—the best-case scenario.

Worthy of mention in our discussion of space and environments is the *Occupational Therapy Practice Framework*'s (OTPF) guidelines for **context** (AOTA, 2014, p. S28). Context, as well, defines programming "space" but requires us to stretch our concept of space just a bit. Context, where and how intervention may occur, according to the OTPF, includes not only physical concerns, but also cultural, social, personal, spiritual, temporal, and virtual issues. All of these conditions are inter-related and occur within and surrounding the client, and they all influence performance. As we consider all of the factors that may influence our decisions about choosing the most persuasive and appropriate environment for programming, we will remain cognizant of these inter-related contexts.

Exercise 12-1

Identifying the Required Space to Meet the Needs of Your Program Design

1. Consider the space/square footage required for each participant served (i.e., an area that is a 2-foot square will contain 4 square feet). Remember that many service models can be considered, including rotating groups or individuals and weekday, weekend, or evening scheduling.

> The earlier example of the day camp to promote movement and socialization through play could be offered in a number of different ways to accommodate the needs of the community. For example, you could offer two groups per day, each for a half day; four groups per day for shorter periods; groups that rotate on 1- or 2-week schedules; or after-school groups. Depending on space and staffing, perhaps concurrent groups could be accommodated. Neville-Jan, Fazio, Kennedy, and Snyder (1997) described an elementary-to-middle school occupation-centered transition program that utilized scheduling concurrently with the children's academic day (pp. 144–157).

   Note here your anticipated program schedule and the approximate square footage of your space needs (both indoor and outdoor as required by your program):

   _____

   _____

   _____

   _____

   _____

2. Consider the space/square footage for any equipment your goals and objectives require.

> The planner of the day camp, for example, intended to access the program outcomes, objectives, and goal primarily through the sensory-integrative practice frame of reference. Both indoor and outdoor space was considered in accommodating equipment such as the flexible crawl tube and a ball-crawl for a program providing service to six children between the ages of 4 and 5 years.
>
> The parent-child program introduced earlier blended integrated community sites with a classroom-style, table-and-chair work space for both a parent and a child of middle-school age that took into consideration the varying heights and weights of the participants.

   Note here your anticipated space needs for equipment:

   _____

   _____

   _____

   _____

   _____

3. Will your program require space for files, office equipment, and office supplies? If this will be needed, can you anticipate an allocated space for office work in the existing agency/organization? Note here what will be needed and the approximate square footage required:

_____

_____

_____

_____

_____

4. Consider any additional equipment/supplies for your program (including what was already noted) such as assessments, arts and crafts, and so on. What kind of storage will be required? Also, consider office supplies. Will your supplies/equipment require secured (locked) storage? If you need to move supplies from place to place (programming in more than one location), do you need storage for supply carts?

For example, the space for the community garden was dictated by the size of the ground plots available to the program (later negotiation permitted the acquisition of additional space). The acquisition of a secured storage shed for equipment/tools and supplies, however, was not negotiable.

Note here your anticipated storage needs:

_____

_____

_____

_____

_____

Exercise 12-2

Utilities and Plumbing

1. Again, consider the design of your program and the anticipated nature and volume of services to be offered. Consider the toilets and sinks that you will need and their location. What will be the needs of your population for adaptations, for accessibility, and for structural changes to the fixtures? Do you need a bathroom in the intervention area, or will one dual-purpose bathroom serve both the intervention area and perhaps reception? Does the bathroom need to be large enough for diaper/clothing changes? Will you need a tub and/or a shower?

Note here your needs for bathrooms:

_____

_____

_____

_____

_____

2. Will you require water sources and/or sinks in the intervention areas? Will you need a water source/sink for arts and crafts? Will you have specialized needs such as oversized sinks for paper making with the addition of a clay trap in the sink drain or a room for

photography supplies? Will you include orthotics or other treatment procedures requiring plumbing? An outdoor faucet is a necessity for filling inflated swimming pools and for cleaning up children after a day camp activity.

Note here your additional needs for water/sinks:

_____

_____

_____

_____

_____

3. Consider your needs for dedicated telephone lines, Internet access (for intervention and/or staff needs), and utilities. Will you require heavy-duty electrical wiring for equipment? Specialized lighting? Wall and/or floor outlets? Outside outlets?

Note what you will require here:

_____

_____

_____

_____

_____

Exercise 12-3

Safety/Ergonomics

Consider any special requirements to ensure the **safety** of your service population and your staff. Will you require security for the building and/or the parking lot? If you are working with an agency/organization, you might not be able to control this, but it is certainly a question to ask, particularly if your staff will be working evening or weekend hours when other employees might not be present. Will outside areas require security walls or fences (e.g., are you servicing potential "runaways" or victims of trafficking or partner abuse)?

1. Ergonomics is defined as the "science of fitting the task to the worker and not the worker to the task" (Fenton & Gagnon, 2003). Ergonomics structure the interaction of the worker with the equipment, work process, and workstation design. With ergonomics, the worker's well-being is protected and the company/business has far fewer injuries and days lost on the job. What are the ergonomic needs of your clients/employees? Are computer workstations at appropriate heights? Is lighting appropriate? Consider equipment and tasks to ensure safe lifting. Refer to our earlier mention of complex environmental modifications to appreciate the scope of such needs.

Note here what you believe are your needs with regard to these considerations:

_____

_____

_____

_____

_____

2. Do you anticipate facility-specific safety requirements with regard to space design (such as codes or restrictions)? If so, what might be the potential impact on your program? When you survey the existing space, make note of any safety concerns you may want to have addressed.

Note your responses here either now or after you have surveyed the proposed space:

_____

_____

_____

_____

_____

Exercise 12-4

Space and Environment

What kind of environment do you wish to create? Will your intervention require individualized space that is free from distractions? A large space for group intervention that might accommodate games, exercises, music, and maybe dancing? A patio area? A room for parent/family conferences? A waiting area for clients/patients/families? A formal reception area?

1. Consider color, furnishings, windows for natural lighting or more subdued artificial lighting, sound (such as distracting noise), and privacy.

Note here your needs with regard to the creation of an environment that will facilitate the achievement of objectives:

_____

_____

_____

_____

_____

Exercise 12-5

Considering Additional "Contexts"

Thus far in this chapter, our work has been primarily within the physical context. It may seem a quantum leap to go from defining the square footage of a room/environment and concerns of physical space to such considerations as how culture, social, personal, and perhaps spiritual and virtual concerns will affect performance. You may have been considering these factors all along but may not have categorized them. How have these dimensions of "environment" influenced your choices in programming?

_____

_____

_____

_____

_____

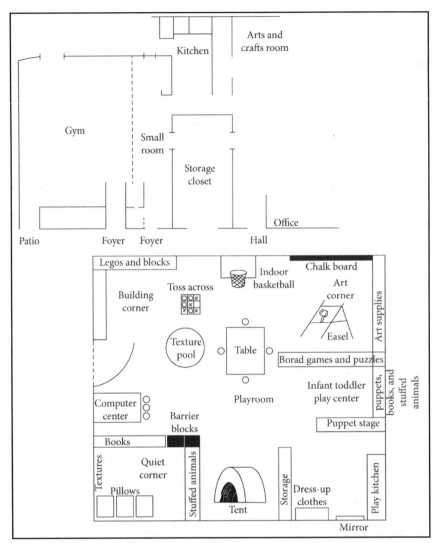

Figure 12-1. Example of a floor/space drawing for a pediatric intervention program.

TAKING A FIRST LOOK AND THEN ANOTHER

You have identified and profiled the agency and/or the community where you will locate your program. You have likely had programming space in mind from your earlier visits; however, if you have not already done so, it is time to take a critical walk-through of the space where you expect to be providing your program. Before this visit, carefully consider your responses to the exercises you just completed with regard to the space requirements deemed necessary to meet the objectives of your program. If necessary, make a second visit; walk the space, and determine the exact square footage that is available to you for intervention and storage. Compare these figures with the results of your earlier exercises. Spend time envisioning how the space will be laid out and how people will get in and out of it. While you are there, also draw a rough floor plan and note the details of the space, including placement of doors/exits, windows, closets, electrical outlets, lighting, telephone lines, and anything else that presently exists in the designated space. For exact square footage, use graph paper to scale (e.g., 1/4" = 1 foot). See Figure 12-1 for an example of a floor/space drawing for a pediatric intervention program.

Exercise 12-6

Comparing Your Rough Space Drawing to Your Original Plan

1. Carefully compare your drawing of the available space with the results of the previous exercises. Discuss any discrepancies you might find. On another sheet of graph paper, note any additions or alterations that meeting your program goal will require. What compromises are you willing to make? Remember that you might be willing to negotiate the mode of service delivery and you might also reconsider your objectives, but you cannot alter your outcome and your goals and still meet the needs of your service population and the community.

> In the planning of the elementary-to-middle school transition program mentioned earlier, the most desirable space (one without distraction) was thought to be a small classroom or meeting room adjacent to the regular classroom. Although it was added later when the program was expanded, such a space initially was not available. The format for programming was redesigned and negotiated to blend and flow with actual classroom and playground activities during the course of the daily round of activities supporting the occupation of "just going to school"/education. The goal of the program accurately reflected the need; thus, negotiation was possible. Without such preliminary work in assessing the need, the assistance of the school administrators and teachers (stakeholders) would not likely have been forthcoming (Neville-Jan et al., 1997, pp. 144–157).

After you have made your comparisons, note here any additions or alterations in the existing space that must be negotiated in order for your program to meet the goals:

_____

_____

_____

_____

_____

Ideal Space

You might want to draft what could be described as an ideal or most desirable space plan to keep in your file for future planning; for now, however, you will need to negotiate from what you require to meet your goals, not necessarily from what might be ideal. Space is a desirable and scarce commodity for most agencies and organizations, particularly if they are not for profit. However, if you have followed through on the previous exercises and have an accurate and detailed assessment of needs, then you will have an informed position from which you can negotiate. Do not settle for less than what you require to satisfy your goals. If you must negotiate for less space (reduced square footage) or less desirable space than you intended (inadequate storage, no windows, and so on), then you may need to alter your objectives and the volume of services you can offer. You will need to be clear about this in your negotiations. Also, consider your bottom line for negotiation. There is always a point from which you might decide that you cannot meet the expected need or cannot do so while offering quality services. Negotiation does not mean compromising ethics, integrity, or quality. If it comes to this, you know to step away and perhaps broker your plan elsewhere in the community.

Designing a New, Remodeled, or Renovated Space for a Private Practice

If you are designing space for a private for-profit practice, you can be more creative in the expression of your needs. However, even if you have substantial freedom in space design, it is critical that you always be realistic in what you must have to meet your expected outcomes, your goals and objectives. If you are successful as you initiate programming and if your outcome measures demonstrate this success, then you will be in a position to negotiate for additional and perhaps more desirable space.

Assuming careful planning and good business savvy (or advice), it is likely that private practices will soon outgrow their space and will find the need to expand into other existing space. It would be advisable to keep this in mind if you anticipate leasing space for a free-standing practice. Consider a business building that is zoned appropriately for your practice, with easy access, elevators to upper floors, adequate parking, and with potential to lease adjoining space when the practice grows. This will help in the future to avoid the time, potential client loss, and expense of having to move everything to a new address.

If you are starting a private practice, the space plan must be detailed, accurate, and comprehensive. This is also true if you are "shopping" for existing space to remodel or if you are able to design your space as a building is being constructed. As a culture, occupational therapy practitioners have a good sense of space, environment, and design; however, the design of a practice space from the ground up requires the services of an architect and perhaps other design professionals. Certainly, you must carefully collaborate from your area of expertise, which is knowledge about the characteristics and needs of the community, the service needs of your population, attention to multiple contexts, and the characteristics of adapted environments.

There are a few other points to consider if you intend to design and plan a private practice. Just as we discussed previously, conduct all steps of the programming process, including the needs assessment, trends analysis, and the community profile. Although you might believe that you know the community, it is likely that you know it only from your own perspective (i.e., the environment that supports your chosen occupations). Of course, place your practice within the community you wish to serve, with consideration for the round of activities that your targeted client/patient population engages in daily and weekly. If your program's targeted population includes children with learning and/or emotional disorders who are seen after school or on Saturdays, consider the daily occupations of the parents and families and place your practice close to areas such as schools, athletic fields, and shopping.

If a mother or father is able to first drop off one child for soccer practice, another for an after-school music lesson, and another for therapy and will then go and shop for dinner, your practice will be more successful than one that is located outside of his or her round of daily activity. Convenience is also a factor for adults who come for their own therapy before or after work or during their lunch hours. "Mapping" your community and the daily occupations of your targeted population and their families and using this map to locate your practice and develop your programming hours will be a long-standing advantage to you. While it might seem to be common sense, placing your practice convenient to the occupational routines of your client/patient population is also a sophisticated marketing strategy.

These considerations also hold true for the planning of day camps for children with special needs. Again, parents may have to balance the schedules of other children, their own work schedules, and the therapeutic needs of the child receiving services. In the case of a day camp, offering low-cost transportation is a real plus, but sometimes simply offering a small space for parents and caregivers to have a cup of coffee, chat with others, and relax is enough to get children there when otherwise they might not have been included. Anticipating and addressing the needs of a caregiver while providing intervention to the client/patient/camper permits the planner to meet several objectives. In addition, if our camp example also includes the siblings of the service population, several needs may be satisfied. Additional programming for these caregivers through focused "help" sessions while their children are receiving services might be a wise marketing tool or, in some cases, another point of potentially profitable service.

The wise utilization of space—whether of a room, a building, or a location within a community—is often key to the success of a program. As stated by Ryan, Ray, and Hiduke (1999), "one of the most important decisions an entrepreneur has to make is where to locate his or her business … location, location, location" (p. 119).

FURNISHINGS, EQUIPMENT, AND SUPPLIES

Now that you have accomplished your preliminary planning and have identified your space/programming environment, it is time to furnish it. Again, revisit your expected outcomes, goals, and objectives. It seems redundant by now, but your well-crafted and informed goals and objectives structure every plan and every decision that you make as you develop your program. We have all witnessed programs where there is an apparent lack of planning, direction, and structure. Consider, for example, treatment rooms filled with laundry lists of supplies and equipment because they were assumed to be important to an occupational therapy practice. This particularly happens when a planner solicits donated items without a clear sense of the program's direction. To avoid making a generic list of, for example, 12 reachers, five boxes of raffia, five inflatable swimming pools, or four computers with cognitive retraining software, let us begin by defining exactly what we want to accomplish.

As we have already noted, our first considerations include our programming goal, our accompanying objectives, and our population to be served. In Chapter 10, you developed the theoretical orientation that you would use to structure your intervention. The **volume of services**—or how many clients/patients/members you would see in the course of 1 day, week, or month—was established as you considered the needs of your population and the number of staff, their qualifications, and their skills. These considerations also helped you select and plan the space where the program would take place. As summarized in the following equation, all of these considerations form the pieces of a puzzle that will lead you to the furnishings, equipment, and supplies that you will need to operate the program:

Outcomes/goals/objectives + target population + theoretical orientation/models + staff + space + service volume = furnishings, equipment and supplies

Let us examine how all of these considerations come together to result in our recommended inventory of furnishings, equipment, and supplies. You will recall that earlier we reviewed the space needs for a day camp example.

The goal of the day camp was to promote movement and socialization through play, and the sensory-integrative frame of reference was selected to facilitate the objectives designed to accomplish the goal. The outcome for such a program might be a happy, engaged child who was able to enjoy a friendship and play with other children. The available space could easily accommodate the program design to offer services for six children between the ages of 4 and 5 years, 4 days per week from 10 a.m. to 3 p.m., for 2 weeks. This service model was then repeated for new groups of children. Children require attention both to facilitate the achievement of intervention objectives and to guarantee safety. For the six children, there were two occupational therapists, one occupational therapy assistant, and two student volunteers. In addition to direct service, administrative tasks and marketing/promotion were shared by the two occupational therapists.

(continued)

The program was conducted both indoors and outdoors. The outdoor area combined a large sand strip with a grassy area for sensory-integrative games and activities. An awning covered four picnic tables for lunch, snacks, and arts and crafts. A smaller indoor area was available for the occasional rainy day and was used primarily for storage.

This service-delivery model could be expanded if the children came to camp for only half days or if two camps were run simultaneously. Such decisions would require that the planners revisit their objectives and their goal. Could the campers meet their objectives in only half-day visits? How would this decision affect the staffing pattern, and what would happen if two camps were run simultaneously? Would more space be required? More supplies and equipment? How would this decision affect the staffing pattern? Could the objectives continue to be satisfied? Would new objectives be required to meet the goal? Would these potential changes in the service-delivery model continue to meet the needs as expressed by referring community therapists, teachers, and parents? (See Figure 12-2 for a partial supply list for this program).

This example demonstrates several things. The equation we have offered to take us to our decision of what equipment and supplies we will need to provide the program is certainly not linear. With each option we might consider, there are pros and cons. It is our clinical reasoning that permits us to integrate all of these potential choices into a best-case scenario for the child/camper. Certainly adding more children to the camp while hiring fewer staff and not increasing supplies or equipment has the potential to "make more money," or does it? Can we consider that offering the very best services (that through our evaluation process we can guarantee are effective) may be more lucrative over time?

HOW DO YOU FIND WHAT YOU NEED FOR YOUR PROGRAM?

We have mentioned several service items in our day camp example that will have to be purchased, including picnic tables, games and activities, and arts and crafts supplies. The picnic tables and perhaps the games will be a one-time purchase, but the supplies for arts and crafts will require continuous replacement. If you are a practicing therapist, choosing the furnishings, equipment, and supplies for your program will not be difficult. On the other hand, if you are a student, you will first need to peruse the catalogues and/or websites of suppliers that occupational therapy practitioners use to furnish their practices. Although some of the supplies and equipment surround you in your classrooms, until now, you may not have been aware of how and where they were obtained or how much they cost. (See the partial list at the end of this chapter for companies that provide equipment and supplies suitable for occupational therapy practices.)

The issue of cost brings us to another important consideration: we have not yet established a budget for our program (that will come in the next chapter). Depending on how you have become accustomed to handling your personal budget, you might be a little confused about designing a program without knowing what you can afford. If you are a student, you should use what might be described as *optimistic budgeting*, or designing the best-case scenario of what the program should be. When you know what you want and what it will cost, then you target the funding. If you are unable to acquire enough financing to run the program exactly the way you want, you can make reductions in a number of areas (such as volume of services, staff, equipment, and supplies) before start-up and during the first year, while still meeting your needs/goals. As you become a more experienced planner, you will always have a funding source and a "ballpark" figure for funding in mind. You then will match each step of the process to the anticipated source and potential amount for funding.

SAMPLE COST SHEET FOR A DAY CAMP

This particular day camp program is a variation of the one described earlier. It is an extension of a pediatric not-for-profit practice, but it also welcomes the siblings of clients. It is staffed by full-time employees of the practice during the 3 summer months. The following is the service provision formula: two 4-day weeks = one camp session × 3 summer months = six sessions × 10 day campers each session = a total of 60 children serviced. The following is a partial cost sheet for the program. *Items marked with an asterisk (*) indicate a partial list.*

1. STAFFING
   a. Full-time camp: registered occupational therapist, entry-level
   Yearly gross salary = $72,000
   b. Part-time camp, part-time practice: registered occupational therapist, 6 years experience, sensory integration certification
   Yearly gross salary = $92,000
   c. Part-time camp, part-time practice: certified occupational therapy assistant, 1 year experience
   Yearly gross salary = $46,000
   Total yearly professional salaries = $210,000
   Approximate combined benefit packages × 20% = $42,000
   Total professional employee cost to company = $252,000
   d. Part-time camp, part-time practice: office assistant
   Yearly gross salary = $28,000
   Approximate benefit package × 20% = $5,600
   Total administrative staff cost to company = $33,600

2. MARKETING
   a. Computer-generated flyers hand-distributed by practice professional staff to parents of children already being seen in the practice and to regional center offices. Approximately 200 flyers distributed at a cost of $.02 per flyer = $4.
   Sixty registrations and deposits were received, and a waiting list was quickly generated that exceeded the capacity of the camp. Thus, no further marketing to obtain campers was required.
   b. Personal marketing to local businesses and companies to obtain donated equipment and supplies and tuition scholarships was part of the responsibility of the therapists who were 100% camp time. An end-of-summer "thank you" picnic lunch for donors and full-time campers was donated by a local caterer.

3. OVERHEAD
   a. Utilities: Water and trash pickup were the only requirements and were at an approximate cost of $102.00 for the summer (absorbed into the larger practice bills).
   b. Van rental (1 × each week of camp) = 12 × $25 = $300

4. EQUIPMENT (Capital)
   a. None required

Figure 12-2. Sample cost sheet for a day camp. *(continued)*

5. EQUIPMENT* (Noncapital): Purchased locally, so no shipping charges.

    a. 4 picnic tables with attached benches (ea. $210) = $840

    b. 4 large inflatable wading pools (ea. $42) = $168

    c. 3 kinder chutes (ea. $49.95) = $149.85

    d. 3 soft ring-toss games (ea. $18) = $54

    e. 1 parachute = $215

    f. 15 beach balls (ea. $1.99) = $29.85

    Total cost of equipment if purchased*: $1,456.70

    Items (a), (b), and (e) were donated: –$1,223.00

    Actual cost of equipment to company: $233.70

6. NONEXPENDABLE SUPPLIES* (purchased for full summer)

    a. 1 class-pack scissors—included 36, left- and right-handed (ea. $32) = $32

    b. 1 class-pack paint brushes—100 assorted (ea. $28) = $28

    c. 3 packs printmaking sponges—35 assorted shapes (ea. $15) = $45

    Total cost of nonexpendable supplies for summer*: $105

7. EXPENDABLE SUPPLIES* (figured for one 2-week session × 6 sessions)

    a. 10 1.7-fl oz nontoxic, nonflammable glue sticks × $.99 ea. = $9.90 × 6 sessions = $59.94 Note: bulk of 100 glue sticks at a cost of $.52 ea. offered a savings of $.47 per stick = total cost of $52.00.

    b. 2 class-pack assorted construction paper—500 sheets × $4.72 ea. = $9.44 Bulk savings of approximately $.03 per sheet over smaller package.

    c. Crayola washable paints in nine colors: 1 gallon each × $15.95 gallon = $143.55

    d. 500 paper paint pans = $9

    Total cost of expendable supplies for summer* (six sessions) = $213.99

    Total cost of expendable supplies for summer* (divided by six sessions) = $35.67 approximate supply cost for each session (divided by 10 children per session) = $3.57 approximate supply cost per child.

Considerations for Establishing Fees and Funding Camp Tuitions

If we had generated a complete list of equipment and supplies for this example (as you will for the program you are designing), we would be able to closely figure the cost of the program for each participant. Knowing this exact figure will help us establish tuition costs for each camper in this program and would also help us estimate the costs of adding more sessions or more children per session. For programs such as this, some planners/managers also figure a break-down of salary/equipment/overhead charges per client along with supplies in order to arrive at a per-person cost.

If the campers require extremely close attention for effective intervention and for safety (e.g., children with behavior disorders or other special problems), we might need to hire more staff and perhaps additional time of specialized professional staff. The cost of higher levels of staff expertise and more personal attention are generally figured into the client's costs. We might also consider training volunteers for the program or adding students. Both volunteers and students require professional time for supervision; these costs must be included in the financial mix but are not generally included in the client's costs.

Funding options for a camp such as the one described in this example include the following:

    1. Private pay (may be considered day care for tax purposes)

    2. Regional centers or other avenues of pay already established for the child's therapy

    3. Donated "scholarships" based on financial need

Figure 12-2 (continued). Sample cost sheet for a day camp.

Furnishing Your Program

The term **furnishings** refers to the furniture we will need to provide the program that will help our clients/patients/members meet their objectives and the goal or goals of the program. What will be required to furnish a welcoming environment? Will you require work tables, chairs, lamps, a computer, television, VCR, a DVD player, a radio, a sofa, a bed, and so on? Many of the programs described in this text have operated on little more than this list. Most have required minimal supplies, and a few have required some equipment; however, equipment for therapeutic purposes has seldom been included. From our examples, you might think that community-based programs are always low-budget, "shoestring" ventures that seldom, if ever, require expensive furnishings or equipment. However, keep in mind that the furnishings, equipment, and supplies are dictated by your goal or goals and your objectives and the needs of your target population, not by their placement in the community. While not intended to be therapeutic, a riding garden tiller that would permit several of the community gardeners in our earlier example with physical limitations to be central to the development of new garden space was a fairly high-end expense.

If you are designing a private practice, the way you furnish it will be extremely important to how you market and promote your practice to your selected population. While the primary aim in some of our community examples was a comfortable, inviting, and safe environment, the private practice will certainly provide all of these things and more. A well-appointed reception area and intervention environment, for example, contributes more than comfort to a practice setting; it must appeal to the senses of the consumer, and it enhances the quality of the intervention. Think about what you have learned about the multiple "contexts" that influence outcomes of intervention. Consider, also, how much the environment and furnishings contribute to your acceptance of practicing professionals (such as your doctor, dentist, counselor, or therapist), assuming that the quality of services is equal.

Exercise 12-7

How Will You Furnish Your Program?

1. Consider what furnishings you will require to meet the set objectives and goals of your program. Consider the volume of services and the age and differing abilities of your target population (e.g., will adaptations be required in furnishings?). List here the furnishings you will need along with costs from your selected catalogue and website sources (such as Sears, J.C. Penny, Ikea, or others of your choice):

Furnishings	Source	Anticipated Cost

EQUIPMENT

Equipment is categorized in terms of cost and useful life (the length of time the equipment is expected to be in service, usually 2 years or longer). The designation of equipment varies from one agency or institution to another and may be specified by granting/funding sources. Braveman (2016), in discussions of financial planning and budgeting for clinical departments, defines capital equipment as a single piece of equipment that exceeds a predetermined amount (e.g., $5,000) and a life span of longer than a predetermined period (e.g., 1 year) (p. 278). In general, for community programming, capital equipment includes amounts of $1,000 or above. For our purposes in developing our budgets, we will consider any equipment needed to support the programming at a cost of $1,000 or more to be in the category of **capital equipment**. Equipment may be intended exclusively for therapeutic purposes (such as adaptive playground equipment or work hardening equipment), but our garden tiller is also equipment that would fall into this category even though its intended purpose is not to provide therapy. Standard playground equipment and many kitchen appliances would also be considered as capital equipment (unless the umbrella/partnering agency or funding source places such things in the category of furnishings, which is something you will determine when you actually do your budget). We consider most equipment to be nonexpendable; that is, we will expect to use it many times and for many clients/patients/members. Of course, eventually the equipment will wear out and will need to be repaired and/or replaced, and such replacement costs will be anticipated in our long-range budget planning, as will service contracts for repairs. Any equipment below the cost of $1,000 is considered **noncapital equipment** and is also included in the category of nonexpendable.

Exercise 12-8

Selecting Equipment for Your Program

1. List here all of the equipment you will need for your program (if you will not need equipment, simply indicate "none"):

_____

_____

_____

_____

_____

2. When you have completed your equipment list, refer to the catalogues and/or websites and determine the source and the cost of each piece of desired equipment. Note these items here and place an asterisk beside the equipment that is in excess of $1,000 (capital equipment):

Equipment	Source	Anticipated Cost

3. You can now make two lists of equipment, one for capital equipment and one for noncapital equipment:

Capital Equipment	Noncapital Equipment

In fact, you might not have to purchase all or any of the furnishings or equipment for your program. If the agency is providing a space, it might also provide the loan of furnishings and equipment. In many of our examples, the tables, chairs, computers, and kitchens of the facility/agency were used. However, it is always good to know all of the costs should you wish to recreate the program elsewhere. Some facilities/agencies will also expect that you replace any equipment that is stolen or damaged because of negligence or misuse by you or your clients/members. Although we expect that this would not occur, knowing the cost sometimes helps programmers to be more aware of security and maintenance.

Supplies

Now consider **supplies** needed to support the services provided by your program (such as computer software, arts and crafts, paper, pencils, toys, garden seeds, cooking ingredients, etc.). Consider supplies needed per client/patient/member on a daily/weekly basis. Also consider what supplies are **expendable** (such as masking tape or plant fertilizer, which must be replaced when they are used) or **nonexpendable** (such as scissors, gardening forks, or inflatable wading pools, which can be used several times without replacement). If you have used wading pools in your practice, you know that they are a good example of an item that could be considered either expendable or nonexpendable. They are, in fact, listed as a nonexpendable supply item, but if you purchase the cheap ones, they are extremely vulnerable to rips and punctures and might not last the course of one day. Over the long haul, spending a little more for equipment and nonexpendable supplies is very wise. Again, make your lists from what you want, and decide later where you can cut some corners without jeopardizing your goals and the quality of your program.

Assessments/screening instruments are also generally listed under nonexpendable supplies (except for paper forms, of course). They are included in the combined supplies selected to support your client/patient/member services in the development of the total budget.

Exercise 12-9

Selecting Supplies for Your Program

1. Consider now what nonexpendable supplies you will need to begin your program. To determine the number of items needed, consider the number of clients/patients/members that you will service, the daily or weekly time schedule, and the specific supplies required to provide the program. Consider the following examples:

   a. *Six campers serviced daily = six pairs of right-handed scissors and (to be prepared) three pairs of left-handed scissors*

   b. *Six campers serviced daily = two "quality" inflatable wading pools (three children to each pool with no hard edges to encourage safe movement as well as socialization)*

   c. *12 community gardener/members attending daily = 12 pairs of gardening gloves*

   d. *12 community gardener/members attending daily = four spading forks, four long-handled hoes, and four short-handled hoes*

   Using this formula to help determine quantity, note the nonexpendable supplies you will need for your program and the source, amount, and anticipated cost (remember that if you have sufficient storage, sometimes it is substantially cheaper to order in bulk even though it may be more than you require at the present time). Write your formulas here:

Nonexpendable Supplies	Source	Quantity	Anticipated Cost

2. Decide now what expendable supplies you will need to start your program and to operate it for one cycle of clients/patients/members. Consider the following examples:

   a. Two 4-day weeks = eight 1-hour arts and crafts sessions × six day campers = 12 (1.7 fl oz) nontoxic, nonflammable glue sticks (estimated that gluing would be involved in one-third of the arts and crafts activities, assumed one stick would be used per child per week, and anticipated little waste and better product with the glue stick as opposed to a bottle of less expensive glue.)

   b. The community garden is supplied with expendables in gardening "cycles" to include planting, maintaining, harvesting, and clearing.

   Planting cycle = area of garden × 12 gardeners/members = 72 packets of assorted seeds, 12 spools of row-marking string, 100 row-marker sticks, and five large bags of fertilizer (estimated planting of some individual and some group choices, including annual flowers, herbs, and vegetables for future saleability; assumed that row-marking string and sticks are cheaper in quantity and are easily stored; and assumed that supplies are donated or purchased locally; buying locally whenever possible encourages asset development and capacity building in your community).

   Using the examples as guidelines, note your formula here for determining the expendable supplies that you will need:

   _____

   _____

   _____

   _____

   _____

List here the expendable supplies you will need to provide your program for one cycle:

Expendable Supplies	Source	Quantity	Anticipated Cost

Exercise 12-10

Long-Term Budgeting

Most budgets will be based on 3-month, 6-month, 1-year, and 3-year cycles. This may be referred to as *short-term budgeting* (what you require to operate one cycle of your program) and *long-term budgeting* (what you require for several cycles of your program, usually up to 3 years). Long-term budgeting requires that you make **cost projections**, including a percentage increase for inflation. For our purposes in this chapter, we are only considering the costs associated with furnishings, equipment, and supplies. We will consider other costs in the chapter to follow.

1. Consider the equipment noted in the previous exercise. Will any of it require replacement over the course of a 3-year period? When we figure the final budget later, we will include indirect costs such as the costs of service and maintenance contracts and **overhead** (electricity, telephone, Internet, etc.). For now, however, we are only considering some of our **direct costs**, or those costs for equipment and supplies that will directly support the client/patient/member services. Note here any equipment (capital or noncapital) that you anticipate may need to be replaced during the first 3 years of your program:

Replacement of Capital Equipment   Anticipated Cost (considering inflation)

_____

_____

_____

_____

Replacement of Noncapital Equipment   Anticipated Cost (considering inflation)

_____

_____

_____

_____

For our earlier example, the gardening gloves and the wading pools probably would be the most vulnerable to "short lives." For example, a good pair of gardening gloves with rubber or leather palms would be expected to last the home gardener for perhaps 1 year or more with proper care. Twelve pairs of such gloves would cost about $30 each, or $360 out of a 12-month budget. It is not likely that all of our gardeners/members will wear out gloves equally, so we could cut some corners and spend $7 for a pair of good (but not the best) gloves and anticipate that they would probably last 1 year for some of our less enthusiastic gardeners and 3 or 6 months for others. We could then anticipate glove replacement in increments over 3 months, 6 months, and 1 year. In reality, gloves are items that gardening-supply stores might donate, but we want to know what they cost in the event that we must pay for them.

A durable, inflatable wading pool might last through a summer of 2-week camper rotations or approximately six 8-day cycles (with each of two pools meeting the needs of three children each and with the combined pools sheltering some 288 small bodies over the course of a summer). Although it is possible that these pools will last all summer, it is likely that at least one will require replacement at a cost of around $42 to $45 during the 3-month interval.

---

2. Now consider your nonexpendable supply list. How often will you need to replace these supplies? Make your calculations and note here what nonexpendable supplies you anticipate replacing, how often, and the anticipated (plus inflation) costs:

Nonexpendable Supplies   Replacement Cycle   Anticipated Costs

_____

_____

_____

_____

_____

3. What will be your replacement cycle for expendable supplies? Will you bring in new groups every 2 weeks like our day camp example, or will your cycle be every 1, 3, or 6 months? Will you have new members/patients/clients cycling through your program all the time, or will your expendable supplies be exhausted in cycles like the community garden example?

For the community garden, the most expensive season of the year was the first one—the planting season. Seventy-two packets of seeds cost from $.50 to $2.10 per packet depending on the quantity of seeds per packet (100 to 8000) and how exotic the potential plants were considered to be. The hemp twine for row marking sold for $8.95 per a 200-foot ball, and the wooden markers were $5.00 for 100. The program later received a donation of nonexpendable metal row markers that would have cost $22.95 per 50 if purchased and 10 flats of live seedlings that would have cost approximately $15.00 to $25.00 per flat.

Although starting up the garden each season appeared to be expensive, for most of the year, costs were substantially reduced. Therefore, the budget for the year was heavily influenced by the planting season and was less influenced by the maintenance (fertilizer and mulch) and the harvest and cleanup. The garden was organic, so there were no chemical pesticides to purchase; this also enhanced marketing for produce and floral sales; however, the task of maintenance and removing pests required more attention on a daily basis.

Note here your anticipated expendable supplies and when you will anticipate replacement along with your projections of cost (consider that inflation will also have an impact on the cost of your expendable supplies):

Expendable Supplies	Replacement Cycle	Anticipated Costs

Summary

First, anticipating space needs by matching them closely to program outcomes, goals, and objectives will place the planner in an excellent position to prepare for the necessary negotiation that will take place in the process of locating or sometimes being assigned space for program operations. A detailed analysis of the size and nature of space required for intervention, the plumbing and utilities needed, and considerations for safety and ergonomics place the planner in a good position to review available space with a careful eye toward what negotiations may be made without compromising the goals of the program. Although somewhat different than the space considerations of the planner working in cooperation with an agency/facility, the space needs of those who anticipate initiating a freestanding practice continue to be based on the community and service profiles, the comprehensive assessment of needs, and ongoing reviews of trends that might affect the success of the program.

In preparing to initiate a program, you will need to obtain (and likely purchase) a number of items to facilitate the achievement of objectives and, ultimately, the goals of the program. These items fall under the categories of furnishings, capital and noncapital equipment, and expendable and nonexpendable supplies. Furnishings are those things that we would describe in our households as "furniture," including tables, chairs, sofas, lamps, beds, and dressers. They may be considered part of our indirect services in some cases (such as providing a comfortable reception area) and direct services in others (such as tables and chairs for activities or perhaps a bed for activities of daily living practice). In program design and development, many of these items are intended to add comfort and style to the space where we will carry out our intervention rather than to directly support the intervention itself.

Equipment may be intended for therapeutic purposes such as playground equipment designed specifically to facilitate the sensory-integration aspects of a child's development. On the other hand, it may be used to encourage participation such as the riding tiller or tractor for the community garden. In most settings, equipment is categorized by cost. Although the amount may differ depending on the setting, generally, in our community-based programming, those items over $1,000 are considered to be capital equipment and those under this purchase amount are considered to be noncapital equipment.

Supplies are also categorized, but not usually by cost. They may fall into the category of expendable, or those things that are "used up" by participants in the course of their direct-service program. Items that have a longer life, or are not "used up" in the process of intervention, are termed nonexpendable items. All of these items cost the program money, and they are considered to be a substantial part of the budget process, both short- and long-term. Of course, there are other indirect and direct costs to programming, which are considered in detail in Chapter 13. In this chapter, we have considered all of the costs to operate our program. In the chapter to follow, we will consider how we will pay these costs.

SELECTED COMPANIES THAT PROVIDE EQUIPMENT AND SUPPLIES APPROPRIATE FOR OCCUPATION-CENTERED COMMUNITY PROGRAMMING

- Attainment Company, Inc.
  P.O. Box 930160, Verona, WI 53593-0160, (800) 327-4269
  http://www.attainmentcompany.com/
  *multiple options/supplies for children and adults with special needs
- Best Priced Products, Inc.
  P.O. Box 1174, White Plains, NY 10602, (800) 824-2939
  http://www.bpp2.com/
  *rehabilitation supplies and equipment for adults and children
- Childswork/Childsplay
  P.O. Box 1604, Secaucus, NJ 07096-1604, (800) 962-1141, email: care@GenesisDirect.com
  http://www.childswork.com
  *social and emotional needs of children and adolescents
- Communication Skill Builders
  3830 E. Bellevue, P.O. Box 42050-CS4, Tucson, AZ 85733, (602) 323-7500
  http://www.jacketflap.com/
  *communication supplies for adults and children
- Communication/Therapy Skill Builders (A Division of the Psychological Corporation)
  555 Academic Court, San Antonio, TX 78204-9941, (800) 211-8378
  http://www.skillbuildersonline.com/
  *pediatric and adult assessment and intervention
- Dick Blick Art Materials
  P.O. Box 1267, Galesburg, IL 61402-1267, (800) 828-4548
  http://www.DickBlick.com/
  *arts and crafts supplies for the artist and teacher

- Discount School Supply
  Box 60000, San Francisco, CA 94160-3847, (800) 627-2829
  http://www.DiscountSchoolSupply.com
  *arts and craft supplies, manipulatives, toys, books, language/science; social awareness; active play/dramatic play; furniture for children
- Flaghouse
  601 Flaghouse Drive, Hasbrouck Heights, NJ 07604-3116, (800) 793-7900
  http://www.flaghouse.com/
  *adult and pediatric rehabilitation supplies and equipment; physical education and recreation supplies and equipment (for school, office, institutions, and health care facilities)
- Ikea (United States and Europe)
  Many local stores, and catalogue: http://www.ikea.com/
  *home furnishings
- Imaginart
  307 Arizona Street, Bisbee, AZ 85603, 800-828-1376
  http://www.manta.com/ http://www.amfibi.company/
  *therapy supplies for pediatrics, physical rehabilitation, and mental health
- J.C. Penney (U.S.)
  Local stores and catalogue: http://www.jcpenney.com
  *home furnishings; clothing
- K. Log, Inc.
  P.O. Box 5, Zion, IL 6009-0005, (800) 872-6611
  http://www.K-log.com/
  *furnishings for offices, classrooms, and multipurpose environments
- Lilypons Water Gardens
  6800 Lilypons Road, P.O. Box 10, Buckeystown, MD 21717-0010, (800) 723-7667
  http://www.lilypons.com/
  *supplies, equipment, plants for water gardening, fish, snails, and frogs
- Nasco Arts and Crafts
  Fort Atkinson, WI; Modesto, CA, (800) 558-9595
  http://www.enasco.com/
  *arts and crafts (education and studio quality), educational materials, farm equipment
- North Coast Medical, Inc.
  187 Stauffer Blvd, San Jose, CA 95125-1042, (800) 821-9319
  http://www.ncmedical.com/
  *adult rehabilitation and fitness supplies; hand therapy supplies
- PCI Educational Publishing
  2800 NE Loop 410 Suite 105, San Antonio, TX 78218-1525, (800) 594-4263
  http://www.pcieducation.com/
  *supplies for cognitive and emotional independence
- Sammons Preston Products
  P.O. Box 5071, Bolingbrook, IL 60440-5071, (800) 323-5547
  http://www.allegromedical.com/Sammons_Preston/
  *supplies and equipment for adult rehabilitation
- S & S Worldwide
  P.O. Box 513, Colchester, CT 06415-0517, (800) 243-9232
  http://www.ssww.com
  *arts, crafts, games, and exercise for therapy and rehabilitation

- Sears Home (local stores and catalogue)
  http://www.Sears.com/
  *home furnishings; clothing; small farm and garden equipment
- Sears Home Health Care
  20 Presidential Drive, Roselle, IL 60172, (800) 326-1750 (to request a catalogue)
  *adult rehabilitation equipment
- Shepherd's Garden Seeds
  30 Irene Street, Torrington, CT 06790-6658, (860) 482-3638
  www.shepherdseeds.com/
- Renee's Garden Seeds/California (heirloom seeds)
  http://www.reneesgarden,.com; http://www.amazon.com/patio/
  *garden seeds, ordinary to the exotic; heirloom and gardening supplies
- Smith and Nephew, Inc
  One Quality Drive, P.O. Box 1005, Germantown, WI 53022-8205, (800) 558-8633
  http://www.smith-nephew.com/
  *adult rehabilitation supplies
- Tandy Leather Crafts
  TLC Direct, 1400 Everman Parkway, Fort Worth, TX 76140-5089, (888) 890-1611
  www.tandyleather.com
  *leathercraft kits, Indian Lore; leather hides and tools for the craftsperson and hobbyist
- Wellness Reproductions, Inc.
  23945 Mercantile Road, Suite KM, Beachwood, OH 44122-5924, (800) 669-9208
  http://www.couragetochange.com
  *supplies and resources for mental health facilitators and educators
- Whole Person Associates
  210 W. Michigan, Duluth, MN 55802-1908, (800) 247-6789
  http://www.wholeperson.com
  *stress management, wellness-promotion, and emotional self-care resources

REFERENCES

American Occupational Therapy Association. (2014). *Occupational therapy practice framework: Domain and process* (3rd ed.). Bethesda. MD: American Occupational Therapy Association.

Braveman, B. (2016). Financial planning, management, and budgeting. In B. Braveman (Ed.), *Leading and managing occupational therapy services* (2nd ed., pp. 277- 296). Philadelphia, PA: F. A. Davis.

Fenton, S., & Gagnon, P. (2003) Work activities. In E. Crepeau, E. Cohn, & B. Schell (Eds.), *Willard and Spackman's occupational therapy* (pp. 342- 346). Philadelphia, PA: Lippincott, Williams and Wilkins.

Neville-Jan, A., Fazio, L.S., Kennedy, B., & Snyder., C. (1997). Elementary to middle school transition: Using multi-cultural play activities to develop life skills. In D. Parham & L. S. Fazio (Eds.), *Play in occupational therapy for children* (pp. 144-157). St. Louis, MO: Mosby-Yearbook.

Renda, M., Shamberg, S., & Young, D. (2015). Complex environmental modifications. *American Journal of Occupational Therapy, 69*(Suppl 3), 1-7.

Ryan, J. D., Ray, R., & Hiduke, G. (1999). *Small business: An entrepreneur's plan* (5th ed.). Fort Worth, TX: Dryden Press.

13

Costs of Programming and Projected Funding Needs

Fazio, L. S. *Developing Occupation-Centered Programs With the Community, Third Edition* (pp 213-226).
© 2017 Taylor & Francis Group.

KEY TERMS

1. Budget
2. Budget line/budget narrative/budget justification
3. Budget itemization
4. Revenues
5. For profit/not-for-profit or nonprofit
6. Fee for service
7. Strategic Plan
8. Indirect costs/overhead
9. Direct costs
10. In-kind
11. Insurance
12. Malpractice/professional liability
13. Benefits
14. Hiring/retention
15. Outsourcing

There are two critical dimensions to the community programming proposal. While they are no more or less important than other aspects of the proposal, when it comes to anticipating long-term success of the program, carefully determining the cost and evaluating the effectiveness of the program make the difference in its staying power and funding. Frequently, the programmer least favors developing these two areas, but they also are the areas that separate the daydreamer from the true proactive planner.

If we could maintain our excitement and momentum through the processes of budgeting, evaluation, and planning, we would find evidence of many more successful, long-running, sustainable programs. Sadly, many programming efforts are like sparklers on the 4th of July; on July 5, they have disappeared into the landfill. The idea that will last, on the other hand, is supported by sound money management and the careful evaluation of outcomes. How do we deal with our budgetary concerns? What will this program cost, and how will it be funded? What does it mean to manage the finances of a program?

Braveman (2016) discusses financial planning, management, and budgeting for occupational therapy managers and reminds us that planning and managing a budget requires high-level skills that include a working knowledge of health care systems at all levels, multiple payment and reimbursement structures, human resources systems and costs, equipment and materials purchasing and management, and facilities management and improvement systems (p. 279). Braveman (2016) also discussed the important role of strategic planning alongside financial planning and management (pp. 279-280). Although different in some respects, all of these functions and tasks are also the responsibility of the community programming planner and manager. Smith (1996) has outlined the key categories that an occupational therapy financial manager must be alert to in light of the external environment within which health care organizations function. Her discussions describe the multiple levels of financial accounting and management known to most occupational therapy managers. Focusing largely on service billing, her categories include such tasks as establishing prices and pricing policies and the negotiation of reimbursement contracts with third-party payers and individual payers (pp. 63-100). Although Smith's information may be more suited to what we might describe as a clinic- or hospital-based, treatment-focused practice, her words also ring true for many freestanding practices. Jabri (2003) discusses financial planning and management with an eye for service quality. Focusing on strategic planning to establish a sound financial plan; she alerts the reader to the power of effectively managing a budget in order to manage the service quality of a department or one's business (2003, p. 147). Braveman (2016) and Smith (1996) share with Jabri (2003) considerations of certain aspects of cost accounting, such as strategic planning and monitoring productivity and efficiency as critical to all programming whether as treatment-based interventions, wellness promoting, or prevention. These considerations apply, whether the administrative structure is a for-profit private practice or a not-for-profit program operated under the umbrella of another agency or agencies.

Liebler and McConnell (2012), Jabri (2003), Thomas (1996), and Logigian (1994) discuss cost management as well as the additional roles of the financial manager. *Accountability* is the key word in financial management, whether in health care or the business sector. In terms of accountability in occupation-centered, community-based programs, the linkages between occupation, quality improvement, and program evaluation must be supported and encouraged alongside the present-day concerns for efficiency and cost-effectiveness. We cannot afford to let the current payment systems restrict our creativity, diminish our goals, or compromise our ethics.

COSTS, BUDGETS, AND ANTICIPATED RESOURCES

Figuring costs, budgeting, and anticipating resources can be a challenge. Some program planners prefer to set lofty goals, plan big, and be prepared to scale back; other planners like to start small and expand their thinking later. Starting with a "big" plan is a way of encouraging excitement and creativity; in many ways, it widens the scope of opportunity. However, the big plan is seldom obtainable in the early efforts. As long as the planner is prepared for this and is willing to grow in increments (postponing the larger version for somewhere later on in the three-year time line), planning can progress smoothly. Thus, good management ensures the reality, and for both the conservative and the aggressive approach, a long-range plan is critical. In the process of developing our profiles of the community and identifying assets, stakeholders and potential community partnerships, we acquired information that greatly influences our financial planning. Whether a community has existing resources available and/or potential resources that can be further developed via asset and capacity building, financial planning is critical and consideration of several potential funding streams is necessary.

Budgeting is both a planning and controlling tool. As a plan, the budget is a specific statement of the anticipated results, such as expected revenue to be earned and probable expenses to be incurred in an operation for a future defined period. A budget is a statement of what the organization intends to accomplish, not merely a forecast or a guess (Hiduke & Ryan, 2014; Liebler & McConnell, 2012).

Regardless of the nature of the program and the planned intervention, all programs have expenses that must be funded. In previous chapters, you began the process of outlining your programming costs to include furnishings, supplies, equipment, space, and personnel. These items begin to form lines in your budget. In its simplest form, a **budget** is a fiscal plan for a program that includes an itemized list of anticipated income (revenues) and expenses. Karsh and Fox (2014) caution us that for a grant funding proposal, the budget must reflect as closely as possible the activities and staffing described in the narrative. In other words, the budget must be closely tied to goals, objectives, and programming, and it must be specific and accurate. They go on to define a **budget line** as an item (line) in a budget (e.g., one occupational therapist at a specified salary, or supplies and equipment) (see Figure 13-1 for an example of budget lines).

Line Item	Cost
Staffing	
Occupational Therapist (full-time at $74,000 per year)	$74,000

Line Item	Cost
Operational Expenses	
Postage	$2,700

Figure 13-1. Examples of line-item budgeting.

For most funding applications, a **budget narrative** and **budget justification** is required (Karsh & Fox, 2014; Kiritz & Floersch, 2015). A budget narrative is a verbal description of each line item in the budget, describing how the amount was calculated and how the item relates to the program (justification). For example, in the preceding line item of occupational therapist (full time at $74,000 per year), our narrative justification might be as follows: *A full-time occupational therapist is required to conduct programming and supervise the occupational therapy student program; salary is comparable to what occupational therapists with pediatric and supervisory experience make in this geographical region.* Although the formats may differ, all funding organizations expect to see clearly how the budget costs relate to the activities to be provided. **Budget itemization** also refers to an item-by-item format in the form of a worksheet that may be used by some organizations to provide the planner with guidance about categories of budgeting and expectations such as projected costs for program implementation/personnel. There are numerous resources available to help the planner in preparing budgets for grant applications that are also suitable when you are proposing a program to members of your community, potential partners, or others. The Centers for Disease Control offer direction through their Budget Preparation Guidelines, Procurement and Grants Office (www.cdc.gov/grants/index.html). The Robert Wood Johnson Foundation offers Site Budget Preparation Guidelines to planners and applicants (www.rwjf.org), and the Kellogg Foundation has many helpful resources offered to the program planner to include budget preparation guidelines (https://www.wkkf.org). Additional helpful resources in preparing budgets for granting agencies include the Budget Builder instructions provided by the Fiscal Management Associates (Fiscal Strength for Nonprofits) (fmaonline.net); and sample budget itemization worksheets are offered by the Community Development Block Grant Program (portal.hud.gov). If you anticipate applying for funding to a specific foundation, you will want to use formatting and terms that they recommend. As you are beginning to identify potential grant funders in the following chapter, be sure to look at the recommendations for budget preparations required for their applications.

For our initial learning experience, we will approach the budget process by first drafting a list of all of our anticipated expenses and then making a projection of our needed income from these expenditures. This needed income may come from a number of sources, including **revenues** generated by payment for services, revenues from program-generated products or services, or what we will describe as *general funding* (comprehensive funds for programming from an agency or foundation). For those who are anticipating initiating a for-profit private practice, this list of costs first becomes part of your startup worksheet and then your business plan (Hiduke & Ryan, 2014; Tyson & Schell, 2011).

Before we begin to draft such a cost sheet in the initiation of our budget, however, there are some additional categories of expense that we have not yet considered, including overhead, insurance, and benefits for employees. Whether you are responsible for these expenses will depend on what kind of program you are planning. In all of the areas of financial management, our level of responsibilities and specific tasks will fall along a continuum depending on the nature of the program. There are obviously fewer fiscal (money-related) management responsibilities for the planner/manager who works under the umbrella of another agency or organization than there would be for the planner who is establishing a business/private practice or his or her own nonprofit. Of course, someone must assume the responsibilities—and perhaps liabilities—of financial management, but in many cases, it will be someone other than you. Whether you are responsible or not, it is important that you thoroughly understand the process so that you can anticipate what will be required to ensure the financial success of the program.

THE NATURE OF YOUR PROGRAM

Occupation-centered practitioners may offer their services under many different administrative structures. It is important to distinguish between the kinds of practices we are describing as independent and private versus those that are established under the administrative umbrella of another agency or partners with another organization. If you are an employee, then the contents of this chapter are generally the concern of your employer (the agency/facility). Of course, you would be expected to maintain a budget for your program and generally provide administrative services, but it is not likely that you would be responsible for funding the collective costs of your program—although you might be expected to seek and write grants to obtain supportive funding.

Although it does not have to be, a private practice is usually **for profit;** in other words, it expects to have money left over after expenses are paid. The purpose of a for-profit company is to generate profits for the owners and perhaps shareholders. Revenue for a for-profit business is typically generated through the sale of products or services. In for-profit businesses, profits are usually distributed to the owners or shareholders in the form of dividends (Consumer Dummies, 2015; Entrepreneur Media, 2015; Hiduke & Ryan, 2014; Tyson & Schell, 2011). In many ways, these practices are much different from those that are **not-for-profit** or **nonprofit.** The purpose of a nonprofit (used interchangeably in the literature with not-for-profit) is typically charitable, religious, or educational. A nonprofit is owned by the public. A board of directors directs and operates the nonprofit but does not own it. Sources of revenue are also different. A nonprofit business may choose to sell products or services, but it is also allowed to solicit donations and gifts and apply for grants from private foundations and the government (Hummel, 1996; Pakroo, 2015; Walsh, 2015). Nonprofit businesses can make a profit, meaning that they can accumulate earnings in excess of their expenses. However, these profits are returned to the nonprofit organization, not distributed as dividends. The excess funds can be used to purchase equipment and supplies, train staff, or increase salaries and benefits; or they can be retained for future charitable use (Scott, 2013). Although both kinds of programs may charge their patients/clients fees, the intent to make a profit over expenses or not to is the difference. Whether a program is for profit or not for profit does not necessarily affect the salaries of employees. In fact, salaries may be higher in nonprofit programs than those in for-profit programs, and benefits may be better. Many of the programs described in this text, for example, are partnered with nonprofit organizations and do not charge a **fee for service** (i.e., the clients/members are not charged for the therapist's services). In fact, many of these programs are supported through grant funding and indirectly through student tuition for service learning or fieldwork. In these ways, a preceptor can be paid, any needed equipment and supplies can be purchased, and overhead is paid. In some cases, some revenue is generated (e.g., through the sale of garden produce or handmade craft products); however, these monies are funneled back into the operation of the program. Sometimes, these programs require a trial period of several months (or maybe longer) in order for the program staff and participants to establish a firm rapport with the community and to evaluate the effectiveness of the program. A small startup grant or gift may be appropriate during this "pilot" period of becoming established; however, more funds would likely be available if applied for after the program has been evaluated for effectiveness. Even though a program is not for profit, it is important to remember that no program is "free." Someone pays, but how much and in what way can be very convoluted.

Scott (2013) speaks to the importance of designing a sustainable funding plan for the nonprofit. She cautions the planner not to put all of his or her eggs in one basket when it comes to raising money. Funding plans should incorporate many different strategies, reaching out to different constituents in different ways and at different times of the year. First and foremost is "visibility in the community, and credibility through alliances" (Scott, 2015, pp. 159-160). We started this process the day we first began to talk about programming and as we identified our population, stakeholders, and our partners.

Even before looking closely at funding, Pakroo (2015) stresses the importance of a strong **strategic plan.** The strategic plan is a working document that will chart your nonprofit's course through the coming years (Pakroo, 2015, pp. 37-48). This plan (equally important to for-profit planning) identifies your goals for generally 1 to 5 years and outlines how you will achieve them. Drafting a plan transforms abstract ideas into specific "to do" items (Scott, 2013). Of course, in our proposal development, we have been doing this from the beginning. Through detailed profiles, literature review, goal setting, and attention to impact, we have developed a well-grounded plan that can easily be expanded into the future.

If you are a student just beginning to learn about programming and funding, it is important to remember that everything is accounted for in your program cost sheet and budget, from the needs of your employees to each piece of paper and pencil that you may use to provide your program. Whether you have assured funding before you begin, perhaps from your collaborators/agencies/ partners or you intend to seek it as part of the planning process, nothing will happen unless you know exactly how much money will be required. It may be helpful to review Figure 12-2 in Chapter 12 for a sample cost sheet developed for a variation of our earlier day camp example.

INDIRECT COSTS, OVERHEAD, DIRECT COSTS, AND IN-KIND

Identifying the various categories of costs is important for planning and for grant applications. **Indirect costs** (often called **overhead**) refer to cost items such as utilities (electric, gas, water, telephone, and Internet access), lease/rent payments, maintenance costs, and sometimes insurance premiums that collectively support your program. If you are starting a private practice, overhead has to be carefully accounted for and usually begins immediately when you obtain space. When you apply for grant funding to support a not-for-profit or a pilot program, overhead costs generally are grouped and included as a percentage of costs in the amount prescribed by the particular granting agency. You would be able to obtain this information from the granting agency and the prospectus for the specific grant. This will be discussed further in the following chapter. There may be other expenses to consider associated with licensing, certification, or accreditation, depending on the nature of your services.

Direct costs are those expenses for services and products that you need for the program and are not otherwise available at your facility/organization. You may or may not see this term in funding application packages (also true for the term *indirect costs*). The **in-kind** budget line is a term associated with grant funding applications and is where you list any financial contributions that your partnering agency/organization will make available to the grant-funded program. In-kind support or contributions may include such things as staff time, space and utilities, and possibly volunteer hours. You would, then, not include these items in your funding request.

REDUCING RISKS: INSURANCE

For occupation-centered community-based programs, at least three kinds of **insurance** must be considered. The private-practice planner generally will be responsible for all of these. The first is the insurance for your practice or company. Insurance, which is always about managing risk, can protect your practice from loss due to fire, public liability, and crime, among other things. In considering insurance for your company, you must first decide on the type of insurance you will need, then you must decide on the amount of coverage. As a general rule, do not risk more than you can afford to lose. You should also talk to several insurance agents who are accustomed to offering policies to similar practices.

The second type of insurance is **malpractice** or **professional liability** insurance. Malpractice insurance covers against claims from clients/patients who suffer damages as a result of services you or your employees perform. You may wish to offer employees this insurance coverage as part of their employee **benefit** package, although many companies require that employees provide their own malpractice insurance. Students are already familiar with malpractice or professional liability insurance since they all receive this coverage when they enter their occupational therapy clinical program. Some people mistakenly believe that malpractice insurance is only appropriate when you are "learning" to be a practitioner and that when you actually become a practitioner, you no longer require it. However, the reality is that in today's litigious climate, the more you know, the more you acquire responsibilities—and the more malpractice coverage you require!

The third category of insurance is also the responsibility of the private practitioners or those who will be responsible for employees. There are three categories of insurances that help employees manage risk and therefore help employers maintain their businesses. Providing health insurance for yourself and your employees may seem to be a big expense when you are establishing your business plan, but consider how much work might be lost if you do not provide it. You can always offer a better insurance package than your employees could find on their own. In order to keep their employees healthy and to help them balance life at home with life at work, many small businesses offer incentives such as limited child care, exercise programs, and weight management/substance abuse programs. Occupation-centered practitioners who own businesses should be the first ones to consider these prevention and wellness benefits for their employees.

You will also want to include disability insurance, life insurance, and worker's compensation insurance. If you are the owner of the business, disability insurance is critical, and you may also wish to offer it to employees. Ryan, Ray, and Hiduke (1999) suggest that disability for a business owner is a much greater risk than death. While life insurance may not offer a direct advantage to the owner of a practice, it is a service to the employee and the employee's family, and it is generally not as costly as the other insurances. Worker's compensation protects employees if they are injured while on the job. As mentioned previously, occupational therapy practitioners must be aware of ergonomics and should ensure that the workplace does not provide risks to the safety and well-being of employees.

THE POTENTIAL COSTS OF EMPLOYEES

There are several questions that come to mind when we hire employees to assist with our program. In Chapter 11, we discussed the various roles of the professional and nonprofessional staff you might wish to hire to support the services of your program. We also discussed how to develop a job description and an advertisement to initiate the employee search. This was the easy part. The **hiring** and **retention** of employees make up a large part of your anticipated labor and budget. We have already discussed the insurances and other benefits you may wish to provide, but there are additional considerations that will affect your finances if you decide to become the owner of a practice.

First, you must decide when you will hire your employees. Will you hire them before your first client or concurrently? If they are hired concurrently with the arrival of clients, how will the preparation and final planning be accomplished? Will you do it? Perhaps you can hire some temporary or part-time employees. In this case, you are able to delay paying benefits during the preparation phase. Although the percentages vary, many employers provide certain benefits only to employees who work more than 80 percent of a full-time work schedule. However, consider that you might require a high level of professional experience and expertise to assist with the final preparations, perhaps expertise that you do not have. In this case, you will want to offer all of the potential options you can to attract the person you need. If you are starting a for-profit practice, you may wish to offer this first employee stock options or profit sharing as an incentive to help with the final preparations. Hiring and then keeping (retaining) good employees is the key to any successful practice. All of these questions must be considered before you prepare to hire. In addition, you must budget the cost of placing employment advertisements and any costs that may be incurred for recruitment. Not only is this true in the beginning, but it must be anticipated as the program begins to grow. Of course, salary must be considered, as well as employment taxes (social security, unemployment, and Medicare) and additional benefits such as retirement, vacation, sick leave, and family leave.

The best way to determine professional salaries is to talk to other managers in your area to obtain a range for the kinds of services you wish to provide. This is another reason to network and to belong to your professional organizations. The professional organizations may also be able to provide you with salary ranges but will not likely be as current as your colleagues. For other staff, you can find salary comparison data on the Internet at http://recruitmentextra.com/salarysurveys.html and at www.wageweb.com. When you have decided exactly what kind of employees you want and when you wish to hire them, it is time to place the advertisement and to begin the screening and interview process.

SCREENING OF POTENTIAL EMPLOYEES, INTERVIEWS, AND HIRING: MAINTAINING COMPLIANCE

As with many of the planning tasks we have discussed, this is yet another area where you may have differing levels of responsibility depending on whether you are starting your own practice/program or whether you are only assisting the company you work for in the employee hiring process. Screening may include a number of measures to verify that your potential employee has provided you with truthful information. A careful review of the resume initiates the process, which is followed by contacting references and verifying state and national certifications and licenses. The next steps can include pre-employment medical examinations, finger printing, and drug screenings. One or more in-person interviews are employed and, in addition to standard interview questions, role-playing of intervention scenarios particular to your program might be appropriate. In some cases, you may wish to conduct your interview online.

If hiring is your responsibility, you should review legal and illegal pre-employment inquiries before you schedule an interview. You can obtain these from http://www.nolo.com. Also, contact the civil rights office for your state and your state's department of industrial relations for guidelines they may provide. Refer to the list at the close of this chapter for other sources that may be helpful.

When you have completed the interview process and are prepared to make an offer, you should check to see that your new employee can legally work in the United States and have that person complete an Employment and Eligibility Verification Form (I-9); you must also be familiar with the requirements for complying with the Americans with Disabilities Act (ADA). As an occupational therapy practitioner, you should be familiar with the *ADA Title I: Employment provision* and may, in fact, have encountered it in the workplace. As an employer, your responsibilities are even greater. Refer to the ADA and also to Regulations to Implement the Equal Employment Provisions of the Americans with Disabilities Act. Since the 9-11 incident threatening national security, and the resulting *Homeland Security Act*, foreign-trained therapists are more stringently monitored.

Contact the National Board for Certification in Occupational Therapy website for updates if considering the services of a foreign-trained therapist. Organizations and managers must continue to be alert to changes in the practice environment. Some of these to follow closely are the continuing implementation and emerging implications of the Health Insurance Portability and Accountability Act; continuing developments concerning electronic health record initiatives; and some of the emerging implications of the Patient Protection and Affordable Care Act of 2010/2013 (Liebler & McConnell, 2012).

As the owner of a practice, you also must be compliant with all labor laws and all tax laws with regard to employees. It is recommended that you become familiar with the U.S. Department of Labor Statutes, the Fair Labor Standards Act, the Immigration and Nationality Act, the Occupational Safety and Health Act, and the Employee Retirement Income Security Act. (See the references at the close of this chapter for more information.)

If you find it necessary to dismiss an employee, it may be equally problematic. Consider the above resources should firing become necessary, and spell out all procedures on the first day of hire in an employee handbook or manual.

Employee Records

If you are the owner or soon-to-be owner of a practice, you must maintain records for all employees. These include all of the basic information (such as name, address, social security number, and so on) as well as the original application and the results of any prehire inquiries. As the employee continues with your company, you add performance reviews, continuing education, and notations of any disciplinary action. Your state fair employment office can provide you with additional information for what must be maintained in an employee's file and for how long. Human resource files are considered legal documents and may be requested in any malpractice suit or other legal action, so it is best to be proactive by being sure that they are complete. For nonprofits' employee files, the inclusion of updated resumes will make the process of grant application and reporting more efficient.

Summing Up Costs

Now that we have considered expenses related to employees, we have covered the standard cost items. As you think of other items that are indirectly or directly related to client/patient services, remember to consider all associated costs. For instance, perhaps you anticipate the need to lease a van for transportation. Remember that if you transport clients/patients, you will need additional insurance coverage and an appropriate driver's license. An occasional trip might be accommodated less expensively by hiring outside vans or buses (i.e., **outsourcing** transportation).

Once you have listed your startup costs and the costs for one cycle of your program, you can project these for extended periods of time. These extensions of time from 1 year up to 3 or 5 years will include areas where you wish to grow (such as more or different staff, perhaps more space, or additional equipment).

The next chapter is intended to provide you with some direction for how your services might be paid for or how to seek funding. It is not intended to provide you with specific directions for who and how to bill for services or exact resources where you might find loans for a private practice or a grant to initiate a program, but enough information is provided to guide you to the specific information and resources that you will need to make these decisions. If you are a student, you will have (or have had) coursework complementary to this text. This coursework will guide you in the specifics of such traditional management responsibilities as determining costs for services, anticipating and projecting revenue, developing an actual bill, and determining how to interface your interventions with appropriate payment services.

Exercise 13-1

What Kind of Program Do You Plan to Have?

1. Discuss with your classmates, colleagues, or partners whether your program will be free-standing or under the management umbrella of another agency or organization. Is your program intended to be for profit, not-for-profit, or a service-learning component of an academic program or community agency? Is that agency a nonprofit?

   To help you define your responsibilities, you must decide if you will be the planner and manager of a program as an employee of an agency or institution or if you will be owner and manager. Maybe you see your role differently—as a consultant or something else.

   Note here what kind of program you have and why you believe this to be the case:

   _____

   _____

   _____

   _____

   _____

2. With regard to the characteristics of your program, write here what your responsibilities will likely be with regard to selection, hiring, and retention of employees; purchase and maintenance of furnishings, equipment, and supplies; the marketing of the program; and management of the budget.

   Selection, hiring, and retention of employees:

   _____

   _____

   _____

   _____

   Purchase and maintenance of furnishings, equipment, and supplies:

   _____

   _____

   _____

   _____

   Marketing of the program (to the community and potential consumers):

   _____

   _____

   _____

   _____

   Managing the budget for the program:

   _____

   _____

   _____

   _____

Exercise 13-2

Developing a Cost Sheet for Startup, One Year, and Three Years of the Program

You have already accomplished a large part of the task of developing a cost sheet in the exercises you completed for Chapters 11 and 12. When you have completed this chapter, you will have all of the projected costs for the program and the structure of a budget.

Return to your lists of furnishings, equipment, and supplies and your staffing requirements. Using the structure provided by the example, define your costs in the following exercises.

Startup, One-Month, and Yearly Costs

Our first consideration will be the professional and nonprofessional staff that we will require to run the day-to-day programming. Revisit the discussion in Chapter 11. To first determine your staffing needs, you must consider the needs and availability of the service population, the physical space where the program will be offered, the nature of the services you expect to provide, and the configuration of service delivery. Because professional staff can be expensive, you should also begin to give some attention to your anticipated budget and your potential funding, although you must first consider your program goal and the needs of your target population. Although you must be able to justify your costs, it is always important that you do not jeopardize the quality of your program by seeking to reduce costs too soon.

1. Consider your costs for staffing (including the cost of advertising, salary, and benefits for full-time employees). For company-paid benefits, you can estimate approximately 20% of the salary figure, but realize that this can vary substantially):

Staff Position	Percent of Time	Monthly/Yearly Gross Salary	Benefits

Total cost of staff salaries and benefits:

For 1 month: _____   For 1 year: _____

Total costs of startup hiring: _____

Total staff associated costs (advertising positions, salaries, and estimated benefits): _____

2. Return to the exercises in Chapter 12 for your estimated cost lists for furnishings, equipment, and supplies. Finalize all estimated costs (including shipping) for startup and for one cycle of your program (e.g., 1 month, 3 months, etc.). Note below your total costs for each of these categories:

Total cost of capital equipment for startup: _____

Total cost of noncapital equipment for startup: _____

Note any replacement of equipment that may be required over a 3-year period and anticipated cost:

_____

_____

_____

_____

Total cost of furnishings for startup: _____

Note any replacement of furnishings that may be required over a 3-year period and antici-pated cost:

_____

_____

_____

_____

Total cost of nonexpendable supplies for startup: _____
(Remember to include any assessment materials here or in the question that follows.)
Note any replacement of nonexpendable supplies and the estimated cost (what are the anticipated cycles for replacement—6 months? 1 year? more?):

_____

_____

_____

_____

Total cost of expendable supplies for one programming cycle: _____
What is the anticipated cycle for replacement of supplies? _____
What are the resulting 3-month, 6-month, and/or yearly total costs of supplies? _____

3. Note here your estimated overhead for 1 month and for 1 year (carefully consider how you will operate your program, seasonal changes, anticipated fluctuations in service volume, and how this may affect overhead):
Utilities (gas, electric, water, trash disposal, other)

Monthly Estimate   Yearly Estimate

_____

_____

_____

_____

Other overhead costs you may anticipate (such as equipment maintenance contracts, secu-rity, transportation, and so on):

_____

_____

_____

_____

Total estimates of overhead for: 1 month: _____   1 year: _____

4. A detailed marketing plan will be developed in Chapter 15, and you will wish to return to this exercise to record specific costs. For now, provide a rough estimate of what you may wish to spend for such things as brochures, business cards, a website, a website designer, etc. See Pakroo (2015) for online resources and practical assistance with marketing and media. You can finalize the costs later. Record your estimates here:

Marketing Methods   Cost for Startup   Yearly Cost

_____

_____

_____

_____

5. Carefully review your developing program proposal for any anticipated costs that you may have forgotten to include. If you find additional costs, record them in the appropriate categories.

6. Add all of the above totals to determine an estimated figure of operating costs for your program for 1 year and for 3 years.

Total operating costs for 1 year: _____

Total operating costs for 3 years (remember that this figure will reflect inflation and will not necessarily include all of the categories in your startup and 1-year costs): _____

These exercises will help you with all of the cost questions that you will need to answer in order to operate your program and likely to meet any application requirements of a granting organization. It is better to have a very comprehensive financial plan from which you can then select the budgetary information required by grant applications. Granting organizations most often want a summary.

SUMMARY

The strength of your program evaluation plan and the accuracy of your cost sheet are critical to the funding success of your program. Through this process of planning program evaluation and anticipating costs and, later, funding, you must maintain the importance of occupation and the more qualitative aspects of meaning in your program design and plan. In the potentially restrictive environments of todays' health care, it is important to not lose sight of the goal and purpose of your program.

This chapter has proposed numerous resources for you to explore as you develop your budget and your financial plan. You have completed a brief review of your plan, and you have decided exactly what you hope to accomplish and how you aim to do it. Your careful analysis of what will be needed to operate your program in previous chapter exercises has now resulted in the combined estimated costs of your program. In the chapter to follow, you will choose the direction in which you hope to go and identify your proposed funding sources.

REFERENCES

Braveman, B. (2016). Financial planning, management, and budgeting. In B. Braveman (Ed.), *Leading and managing occupational therapy services* (2nd ed., pp. 277-296). Philadelphia, PA: F. A. Davis.

Consumer Dummies. (2015). *Starting a business all-in-one for dummies.* Hoboken, NJ: John Wiley and Sons.

Entrepreneur Media. (2015). *Start your own business* (6th ed.). Irvine, CA: Entrepreneur Press.

Hiduke, G., & Ryan, J. (2014). *Small business: An entrepreneur's business plan* (9th ed.). Boston, MA: Cengage Learning.

Hummel, J. (1996). *Starting and running a nonprofit organization* (2nd ed.). Minneapolis, MI: Center for Nonprofit Management, Graduate School of Business, University of St. Thomas, University of Minnesota Press.

Jabri, J. (2003). Financial planning and management. In G. McCormack, E. Jaffe, & M. Goodman-Lavey (Eds.), *The occupational therapy manager* (pp. 147-176). Bethesda, MD: American Occupational Therapy Association.

Karsh, E., & Fox, A. (2014). *The only grant-writing book you'll ever need.* New York, NY: Perseus, Basic Books.

Kiritz, N., & Floersch, B. (2015). *Grantsmanship: Program planning and proposal writing.* Los Angeles, CA: The Grantsmanship Center.

Liebler, J., & McConnell, C. (2012). *Management principles for health professionals.* Sudbury, MA: Jones and Bartlett.

Logigian, M. (1994). Cost management. In K. Jacobs & M. Logigian (Eds.), *Functions of a manager in occupational therapy* (pp. 99-121). Thorofare, NJ: SLACK Incorporated.

Pakroo, P. (2015). *Starting and building a nonprofit: A practical guide* (6th ed.). Berkeley, CA: Nolo Press.

Ryan, J. D., Ray, R., & Hiduke, G. (1999). *Small business: An entrepreneur's plan.* Philadelphia, PA: Dryden Press.

Scott, L. (2013). *From passion to execution: How to start and grow an effective nonprofit organization.* Boston, MA: Cengage Learning.

Smith, N. (1996). Financial management. In M. Johnson (Ed.), *The occupational therapy manager* (pp. 63-100). Bethesda, MD: American Occupational Therapy Association.

Thomas, V. (1996). Evolving healthcare systems: Payment for occupational therapy services. In M. Johnson (Ed.), *The occupational therapy manager* (pp. 577-602). Bethesda, MD: American Occupational Therapy Association.

Tyson, E., & Schell, J. (2011). *Small business for dummies*. Hoboken, NJ: John Wiley and Sons.

Walsh, L. (2015). *How to start a nonprofit*. Middletown, DE: Made in the USA Press.

Internet Sources

American Occupational Therapy Association: http://www. AOTA.org

Center for Disease Control (CDC). Budget Preparation Guidelines, Procurement and Grants Office: www.cdc.gov/grants/index.html

Community Development Block Grant Program: portal.hud.gov

Department of Labor: www.dol.gov

Equal Employment Opportunity Commission (EEOC) (202-663-4900): www.eeoc.gov/smallbus.html

Fiscal Management Associates: fmaonline.net

General Business Salary Comparisons:

   Recruitment Extra!: http://recruitmentextra.com/salarysurveys.html

   Wage Web: www.wageweb.com

HIPPA: www.elastica.net/compliance

Immigration and Naturalization Service: www.ins.usdoj.gov/employer/index.html

Internal Revenue Service (IRS): www.irs.gov

Kellogg Foundation: https://www.wkkf.org

Legal and Illegal Pre-Employment Inquiries: http://www.nolo.com

National Association of Women Business Owners (NAWBO): www.nfwbo.org

National Board for Certification of Occupational Therapy (NBCOT): http://www.nbcot.org

Occupational Safety and Health Administration (OSHA): www.osha.gov

Patient Protection and Affordable Care Act: smallbusiness.house.gov/uploadedfiles/affordable_care_act

Robert Wood Johnson Foundation: www.rwjf.org

U.S. Department of Justice, Americans with Disabilities (800-514-0301; 202-514-0301): www.usdoj.gov/crt/ada

14

Funding Your Program

LEARNING OBJECTIVES

1. To investigate the multiple ways to fund sustainable community practices
2. To explore the nature of one's practice in relation to funding sources
3. To learn the vocabulary of "funding"
4. To understand the process of grant preparation and application
5. To distinguish the structure and function of the various funding agencies

KEY TERMS

1. Public and private funding
2. Private payer/pay out of pocket
3. Gift tuitions/matched funding
4. Collection agency
5. Cash flow
6. Sliding scale
7. Fundraising
8. Proposals
9. Grants
10. 501(c)(3)/determination letter
11. Pilot program
12. Regional association of grant makers (RAG)/requests for proposals (RFPs), applications (RFAs), statement of qualifications (RFSQ), information (RFIs)
13. Foundations
14. Letter of inquiry/letter of intent (LOI)
15. Cover letter/abstract/executive summary
16. Capital
17. Business plan

Fazio, L. S. *Developing Occupation-Centered Programs
With the Community, Third Edition* (pp 227-243).
© 2017 Taylor & Francis Group.

What Kinds of Funding Are Appropriate for Community-Based Programs and What Kinds of Funding Are Appropriate for "My" Program?

In order to answer this question, you must first consider who you are as a service entity and just what it is that you want to do. This was where we started the program development process. What is the impact you want to make? What is the outcome(s) you wish to achieve? Working backwards from impact and outcome, what is the problem that you (and/or your organization) want to solve, what do you need to do to solve it, and what will it cost? Cost may be one of the last things considered, but in this chapter, it is the motivator. Answers to these questions and others as you develop your ideas and your proposal will help you determine what kind of funding you will need to operate your program and what preparation you will need to make to find and obtain that funding.

As noted in the previous chapter and depending on the services you wish to provide, you may rely on private and public insurers for individual clients and patients. You may also look toward federal legislation for persons with disabilities, both adults and children. Occupational therapy practitioners must remain abreast of past and current legislation that will benefit their particular clients. There is federal funding for programs that are designed to help disabled persons successfully integrate into the community through education, vocational training, social skills, medical services, and independent living skills. Reed (1992; reprinted in Merryman & Van Slyke, 2014) provides a classic historical account of federal legislation beginning with World War I and encourages all practitioners to be alert to legislation (past, present, and future) that will benefit his or her clients, saying "this is one of the reasons we track trends, and trending issues…trends often predict political action and resulting legislation. It is also necessary that practitioners advocate for client/patient access to present legislation through knowledge of public laws as well as assume advocacy roles for needed future legislation" (p. 399).

Most of the programs described in this text are designed to promote health and well-being and to prevent illness or injury for the individual and/or for the larger community. Programming of this nature requires the occupational therapy practitioner to constantly explore and expand differing and varied funding sources. In a 1998 special issue of the *American Journal of Occupational Therapy* devoted to community health, Brownson noted that we are looking at health from an ecological perspective and health care as a continuum from health promotion to tertiary prevention, maintaining that the expansion of occupational therapy roles in this way will require the exploration of new and different sources of funding (p. 64). We have seen this evolution as we have followed the agendas provided by the U. S. Department of Health and Human Services (HHS) from the publication of *Healthy People* in 1979 to *Healthy People 2000* (HHS, 1990), *Healthy People 2010* (HHS, 2000), and, most recently, *Healthy People 2020* (HHS, 2010). Each of these publications focuses on health disparities and access to quality of life, issues requiring creative and resourceful funding streams.

As you ask yourself these questions, you may determine that you will require grant funding of some kind, particularly to get started, but discovering the need for grant funding is not where you begin. "The most successful programs are mission driven, not grant driven" (Karsh & Fox, 2003, p. 13). According to these authors, you do not develop your program simply to obtain funding, but if you need funding, you will likely find a granting organization interested in your program.

Potential Funding Sources

Public and Private Funding Sources

At the close of the previous chapter and in this one, you will find a number of resources that can help you make your way through the potentially confusing maze of anticipating and covering your costs. While these resources describe structurally sound systems, specifics are usually a bit behind what is actually happening in the rapidly changing world of today's health care. Always seek out the most current information.

What might be described as **public funding** for occupational therapy services includes both insurance and grant-based programs. Federal and state insurance programs such as Medicare, Medicaid, and worker's compensation require constant attention to updated policies and procedures. Membership in your professional organizations can greatly facilitate this process, such as the American Occupational Therapy Association's (AOTA's) *One-Minute-Update* and other electronic venues for maintaining currency. Examples of grant-based public funding programs include the Individuals with Disabilities Education Act (2004) and the Older Americans Act (O'Shaughnessy, 2012). We also must remain attentive to the policies of **private funding** sources; insurance benefit programs such as Blue Cross/Blue Shield, managed care organizations, and other commercial insurers. If you plan to bill Medicare or private insurances as an independent practitioner, it is recommended that you work as an employee within a system that receives some of their compensation from these agencies before you try it on your own; or perhaps hire a consultant early on to assist with the provider applications and advanced preparation. Once you understand the systems and know the correct coding for billing required by the particular carrier or agency to facilitate payment, you can likely do it on your own. You can also access the websites of your particular carriers for the latest updates. The AOTA also provides updates to members regarding the latest summaries of frequently utilized Current Procedural Terminology codes and Medicare fee schedules (http://www.aota.org/).

Even though substantial preparation is required to receive payment for services through public and private insurances, many occupational therapy practitioners who engage in community programming believe it is to the community's advantage to fit their services into the more conventional payment models just described. However, there are many ways to access funding options. Being responsive to trends will also assist the programmer in utilizing the appropriate language and descriptions to better position him or her for funding. The clinical psychologist Patrick Vega (1998) provides one example when he describes a developing trend in the middle 1990s toward interest in behavioral disease management, which is also an area of interest to occupation-centered practitioners and continues to be. He encourages psychology practitioners who wish to engage in this kind of programming to go directly to local hospitals with their well-developed educational programs targeting the facility's wellness programs and cardiac units. There is a message for occupation-centered practitioners here as well as we also promote education/skills-based wellness programming. Vega goes on to propose that disease management, whether somatic or behavioral, will target those diseases that have high cost, high frequency, and high chronicity. As a nation, we remain concerned about cancer, diabetes, heart disease, asthma, and obesity. Cost savings for purchasers of insurance coverage is the key to the future. Avoiding stress injuries in the workplace through the practice of ergonomics is a current example, responsive to trend, and is rich with opportunity for occupational therapy practitioners, as is multicontextual programming promoting safety for all ages. As you investigate need and opportunities, it will be wise to do the following:

1. Be flexible in the way you offer programming and be able to match the need and try to do so by utilizing community assets.

2. Propose what you think (know) you can do based on what you have done (programming effectiveness, yours or that of others before you, published evidence).

3. Look for opportunities to partner, collaborate, and work as part of a team.

If these ideas match your interests as an occupation-centered program planner, you can tailor the development of your proposals toward these ends. Although licensure laws for some payment systems attempt to and do "carve out" territories for practitioners, few of the caregiving professions really "own" anything today. The market share goes to those who have the skills and information to do the job cost-effectively and to those who demonstrate that they can do what they claim. None of the health/wellness-oriented professions have a secure foothold in today's market; they all are searching for opportunities.

Private Payers

If you anticipate operating a practice as a for-profit business, the first professional relationships you must establish are with an attorney and/or a tax advisor. The next and most lasting relationship is with an accountant/bookkeeper. You will likely need help in setting up monthly profit-and-loss statements and certainly to keep track of accounts payable and receivable. There are computer software programs (such as Intuit's QuickBooks) to help you if you decide to handle your own finances, which you may want to consider, at least in the early stages before your business grows. How will you know whether you can make it on your own? Consider the size of your startup practice, and look at how you manage your personal finances; these two things will help you make the choice of whether to try to manage the "business" side of your practice or to hire someone to assist you. Also remember that "on your own" does not necessarily mean alone; working with partners, establishing collaborations, and utilizing personal resources are the keys to successful programs and practices.

This brings us to another form of payment for services in which the client/patient, or **private payer**, pays "**out of pocket**." In many of the developing community-based practices, it is not uncommon that clients/patients/parents pay directly for the services provided. Many parents are accustomed to paying for special classes, music lessons, sports, and camp fees; paying for occupation-centered intervention for their children is seen as being of little difference, particularly if it grants access to opportunities—access they were excluded from before engaging in programming. Older clients are accustomed to paying for classes, sports club memberships, and prevention programs (such as Weight Watchers; http://www.weightwatchers.com). Many occupation-centered wellness and prevention programs are similar in structure. Often, as in a camp program, there may be many forms of payment, including private pay for those who can, donation-based **gift tuitions** for those who cannot, and public and private funding for those who are eligible. Donated "gift tuitions" or "scholarships" for children who cannot afford a camp fee may be obtained from local fire departments, police departments, or other community service providers and businesses. Seeking such funding from professional sports organizations and larger companies is also a good idea. Some organizations/businesses will provide **matched funding** for programs. For every dollar (or tuition/programming fee) that you raise through small funding activities such as bake sales, garage sales, car washes, etc., they will offer a matching donation/gift of their own. Restaurants will sometimes offer a fundraising evening where a percentage of the proceeds is donated to a particular organization. Remember that the tax advantage for these organizations or individuals is to restrict their "gifts" to nonprofit organizations.

If you anticipate receiving out-of-pocket payment for services, you may require the assistance of a **collection agency**. For a fee, these agencies will help you retrieve payment from clients who are past due in their accounts. For a specified time, your bookkeeper will follow those who are delinquent (usually 30 days), then the bill is turned over to a collection agency. Sometimes, insurance companies take a period of time to pay for a service, but usually you can anticipate receiving payment; that may not be the case with private payers. Depending on the volume of services you offer, this could present a substantial problem for your **cash flow**. Cash flow is the actual money you have on hand to operate your business. Remember that you can be turning a profit in a private practice but still have no money on hand; perhaps this is another reason to hire an accountant. For programs/businesses that rely on out-of-pocket payment, it is strongly recommended that a receptionist (not the therapist) collect the fee from the client before intervention. Although there is an associated cost, making arrangements to accept credit card payments will facilitate the payment process; however, it also means that a client may have to be turned away. Most therapists are reluctant to refuse treatment, particularly for children, so a **sliding-scale** fee structure may help. This means that fees are set based on the income, or ability to pay, of the client/parent. The top of the fee scale is for those who can pay more, with adjusted increments for those with fewer resources. Remember, though, that for a private practice, there is always a bottom line—an amount of revenue that you must generate to keep your business solvent and ultimately profitable.

A word about **fundraising**: this is a critical process to nonprofits, which devote considerable time and expertise to it. Pakroo (2015) provides some basic fundraising rules (pp. 105-109): building relationships with potential donors is the first. Committed supporters are essential to a non-profit's success (Bray, 2015; Pakroo, 2015). Contributors can provide more than money. They can also offer positive word of mouth, willingness to volunteer, and networking with their own contacts. Pakroo (2015) goes on to emphasize the importance of building a compelling and detailed case for why a potential donor should support your organization. Here is where your passion comes together with logic. Also, put your stakeholders and board of directors to work. If you have selected this group carefully and strategically, as has been recommended, they become crucial to the fundraising process. This is a very basic discussion and there is much more to be considered. In discussions of fundraising as well as other concerns of nonprofits, it is recommended that you take advantage of the previously mentioned authors as well as others in the Nolo publisher series (http//www.nolo.com/).

Public and Private Grant Funding

According to Karsh and Fox (2003) (both seasoned grant writers), "Grant writing is one of those seemingly benign terms that tap into about every neurosis imaginable" (p. ix). Can I get one? Do I know enough? If I get one, what will I do with it? By the way, as Karsh and Fox and others remind us, we do not "write grants"; we write **proposals** in order to win **grants** (Brown & Brown, 2001; Karsh & Fox, 2003, 2014; Kiritz & Floersch, 2015; Smith & Tremore, 2003). This is exactly what you are doing if you have followed the process in this text—you are creating a proposal. In order to seek grant funding, some tweaking and perhaps additional development will be necessary, but you will have accomplished some work in all of the areas of program design that a granting/funding agency is interested in.

Perhaps a few additional cautions are required. Although writing grant proposals is the primary fundraising tool for organizations that provide essential services to a community, the process is extremely competitive. People use the phrase "to win a grant" because that is how it works, and not everyone "wins." However, regardless of the granting agency, to even be in the competition you must have a proposal of extremely high quality. The elements of a proposal are basically the same no matter who the grant maker is or how much money the grant provides. The proposal will convince the grant maker of your capacity to identify and then implement and sustain a quality program. Most experienced grant writers would agree that submitting a poorly thought out, poorly developed, poorly written proposal is sometimes the most damaging thing you can do to your long-term prospects. The message is, "If you are not ready, do not submit a proposal." Smith and Tremore (2003) emphasize the need for "good writing." They offer some general hints: (1) use everyday language, (2) avoid jargon, (3) be politically correct, (4) avoid sexist language, (5) explain acronyms and terms, (6) use strong, active verbs, and (7) speak with authority. Whatever you do, do not adopt the tone that "We can do this…only if you give us the money." If the work is important, you will figure out a way to do it (Smith & Tremore, 2003, pp. 185-191). You are giving the agency the opportunity to fund your program; you are not begging. Good writing and good "presentation" are of equal importance when you are presenting your proposal to an organization or a board of directors who represent your larger community. See Chapter 3 for ideas regarding the skills that are required to build a positive interface with your community.

Who am I and what do I want to do? What difference do I want to make? These questions were asked earlier in this chapter, and the answers are of particular importance now that we are considering applying for grant funding. Knowing who you are and what you want to do determines where you go for your money. Organizations that seek funding fall into three or four general categories. According to Karsh and Fox (2003, 2014), these are (1) grassroots organizations, (2) social service agencies and other service providers, (3) advocacy groups, and (4) individuals. Grassroots organizations may range from neighborhood improvement groups (managing graffiti) to obtaining uniforms for the Little League baseball team, and they may be the organizations you decide to help achieve their goals. Social service agencies and service providers are logical partners and collaborators for many of our interests. Advocacy groups are interested in specific issues—such as funding for special schools or trying to raise awareness for various sociopolitical forums such as rights for individuals with disability (two of many examples)—and again they are good partners for you. Individuals may seek grants to fund their projects. Artists, writers, filmmakers, and scholars make up this group. Sometimes the projects are small and sometimes large. Consider this direction as you examine your interests and the impact you wish to make. Many occupational therapy practitioners have strong interests and talents in the arts and could readily lead a community initiative in this area.

SOCIAL SERVICE AGENCIES AND OTHER SERVICE PROVIDERS

We may want to look more carefully at this category of provider, where we often choose to partner. These organizations are either nonprofit organizations or local government agencies set up to address the needs of groups of people of all ages and types: children's day care, after-school programs, violence prevention, pregnancy and substance-use prevention for teenagers, immigration counseling, domestic violence prevention for families, health, sanitation, and perhaps housing needs of a community and many other similar examples (Barbato & Furlich, 2000; Karsh & Fox, 2003, 2014). Very likely your developing proposal will target one of these populations. Not-for-profit social service organizations may each operate one small program, perhaps providing services for a small group of children. Larger nonprofits and government agencies may run many programs for all ages and needs. Funding needs may run from a few hundred dollars to a few million, and funding sources may include individual donors, private foundations, corporations, and government funding agencies. When we talk about programming intended to develop communities and to build assets and capacities, it is often this category of organization or "grassroots" organizations that we mean.

If service providers are nonprofit, as opposed to government agencies, they are usually incorporated under state laws and receive tax-exempt status from the Internal Revenue Service (IRS). The term **501(c)(3)** refers to the section of the Internal Revenue Code that authorizes this type of organization, like the term **determination letter**, which refers to the document from the IRS stating that your organization is tax-exempt. Karsh and Fox (2003, 2014) describe the process of using state incorporation papers or an IRS determination letter to prove that you are a nonprofit because most foundations and government funders give only to such organizations. The term *not-for-profit* (as opposed to nonprofit) is the technical term in the law and recognizes that the *purpose* of an organization is "not for profit," although the organization could show a budget surplus, but not likely. As an aside, if you are a for-profit practice and show a deficit, it does not automatically make you a nonprofit organization.

Contributions to a 501(c)(3) are tax-deductible, so individual donors as well as foundations and government entities are more inclined to fund this type of organization, although there are grants for for-profit organizations and small businesses as well. If you are not already working under the umbrella of a not-for-profit agency (and you need to know this), the process will involve a lawyer and substantial paperwork to form the nonprofit corporation. In some communities, a private attorney may provide this service at low cost or for free (*pro bono*). It will take several months to prepare the paperwork and to wait for the IRS to review the documentation; allow sufficient time on your *timeline* before you prepare to seek funding.

Even though you receive a nonprofit status, it may take time to win grant funding. Although some foundations are interested in brand-new organizations, most funding agencies expect to see a significant track record of service with some funding, a committed board of directors, sound fiscal health, good leadership, a clear vision/mission, the proven capacity to implement programs, and the ability to sustain projects, activities, staff, and programs (Barbato & Furlich, 2000; Brown & Brown, 2001; Karsh & Fox, 2003, 2014; Knowles, 2002). In most cases, a substantial amount of work has to be done before you seek a grant. Operating your program with a small number of participants for a period of time will permit you to work through any problems and to evaluate early outcomes. This **pilot program** may offer you enough data and experience to apply to some granting agencies.

THE FUNDERS—WHO ARE THEY?

The federal government gives grants. State and local governments give grant-like funding in the form of contracts. Private foundations, corporations, and individuals (through a fund or trust) give grants. In some parts of the country, a **regional association of grant makers (RAG)** may publish a standard or common application form that grant seekers can use for all participating foundations in that area. Some RAGs also publish a common report form.

Government grants are generally announced through **requests for proposals (RFPs)**. These may also be called **requests for applications (RFAs)**. You may also see **requests for statement of qualifications (RFSQs)**, and **requests for information (RFIs)**. These communications tell the applicant the nature and cost of the program to be proposed. They include guidelines, due dates, and other information. For examples of RFPs, you might wish to view the Foundation Center's weekly *RFP Bulletin*. This is a free e-mail subscription, arriving weekly and containing over a dozen weekly grant announcements with links to the relevant websites. The websites contain guidelines, application forms, and other announcements. Brown and Brown (2001) provide substantial information about funders, generating leads, foundation resources, guides to funding periodicals, and funding opportunities on the Internet (pp. 77-93).

FOUNDATIONS

Foundations are nongovernmental and are established as nonprofit corporations or charitable trusts. They range in size from very small family foundations (grant decisions made by family members) and small budgets under $100,000 to enormous organizations that have many staff members and give away millions of dollars each year. Examples of such large foundations are the Robert Wood Johnson Foundation, the Carnegie Corporation, the Kellogg Foundation, the Kresge Foundation, the Bill and Melinda Gates Foundation, and the Ford Foundation. Large foundations publish requirements that are as specific as the RFP for government grants, but smaller foundations are far less prescriptive. Examples of other foundations include the Martha Stewart Foundation, the Mark Wahlberg Foundation, and the Magic Johnson Foundation.

In general, family foundations have specific and narrowly focused giving patterns based on the intentions of the donor or the interests of current family members who are the officers or trustees. Independent private foundations will usually have at least a small professional staff and often began as a family foundation but are no longer controlled by the original donor or the donor's family. Even though there may be a separation from the origin of the foundation, Karsh and Fox (2003, 2014) tell us that private foundations remain ethically and, in most cases, legally bound to follow the donor's intent. If the original endowment or bequest said the money was to be used for the protection of Siamese cats or the training of potential opera singers (female, ages 9 to 15 years), then that is what it is used for. In most cases, though, the parameters are broader; for example, "health services for children of poverty-level families."

United Way is an example of a federated fund. Such funds were created to benefit the community by pooling donations from individuals and businesses and using those funds to support nonprofit organizations. Unlike most other foundations, federated funds devote a large portion of their resources to ongoing fundraising efforts.

Corporate foundations, or company-sponsored foundations, are independent foundations created by a large corporation with funds from the business itself. In most cases, the foundation functions like other foundations, receiving proposals and making grants, but giving may be tied to the corporation's own goals. Examples of corporate foundations are Bank of America, Starbucks, Target, Toyota, Verizon, Walmart, and the Ford Foundation.

Community foundations, or community trusts, occupy a place in every state and Puerto Rico; usually, there are several of these local foundations. Karsh and Fox (2003, 2014) provide an extensive list by state. Three random examples are the Cesar E. Chavez Community Development Fund, in Keene, CA; the New York Community Trust, in New York, NY; and the Community Foundation of the Texas Hill Country, in Kerrville, TX. Community foundations have been set up to administer individual trust funds or pools of funds from individual donors who do not want to create a new foundation but do want to benefit their communities in some way. To determine if there is a community foundation in your area, go to your local library, the Internet, or a listing at the Foundation Center's website (http://www.foundationcenter.org).

Financial institutions have always administered charitable trusts set up according to a donor's instructions, and they continue to do so. Proposals to a trust held by a financial institution are much the same as proposals to other foundations.

How Do You Find Foundations?

The Foundation Center is a national organization that provides support to foundations and information to the potential grant seeker. There are Foundation Center Libraries in five cities across the United States: New York, Atlanta, Cleveland, Washington, D.C., and San Francisco. In many other locations, a public library or nonprofit organization is designated as a Foundation Center Cooperating Collection. (See website address at the end of this chapter for more information.)

The Foundation Directory is perhaps the most important resource for potential grant seekers, but there are many other directories that describe foundations and corporations by location, program interests, size of grants given, and many other characteristics. *The Foundation Directory* reports on foundations with assets in excess of $2 million or annual giving of at least $200,000. Other versions of the directory provide information for those private and community foundations in the United States holding assets from $1 million to $2 million or with annual granting programs from $50,000 to $200,000. A companion document, available from the Foundation Center (see website at the end of this chapter) and titled the *Guide to U.S. Foundations, Their Trustees, Officers, and Donors*, provides brief data on foundations with assets below $1 million and giving programs of less than $50,000 annually. The Foundation Center Libraries also maintain foundation annual reports. The foundation annual reports will provide helpful clues to the kinds of activities the foundation prefers to fund, the dollar amounts offered, and other characteristics of eligibility. *The Foundation Directory Online* can be subscribed to, but first check your library; it may already subscribe.

Before submitting a proposal to a foundation, you would be wise to call or write (or access their website) for their annual report, grant application form or guidelines (some may not offer guidelines), descriptions of programs funded, and any other information that you can get. The more information you have, the better your chance of submitting an acceptable proposal. Generally, your application/proposal will be rejected outright if it does not meet the recipient's guidelines. Another source of information about a particular foundation is their tax return (referred to as a 990). These tax returns will almost always include a list of organizations funded and the amount of money given to each. Some may indicate the particular program funded. The 990s are usually available through a website called *GrantSmart* (http://www.GrantSmart.com/).

Corporations and local businesses may fulfill their civic responsibilities through grants and sponsorships to nonprofit organizations. As an example of a private funding organization, the Pfizer pharmaceutical company's corporate philanthropy includes, among many other agendas, maternal and child health programs to help low-income, high-risk parents get prenatal and well-baby care and information. Occupation-centered community nonprofit programs such as those targeting skills for teen mothers, those designed to encourage nurturing mother-baby shared occupations, or those providing screening for developmental milestones in infants and children would be appropriate for this organization (Klinko, 2015).

Business donors or sponsors in the local community are often the best place for a small organization to begin seeking funding and to establish a successful track record in using these gifts. This is one of the things you will be alert to when you are doing your profile, particularly if you do a walk and/or drive survey. Start with a local bank, or perhaps a retail store. Ask the manager if they provide assistance to a group like yours and what you have to do to apply for it. Ask if he or she would look at your proposal and give you an opportunity to talk about it. Wherever your community is located, urban or rural, it is likely that a Walmart retail store is somewhere at the heart of it. If you are looking for a small amount of matching money (up to $2,000 to double what you already have) for your children and youth program, consider this organization. Civic associations in which local businesspeople participate—such as the Chamber of Commerce, Lions Club, Rotary, and Kiwanis—often have giving programs or provide sponsorships for local organizations or programs. Each association will have its own priorities and most gifts will be small, but it is a way to partially fund your pilot program in preparation for seeking larger amounts of funding. Although, maybe it is all you need.

FEDERAL GRANTS

The federal government awards many billions of dollars in grant funds each year. A federal grant is an award of federal money made to accomplish some general public purpose (Karsh & Fox, 2003, 2014). The nature of the grant, who is eligible, how the award is given, and the terms and conditions are specified in the legislation that creates each grant program and in detailed regulations (regs). The legislation provides the structure for any restrictions or limitations and for the extensive reporting requirements that are generally required.

Just as the *Foundation Directory* provides information about foundation funding, the *Federal Register* does the same thing for federal granting monies. The *Federal Register* is a daily publication that reports on official federal actions, including all federal funding opportunities. Announcements for grant programs, often with the whole application package, appear in the *Federal Register*. Occasionally, the announcement will appear as part of a department's grant-making plans for the year; which provides substantial lead time for your application. It is more likely, though, that notification will allow 30 to 90 days for an application response. Without access to the *Federal Register*, you will not be able to make competitive federal applications for funding. As with other funding announcement documents mentioned earlier, you can likely find a copy at your library or obtain Internet access. Karsh and Fox (2003, 2014) provide a "guide" to searching the *Federal Register Online*. Many federal agencies have their own websites where they publish grant information. You will want to access these sites as well. Some examples of interest to occupation-centered practitioners are the Department of Health and Human Services (related sites: Administration for Children and Families; National Institutes of Health, and Substance Abuse and Mental Health Administration) and the Department of Education (see end of chapter for websites).

In general, federal (also state and local) grant proposals are complex and time-consuming to prepare. It is virtually impossible to develop and write a comprehensive, technical grant application in the short window of time that most federal programs offer between announcement and due date. This is one of the reasons it is important to develop your proposal far in advance. Brown and Brown (2001) suggest that the grant seeker develop a system of year-round grant seeking. These authors propose that one can demystify grant seeking by "organizing your office and practicing the right work habits so you can get more and better grant proposals out the door and more money coming in without suffering (Brown & Brown, 2001, p. xix). Many organizations devote key personnel to the year-round process of seeking funding. According to Brown and Brown (2001), there is a "grant-seeking" cycle that first involves the meticulously prepared proposal with comprehensive files containing all of the collected information for each component of the proposal—from goals and objectives for programming, to the results of outcome evaluations, to staff job descriptions and resumes. Therefore, when you prepare a proposal, regardless of the agency, make sure that you have everything they could possibly ask for.

DEALING WITH THE APPLICATION

Many first-time grant seekers skim or speed-read the application. They are generally interested in how much money they can get, the questions that must be answered in the proposal, and the absolute midnight deadline when the proposal has to be driven to the local FedEx. In fact, if you hope to be successful, the whole package must be read carefully and more than once.

Successful grant writers (Barbato & Furlich, 2000; Karsh & Fox, 2003, 2014; Knowles, 2002; Smith & Tremore, 2003) suggest that as you become familiar with the application (and, they do not all look the same), you should ask yourself the following questions:

- Am I (or is my organization) even eligible to apply for the grant described in the package?
- Does my idea for a grant mesh with the grant maker's? Does our mission align with that of the grant maker? Can I create a connection between the two?
- What kinds of projects has the grant maker funded recently? What is the funding cycle? When do they accept applications?
- How much money is the grant for, and will it cover my expenses? Most grant applications stipulate the approximate amount of funding that will be awarded. Some only tell you what the total amount will be and approximately how many grants will be given; others give a maximum possible award, or an average.
- Do I really have to answer all of the questions? Yes! Most grant applications include a list of questions or topics that you must address in a specific number of pages; some may restrict the number of words per question. You must answer all of the questions or address every topic that is included in the application and with the number of pages/words specified.
- What if there are no real questions? Foundations, particularly, may simply describe what they want you to tell them without asking specific questions, or they may suggest what they would like to see in the proposal. They may say something such as, "we are interested in learning as much as possible about the applicant…this includes budget (past, current, projected), audited financial statements, an IRS letter explaining tax status, and examples of past accomplishment…the main body of the application should not exceed 15 pages" (Karsh & Fox, 2003, p. 290). Your task is to focus your writing/proposal so that the source clearly understands your vision of what you want to achieve.
- I do not find any guidelines, instructions, or specific questions. In this case, you may wish to write a **letter of inquiry (LOI)**. Something like an abstract (discussed a bit later), this letter is a brief summary of your organization, its purpose, the need you wish to address, your program to address the need, the cost of your program, and the amount you're requesting. You will also want to include why you selected this particular funder and how your program will fit their overall interests. Follow this with a telephone call. The LOI refers to both a letter of inquiry and a **letter of intent**.

- A letter of intent is requested by some funders to determine approximately how many applicants they may expect to receive applications from.
- What information/documents am I likely to need? You can review the chapters in this text for much of the information you will need: projected outcomes/impact, mission/goals, objectives, programming, staff, space needs, associated trends, the community and population profiles, needs assessments, evaluations, budget, and current funding sources. In addition, you may need personnel policies and procedures, staff resumes, job descriptions, organizational charts, names of board members, evidence of collaboration/partnering with other individuals/disciplines/organizations, certificate of incorporation as a not-for-profit organization, and proof of tax-exempt status. Of more importance all of the time is the question of, "How will you sustain your program when the grant runs out?" This may be where you will also have prepared an assessment of the community's assets and, perhaps, a plan for building assets. In all cases, read the application carefully so that you do not leave anything (asked for) out and, generally, do not put in things that are not asked for.

THE GRANT PROPOSAL

It is important for you to appreciate that grantsmanship refers to the process of collecting information, developing your ideas, and writing. It is a process that you initiated with Chapter 1 in this text. It is much more than just answering a series of questions. Certainly, you may need to answer questions, but you will do so from information collected during the process of developing your program. Knowing yourself and your community will help you establish the context for your work and what you want to accomplish, and it will help you find the best grant maker for your purposes. It is essential that you get the funder to believe in your ideas and to trust that you, as the leader/organizer/collaborator, know what you are doing and have the sense of purpose to do it. The basis for this trust is established alongside the development of your program.

In most cases, the actual "pieces" needed to accompany your proposal for funding will include the following:

- The cover letter
- The cover sheet
- The abstract, or executive summary
- The table of contents
- Appendices (attachments)

You know from the development of your community programming proposal what a table of contents, a cover or title sheet, and an appendix would include, but you may not be familiar with the **cover letter** and/or the **abstract/executive summary.** The abstract/executive summary "summarizes" the entire proposal; it includes key points for each section and highlights how your work fits with a foundation's priorities. It includes only information discussed in your proposal.

A **cover letter** is an introduction and is the first document in a grant application. Most often, it is used on foundation and corporate requests, not in applications for federal or state funding. But again, read the directions to be sure. The letter should be reflective, sincere, and provide only a taste of what is to come in the grant request. Generally, it is best to do the cover letter last, after you have completed the entire grant application. Remember, though, it is not simply a summary. The cover letter must be persuasive, and it is an opportunity to get personal—probably the only appropriate place in a funding proposal. Barbato and Furlich, in their book *Writing for a Good Cause*, outline the process of crafting proposals and what they describe as "other persuasive pieces for nonprofits" (2000, preface). The cover letter is the first line of persuasion; it tells the reader right away whether the proposal is worth reading. Mary Bellor, president of the Philip L. Graham Fund in Washington, D.C., is quoted in Barbato and Furlich (2000) as saying, "I read the cover letter first; I want to see who you are, what you do, who benefits, and why it matters ... I want a preview of what I'm going to find in the proposal, I don't want a summary" (p. 86).

The abstract or executive summary is a brief, one-page overview of what the grant reviewer will find in the full grant application. It is written (or assembled) after the grant application narrative has been entirely written. It should be one page only; Barbato and Furlich (2000) recommend even less than that (p. 93). Browning (2001) recommends lifting key sentences from the following areas of the proposal, keeping them in the same order as they are in the narrative (pp. 119-120):

- Your proposed initiative
- Program design/plan of action
- Problem statement/statement of need
- Goals
- Measurable objectives
- Impact on problem

Other grant writers (Barbato & Furlich, 2000, pp. 92-93) recommend an even more succinct version that includes the following:

- The problem you want to address
- Your proposed solution
- How much your proposal requests

BANKS AND LENDING INSTITUTIONS

If you are planning a for-profit program/practice, then some of your funding needs may fall into the category of a loan. It is generally expected, however, that you have your own **capital**. If you have other sources of income and collateral (home equity, stocks, or bonds), you might be in a position to borrow funds in addition to your own. Of course, there is always some risk that must be considered if the practice struggles. A solid **business plan** with good projections and supporting data is a prerequisite to requesting a startup loan. The following outline (Hiduke & Ryan, 2014; Ryan, Ray, & Hiduke, 1999, p. 6) is suggested for developing a business plan appropriate for seeking funds from a lending agency (you will recognize in their suggested plan many of the components you have already prepared during your planning process):

1. Cover sheet

2. Statement of purpose

3. Table of contents

   - The Business

     A. Description of the business

     B. Marketing

     C. Competition

     D. Operating procedures

     E. Personnel

     F. Business insurance

     G. Financial data

   - Financial data

     A. Loan application

     B. Capital equipment and supply list

      C. Balance sheet

      D. Break-even analysis

      E. *Pro forma* income projections (profit and loss statements)

- Three-year summary
- Detail by month, first year
- Detail by quarters, second and third years
- Assumptions upon which projections were based

      F. Pro forma cash flow

- Follow guidelines for letter E

- Supporting documents

      A. Tax returns of principals for last 3 years

      B. Personal financial statement (forms supplied by lender)

      C. If franchised, a copy of the contract

      D. Copy of proposed lease or purchase agreement for space

      E. Copy of licenses and other legal documents

      F. Copy of resumes of all principals

      G. Copy of letters of intent from suppliers, etc.

These authors also suggest the following website to assist in the preparation of this plan: www.sba.gov/starting/indexbusplans.html. Clearly, going this route is not for the faint of heart, and you still should seek the services of an accountant. It should be comforting to know, however, that the planning you have already accomplished is the foundation on which you can build the additional pieces.

WHAT HAPPENS NEXT?

You submit your application and you wait. You will generally know when the selections will be made and when you can expect notification. You may not hear if you are not selected, so a phone call may be acceptable if the granting date has passed and you have heard nothing.

When the applications arrive at the granting agency (they are never accepted after the deadline), they are evaluated and points are attached to each section of the proposal/application indicating strength/weakness. Generally, in the application information, you will be informed about how the evaluation will be determined. The irony is that sometimes you will receive a high score but receive no funding. Generally, only a few of the best scores can be funded. However, you should note your scores and be pleased with your high scores. You have learned something valuable for the next application. If you have low scores, do better the next time.

If you receive notice that your application has been funded, most often for 3 to 5 years, your work begins. You cannot abandon your program, take the money, and go to Tahiti. You have an unrelenting responsibility to meet the terms of your proposal. Are there strings attached to the grant award? You can be sure of it. All granting organizations expect reporting on a regular basis. They will want to know that your program is making a difference. They will want evaluation results and they will want to know that their money is well spent. Read carefully what kind of reporting is expected, what documents may be needed, and what the reporting deadlines are. Even for small amounts of money, there are expectations that require reporting procedures.

Exercise 14-1

If you are a student, likely this portion of your work will be for learning purposes only. Even though you may make a mock grant application, you will not submit it to an agency. That will come later, when you can devote the necessary time and effort to actually implement and run a program.

What Kind of Program Do You Have?

1. Refer to Exercise 13-1 in the previous chapter. Is your program not-for-profit or is the intention to be for profit? Are you affiliated with either of these entities already?

_____

_____

_____

_____

_____

If you are not-for-profit, review what you would need to do to seek 501(c)(3) status. Remember, if you are working under the umbrella of a nonprofit agency, this work will already have been accomplished. Either way, for the purposes of learning, review the process and information you will need and note it here:

_____

_____

_____

_____

_____

2. Refer to Exercise 13-2 in the previous chapter. Carefully evaluate your costs. It is unlikely for the purposes of your student exercises that you have a budget accurate enough for a grant application; however, you should have all of the pieces and be able make a fairly accurate estimate of the sum you will need in order to operate your program:

Startup _____

1 Year _____

3 Years _____

In what lines of the budget do you think you will need to do additional work to be prepared to make a funding application? Note any areas here:

_____

_____

_____

_____

_____

Identifying Potential Funding Sources

3. Review the potential funding sources noted in this chapter compared with the goal and purpose of your program. If you are working under the umbrella of another not-for-profit organization, ask if they already have grant funded programs and their nature (perhaps they receive a portion of their funding from United Way or other similar organizations).

Will you bill insurances? Will you establish a sliding fee scale and accept out-of-pocket pay? Will you consider a private foundation? Will you want to seek a federal grant? If you intend to be a for-profit organization, you may wish to consider a small business loan. Discuss funding options with your classmates, colleagues, or partners to determine which ones seem most appropriate for your program. Note your choices here:

_____

_____

_____

_____

_____

Learn as Much as Possible About Your Selected Funding Source

4. You are now ready to go to the library, websites, and directories to learn as much as you can about your selected funding source. Find the *best fit* with your purpose, your goal, and your program. Note here what sources you will use:

_____

_____

_____

_____

_____

Obtain a grant application package from the agency you have selected and become familiar with it. Evaluate the requested application information compared with what you have in your proposal. Where will you need to do more work? Some funding sources (such as federal and private organizations and lending agencies) require a fairly lengthy application process. Revisit your timeline developed in Chapter 6 and be sure to include the funding process:

_____

_____

_____

_____

SUMMARY

This chapter has provided you with a general outline of funding sources as you anticipate how you will initiate and maintain your program. You have examined the characteristics of your program and, in that regard, have come to some decisions about potential funding sources. If your venture calls for external funding either through grants or a loan, you must anticipate that early in your planning. It was not the purpose of this chapter or this text to tell you everything you need to know to acquire funding for your program. It provides an overview and some guidance. There are many excellent resources listed in the reference portion at the end of the chapter; use them to fill in any gaps you might find. Remember that you have already been introduced to the W. K. Kellogg Foundation. They offer numerous resources to grant applicants. Select the direction in which you want to go, make a plan, utilize the resources, and move ahead.

REFERENCES

Barbato, J., & Furlich, D. (2000). *Writing for a good cause*. New York, NY: Simon and Schuster.

Bray, I. (2015). *Effective fundraising for nonprofits: Real world strategies that work*. Berkeley, CA: Nolo Press.

Brown, L. G., & Brown, M. J. (2001). *Demystifying grant seeking*. San Francisco, CA: Jossey-Bass Publishers.

Browning, B. (2001). *Grant writing for dummies*. Hoboken, NJ: John Wiley and Sons.

Brownson, C. (1998). Funding community practice: Stage I. *American Journal of Occupational Therapy, 52*(1), 60-64.

Hiduke, G., & Ryan, J. D. (2014). *Small business: An entrepreneur's business plan* (9th ed.). Boston, MA: Southwestern-Cengage Learning.

Individuals with Disabilities Education Act (IDEA). (2004). Retrieved from http://idea-b.ed.gov/explore/home.html

Karsh, E., & Fox, A. (2003). *The only grant-writing book you'll ever need*. New York, NY: Carroll and Graf Publishers.

Karsh, E., & Fox, A. (2014). *The only grant-writing book you'll ever need* (2nd ed.). New York, NY: Basic Books, Perseus.

Kiritz, N., & Floersch, B. (2015). *Program planning and proposal writing*. Los Angeles, CA: The grantsmanship center. http//www.grantsmanshipcenter.com

Klinko, F. (Ed.). (2015). *Children and youth funding report*. Durham, NC: CD Publications. Retrieved from http://www.cdpublications.com/cyf/

Knowles, C., (2002). *The first-time grantwriter's guide to success*. Thousand Oaks, CA: Corwin Press Publishers.

Merryman, M. B., & Van Slyke, N. (2014). "Legislation and policy issues. In M. Scaffa & S. M. Reitz (Eds.), *Occupational therapy in community-based practice settings* (pp. 51-60). Philadelphia, PA: Davis.

O'Shaughnessy, C. (2012). *Older Americans Act of 1965: Programs and funding*. Washington, DC: The George Washington University, National Health Policy Forum. Retrieved from http://www.nhpf.org/library/the-basics/Basics_OlderAmericansAct_02-23-12.pdf

Pakroo, P. (2015). *Starting and building a nonprofit: A practical guide* (6th ed.). Berkeley, CA: Nolo Press.

Reed, K. (1992). History of federal legislation for persons with disabilities. *American Journal of Occupational Therapy, 46*(5), 397-408.

Ryan, J. D., Ray, R., & Hiduke, G. (1999). *Small business: An entrepreneur's plan*. Philadelphia, PA: Dryden Press.

Smith, N., & Tremore, J. (2003). *The everything grant writing book*. Avon, MA: F + W Publications.

U.S. Department of Health and Human Services. (1990). *Healthy People 2000. National health promotion and Disease prevention objectives* (Publication No. 017–001-00474-0). Washington, DC: U.S. Government Printing Office.

U.S. Department of Health and Human Services. (2000). *Healthy People 2010.* (2nd ed.). Washington, DC: U.S. Government Printing Office.

U.S. Department of Health and Human Services. (2010). *Healthy People 2020* (ODPHP Publication No. B0132). http://healthypeople.gov/

Vega, P. (1998). Industry trends in practice strategies: A business guide for behavioral healthcare providers. *Journal of Marriage & Family Therapy, 26*(9): 281-291.

Internet Sources

After-School Program Information: http://www.afterschool.gov

Business Plans: www.sba.gov/starting/indexbusplans.html

Department of Education: http://www.edu.gov http://www.ed.gov/topics/topics.jsp?&top=Grants+%26+Contracts

Department of Health and Human Services: http://www.hhs.gov/agencies/grants.html

    Administration for Children and Families: http://www.acf.hhs.gov/grants.html

    Health Resources and Service Administration: http://www.hrsa.gov/grants.htm

    National Institutes of Health: http://www.nih.gov/grants/guide/index.html

    Substance Abuse and Mental Health Administration: http://www.ssamhsa.gov/grants/grants.html

Federal Grants: http://www.Grants.gov/

Federal Register: http://www.access.gpo.gov/su_docs/aces/aces!40.html

The Foundation Center: http://www.foundation.center.org

    http://fdncenter.org/funders/grantsmart/index.html

    http://fdncenter.org/funders/grantmaker/gws_corp/corpl.html

    http://fdncenter.org/funders/cga/index.html

    http://gtionline.fdncenter.org/

The Grantsmanship Center: http://www.tgci.com/

Grantwriting Resources: http://www.fundsnetservices.com/grantwri.htm

Magic Johnson Foundation: magicjohnson.org (MJF)

Mark Wahlberg Youth Foundation: www.markwahlbergyouthfoundation.com

Martha Stewart Foundation: www.marthastewart.com/martha-foundation

National Association of Women Business Owners (NAWBO): www.nfwbo.org

National Institute of Health: http://www.nih.gov/grants/guide/index.html

Publications and Services of the Foundation Center: http://www.foundation.center.org/

U.S. Census Bureau: http://www.census.gov

U.S. Department of Justice, Americans with Disabilities: www.usdoj.gov/crt/ada; http://www.usdoj.gov/10grants/index.html

General Research Directories

The following are published by the Foundation Center, New York, NY (http://www.foundation.center.org):

The foundation directory, Luller, M., & Luman, N., eds., published annually.

The foundation directory, Part 2, Luller, M., & Luman, N., eds., published annually.

The foundation directory supplement, Luller, M., & Luman, N., eds., published annually.

Guide to U.S. foundations, their trustees, officers, and donors, published annually.

The foundation 1000, published annually.

National directory of corporate giving, published annually.

Corporate foundation profiles, published biennially.

National directory of grantmaking public charities.

Guide to greater Washington D.C. grantmakers (2nd ed.).

New York State foundations: A comprehensive directory, published biennially.

Directory of Missouri grantmakers.

Foundation grants to individuals, published biennially.

Grant Directories

The foundation grants index (most recent edition).

The foundation grants index quarterly (most recent edition).

Who gets grants: Foundation grants to nonprofit organizations.

Guidebooks, Manuals, and Reports

The foundation center's grants classification system indexing manual and thesaurus (newest edition).

The foundation center's user-friendly guide: A grantseeker's guide to resources (most recent edition).

The foundation center's guide to proposal writing (most recent edition).

Program-related investments: A guide to funders and trends.

15

Promoting Your Program
Marketing

Fazio, L. S. *Developing Occupation-Centered Programs*
With the Community, Third Edition (pp 245-253).
© 2017 Taylor & Francis Group.

In the simplest terms, **marketing** is the process of letting your potential consumers know that you have services that may be of interest to them. We may not think that we are selling a "product," but in reality, our product is the attainment of goals and the satisfaction of need. In fact, product is "anything that can be offered to a market for attention, acquisition, use, or consumption and that might satisfy a need or want" (Kotler & Armstrong, 1991, p. 7). Marketing also includes an intent to "sell" the services to the potential market/consumer (even if the services are free). This marketing aspect of selling is often referred to by the more aggressive term **sales promotion**, and those areas that are selected to promote your services are referred to as the **promotional mix**. In her discussions of marketing yourself as an occupational therapy practitioner, Gilkeson (1997) describes this promotional mix as including the three areas of advertising, publicity, and personal selling. Gerson (1991) utilizes a more conventional list preferred by business that includes advertising, public relations, direct selling, and sales promotion. Richmond (2003) would remind us that although "marketing" is often used synonymously with "selling" or "advertising," it is much more than that. Marketing can be defined in terms of exchanging products and values with others; however, unless those products (programs) are visible and accessible to the consumer, the exchange cannot take place (Richmond, 2003, p. 179).

Writing for the potential small business entrepreneur, on the other hand, Ryan, Ray, and Hiduke (1999) include all of these areas in their promotional mix. In their words, mix "refers to all the elements that are blended to maximize communication with the target customer or population" (p. 99). An important aspect of promotion for these authors is the advancement of the "image" of your practice, or displaying for the potential consumer the "quality" of your services.

You may think of marketing and promotion as only associated with a private practice/business, but regardless of the nature of your program and services, people need to know about them, and you will want to link the potential consumer to what you are offering. Scott (2013) encourages us to include marketing in the mix of nonprofit organizational tasks. Alongside development and education, marketing is critical to the success of the nonprofit program, particularly when the organization/program is new. Marketing programs are intended to promote your nonprofit and to increase the public's awareness of your organization. The focus is to highlight your cause and gain support from the community (Pakroo, 2015; Scott, 2013).

Pakroo (2015, p. 177) lists the following as efficient ways to promote your nonprofit:

- Coaching board members and other influential supporters to spread the word
- Networking with other nonprofits, government agencies, and community leaders
- Creating a website and promoting it
- Distributing brochures, flyers, or other literature
- Listing your organization or events in local calendars and directories

Social media are a gift to nonprofit organizations, probably for small businesses as well, because of the minimal financial costs. Scott (2013) and others suggest sharing photos from your programs and events on Flickr, designing and managing an organizational Facebook page, providing interesting information on Twitter, and uploading videos to YouTube. Without a doubt, you will also want a thorough organizational website (Orsburn, 2010; Scott, 2013, p. 176). Pakroo (2015) includes substantial guidance on Web development and building in his book (pp. 206-227).

Advertising, of course, includes all of those marketing methods we have come to take for granted in our lives, such as visual media (television), print media (magazines and newspapers), radio, and the Internet. We hardly notice media ads, billboards, or bus signs yet are influenced by their messages. Advertising means buying space or airtime to deliver a promotional message to the public, and **listings or directories** are things like phone books, online directories, classified ads, or other specialized publications designed to reach a self-selected group of people (Pakroo, 2015, p. 177). **Publicity** may be positive or negative and is usually not targeted by the marketer; rather, it is received by the marketer. The receipt of positive publicity, for example, could be in the form of responses to a public presentation we have done or to a community service event we have organized and/or in which we have participated. Of course, there is also the negative potential of such publicity as the announcement of a malpractice suit or other legal sanctions having to do with unethical or unsafe practices. **Public relations** describes the direct intent of interfacing with your public in such a way that the image of you and your service delivery remains positive.

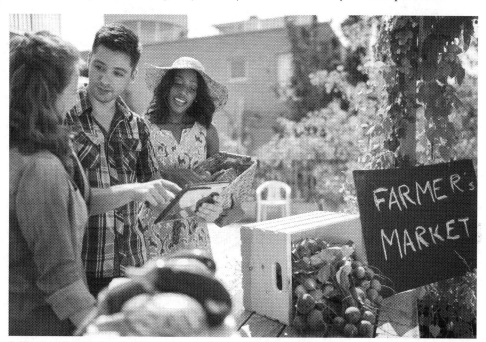

Selling garden produce in the community is not only good for business, it is good public relations for your program.

Personal selling has been emphasized in earlier chapters, and it may begin when we interface with potential partners or collaborators, perhaps earlier. Now let us examine personal selling in consideration of our marketing mix from the perspective of personally going out to make others aware of our program. Drucker (1973) has long been a compelling voice in the wilderness of business management. He suggests that if the marketing process has been well organized and carried out effectively, personal selling might not be necessary. For our purposes, however, personal selling is a critical—perhaps the most critical—part of health promotion, intervention, and the extensive scope of most of the program development described in this text. A few minutes taken to meet the pediatricians, teachers, and parents in your community coupled with the delivery of a well-appointed brochure describing your pediatric occupational therapy services is well worth the time.

Although your new program or practice may represent one of those circumstances where you will open your doors and they will come, this is not likely. If others in the community (your stakeholders) have a vested interest in your program (such as our examples of the cooperative gardening project for the mentally ill who are homeless or the sanctuary program for runaway adolescents), then they will likely assist you in attracting clients and in getting them to you. Anytime you have the enthusiasm, interest, and support of an agency or organization, you will have less marketing to do in order to get your clients through your doors; certainly, your collaborators and your partners will be strong allies in this effort.

As we mentioned earlier in the text, your first marketing task was to sell yourself to the people who required a planner—that is, to the community itself. If they were not yet aware that they needed a planner, then you sold them on the idea. We assume that you have already done this, but the process of selling yourself never quite ends. Even if you have the support of an agency/organization to start the program, you will have to continue "selling" the idea and, more importantly, making people aware of how effective your programming is. As described by Gilkeson (1997), this is **marketing logic,** or the representation of an attitude that supports the principles of selling yourself and the belief in your ideas. It is the belief that you are the "program" and that the program is an extension of you. It represents your beliefs, ideas, and ethics.

If you are developing a new program under the sponsorship of your employer, the marketing task will not be yours alone. It is likely that you have already proven your worth or you would not have been invited to develop a new program. In addition, assuming that the development is responsive to an expressed need, part of the marketing/promotion has probably already been accomplished. In a case such as this, the primary marketing task—as it is for all programs—will be one of proving effectiveness weighed against cost.

Often, a program is initiated because someone else has recognized the need—a member or members of the community—but he or she does not have the expertise or perhaps the commitment to provide it. That person might come to you, or you might hear of it and go to him or her. The marketing task then is to sell yourself as the best one to do the job. Let us consider the following scenario:

You are attending an open house of a new cardiac care unit and happen to overhear one of the attendees ask if there would be a cardiac "wellness" program to complement the surgical practice. You are an astute marketer/planner and later ask one of the cardiac surgeons if you could meet with her regarding your ideas for supplementary services organized around occupation; after all, you are an occupational therapy practitioner (or "therapist," if that is a more marketable term in this environment). Needless to say, after some planning, promotion, and negotiation with the corporation, you will develop a health maintenance and wellness program that may include providers of information and skills in the areas of balanced lifestyle, work, nutrition, relaxation (maybe yoga), graduated exercise, and perhaps sexuality. Your program will also provide personal lifestyle coaching, and you have further marketed it to other cardiac caregivers and surgeons. *This is an example of a success story.*

Of course, you are not finished; you must keep careful formative and summative outcome data to market your program's effectiveness in "lengthening life" and in "enhancing quality of life." The goal of a program such as this could be not only the promotion of longer lives, but also the assurance of longer meaningful lives. This is a burgeoning area of interest and research in occupational therapy, so part of your task is to keep abreast of all of the work that is being done to support the establishment of meaning in one's life and to provide potentially valued options for how one chooses to live, perhaps to include the redesign of one's life (Mandel, Jackson, Zemke, Nelson, & Clark, 1999).

The most challenging marketing task may be for the private practice. Many therapists who initiate private practices do so a bit cautiously while still being employed by other organizations. As we said earlier, a private practice is a business, and there are risks to be considered. If you were an entrepreneur as a child or adolescent and started a successful business (a lemonade stand, babysitting service, or anything else), you know something about marketing and promotion. You may have been selling a product or a service, or maybe both.

For example, neighborhood children might collaborate to climb trees, retrieve mistletoe, package it, and sell it during the holiday season. (The mistletoe was likely hanging on the trees of most of the people who purchased it!) The marketing mix would include an attractively wrapped product and a service (retrieval of the "product" from the trees), and most people would probably buy it. There is little doubt that known neighborhood children are a strong component of the promotional mix regardless of what they are selling. Consider how many subscriptions, boxes of candy or cookies, and holiday cards you have purchased from a neighborhood child at your door. This example may seem a bit remote from our interests as occupation-centered practitioners, but it clearly shows how an effective promotional mix is developed, and it is not unlike what you will do.

You will be selling a product and a service—thoughtful, skilled intervention that is well packaged in a comfortable and welcoming environment. In addition, you can and will prove that this particular intervention makes a difference. Your clients/patients/members may be able to do for themselves some of what you do, but certainly not as effectively or as efficiently. Consider why people go to clubs to exercise when they could exercise at home. Could some of their reasoning also apply to your clientele? You are the professional skilled in understanding and utilizing a meaningful occupation, so your marketing brochures and business card should reflect this. If you find that people misinterpret what you do as an occupational therapist or as an occupational therapy assistant, include a meaningful explanation of your services in a brochure or an explanatory phrase on your business card. You may want these materials to be focused toward the population you wish to serve. For example, a pediatrics program might be described as providing "supportive play through small-group interactions."

In an earlier chapter, we discussed the many levels of assessing need. The term **market analysis** is related in that information is gleaned to "define the market and determine if the organization's perception of the wants and needs of the market are valid" (Shoemaker & Virden, 1992; p. 125). Richmond (2004) reminds us that we must be responsive to the "bottom line"; you must have clients to stay in business. She goes on to describe the target markets that you must be aware of as you conduct your analysis: the clients/potential clients, referral sources, and the payers (Richmond, 2004, pp. 83-86). You might think of the market analysis as a "check" on the validity of your research and your collective needs assessment results. According to Richmond (2003), the market analysis is organized within two main assessment methods: assessment of the organization and assessment of the environment (p. 182). The goals of the analysis incorporate the identification of trends, opportunities, and potential threats as well as competition and the position of the organization offering programming in the market.

THE PROMOTIONAL MIX

What are the choices available to us as we prepare to let others know about our program, and how do we select the options that will be most advantageous? Consider the following possibilities, adapted from Hiduke and Ryan (2014) and Ryan et al. (1999):

Promotional Element	Pros	Cons
1. Paid media advertising (radio, television, Internet, newspapers, and magazines)	Quick, effective	Expensive
2. Direct mail (to your potential consumer)	Affordable, efficient	Can be wasted if you have a fragmented market; difficult to write
3. Professional literature (become a source of information in your specialty and an expert in your field, and write about it)	Little or no cost; respected by colleagues and consumers	Will take work and experience
4. Free ink and free air (reviews, features, interview shows, press releases, newspaper columns to talk about what you do)	No cost and effective	It takes time to "market" to media

(continued)

Promotional Element	Pros	Cons
5. Promotional products (products with the name of your program, such as keychains, pencils, mugs, shirts, etc.)	Targeted and effective; can be very creative	Can be costly
6. Working visibility (develop and maintain a positive presence in the community; stand out from the competitors because you are better)	Common sense	You have to be good!
7. Personal selling and networking (business cards distributed at events, meetings); displays	Personal and effective	Takes time and can be costly

Consider these alternatives as you develop your promotional strategies. For most nonprofit community programs, the planner will rely on those with low cost. Communicating with others in the community about your program is known as **networking**, or getting to know others in the community who can and will help you remain a viable community resource. Sometimes, this is accomplished through very informal means, such as going to the same coffee shop as those you wish to know; spending time in the neighborhood and living in the community is certainly a plus. Networking also might be more formal and can include attending professional meetings or town meetings. Alternatively, if you have a private practice, you may wish to join the local chamber of commerce. Getting free media coverage, or **free ink/free air**, by providing a news item or story is excellent marketing. **Media relations** refers to contacting the media and pitching story ideas in hopes of obtaining editorial coverage. Writing a human-interest story about one of your clients or a client's family and then sending the story along with a photo to the media in the form of a **press release** will not only let the potential consumer know about your services, but it will also let those who may be able to offer financial assistance know as well. A press release can go to a newspaper editor, reporter, and television producers. Always keep in mind working visibility and the process of becoming a professional authority in your specialty; certainly, these are substantial facilitators to a successful private practice. Consider offering to do presentations, workshops, or seminars to parent-teacher associations, Lions or Kiwanis clubs, and community religious groups. These are excellent ways to market your program and give potential consumers a way to see how you work and to know whether they wish to engage your services. You may target some referrals in this way as well. Public service activities such as community health fairs are yet another way to interface with potential consumers and those who may wish to refer consumers to your program.

Promotional Products and Advertising

Regardless of the nature or size of your program, you will likely wish to develop a logo with accompanying business cards and letterhead/envelopes, and perhaps a brochure. You may also want to place your logo on a T-shirt for campers, on the side of a transportation van, or on "Halloween" candy wrappers that your clients give to local businesses in a marketing "reverse trick-or-treat."

Business cards (always carried with you) and brochures (distributed where your potential consumer or family/friends of the consumer will see them) should always be professional. In many ways, these may be considered as print advertising, and they are a representation of your practice.

If they are less than serious, your practice will be assumed to be less than serious. In addition, your informational materials (flyers/brochures) should not be overly dramatic and should never make claims you cannot support. At the next professional meeting you attend that includes an employment fair, pick up the brochures and carefully evaluate them. What do you like? What do you not like? What "messages" are they sending?

Some therapists put advertisements in the Yellow Pages and in newspapers (particularly neighborhood or community newspapers). Again, these must be professional. Brochures, pamphlets, or flyers made available directly to the consumer, to consumers' family members, and to other professionals from whom you may get referrals is sometimes enough to initiate a practice, particularly when startup funding is limited. Physicians will often permit other practitioners to place brochures in their reception areas (after marketing to them and with their approval, of course). A marketing/networking visit to teachers, psychologists, clergy people, and other therapists and a brochure or business card left behind may also generate referrals. Of course, you would not try to advertise in the offices of competitors, but consider whether your services can supplement or complement those of other occupational therapy practitioners (e.g., day camps to complement pediatric practices).

Once you have established programming, consider sending holiday greetings with your logo on the cover. A holiday greeting may be coupled with an end-of-the-tax-year "invitation" for dollars to support programming (such as tuition for camp attendance). If you and your clients/members go into the wider community either as part of your services or to do exhibits and community fairs, a logo on a shirt can go a long way toward making your services known. If you choose to do this, you may wish to remind your clients/members that they are your best advertisements—a very persuasive enabler for a goal of personal efficacy.

Exercise 15-1

Conceptualizing Your Program

1. Think about the program you are designing and developing. How would you like to represent it to potential consumers or other professionals? Referring again to your impact, proposed outcomes, goals, and objectives, write down a few words or phrases that sum up your program in user-friendly terms. Consider what you will do for the client/patient/member, how you will do it (your programming), and who will do it (the expertise of your staff):

_____

_____

_____

_____

_____

2. Consider now what your marketing mix will be. Will you use direct mail and/or personal distribution for brochures? Will you and your employees carry business cards? Will you create some kind of specialty advertising/promotional products? Will you use paid media advertising? Will you rely on free ink/free air? In what ways will you ensure visibility in the community? Note your ideas here:

_____

_____

_____

_____

_____

Now that you have selected your marketing mix, you may find it helpful to collect advertisements from the telephone book or newspapers or a few brochures or promotional items from organizations or professional offices that you visit in your weekly round of activities. Most professionals are finding it necessary to advertise these days. How do they conceptualize the services that they offer? Which ones do you like and why? Which ones do you not like and why?

Exercise 15-2

Developing Marketing Materials for Your Program

Based on the previous exercise, think about a logo that will symbolize your programming. Consider how it will be expressed on your letterhead, envelopes, and business cards. Before you begin, collect some examples and, with your group or colleagues, note why some appeal to you and why some do not. Is there too much information? Not enough? Do you consider the font, color, and paper quality to be professional? What might you do differently?

On a sheet of paper or on your computer, do the following:

1. Sketch some ideas for your logo.
2. Now, consider your letterhead, envelopes, and business cards. How will you use your logo? Will you use any particular terms or phrases to define your services? Sketch how you would like the letterhead, envelopes, and business card to look.
3. Draft some ideas for a brochure, highlighting your program (consider color, photos, and font style as well as the information you will include). Keep it simple, but include everything your potential consumer will need to know.

When you have formulated your ideas, go to your computer and complete the brochure.

SUMMARY

We have explored the elements of marketing a program to the community and to the potential client/consumer. Our first interests are in the "selling" of ourselves as program planners, developers, and practitioners. From this stance of personal selling, we have then gone on to identify ways in which we might promote our program. Several elements of the promotional mix have been identified; they include paid media advertising, direct mail, promotional products, and free ink/free air. We have also described low-cost ways in which we might promote our program, including doing the job well and letting others see what we do (or working visibility). Following the development of our expertise and some accumulated experience, we may also promote ourselves as authorities on a particular element of practice through the professional literature; this is also recommended as a further way of legitimizing our programs and practices. We have also developed a marketing/promotional plan that includes a logo, business card, and brochure to describe our program. With the completion of the marketing plan, we are now ready to firmly establish the timeline for the initiation of our program.

REFERENCES

Drucker, P. F. (1973). *Management, tasks, responsibilities, practices.* New York, NY: Harper and Row.

Gerson, R. F. (1991). *Writing and implementing a marketing plan.* Los Altos, CA: Crisp Publications.

Gilkeson, G. (1997). *Occupational therapy leadership: Marketing yourself, your profession, and your organization.* Philadelphia, PA: F. A. Davis.

Hiduke, G., & Ryan, J.D. (2014). *Small business: An entrepreneur's business plan* (9th ed.). Boston, MA: Cengage Learning.

Kotler, P., & Armstrong, G. (1991). *Principles of marketing* (5th ed.). Englewood Cliffs, NJ: Prentice Hall.

Mandel, D., Jackson, J., Zemke, R., Nelson, L., & Clark, F. (1999). *Lifestyle redesign: Implementing the well elderly program*. Bethesda, MD: American Occupational Therapy Association.

Orsburn, E. M. (2010). *Social media for the CEO: The why and ROI of social media for the CEO of today and tomorrow.* New York, NY: Emerging Media Press. Retrieved from www.social media for the CEO.com.

Pakroo, P. (2015). *Starting and building a nonprofit: A practical guide* (6th ed.). Berkeley, CA: Nolo Press.

Richmond, T. (2003). Marketing. In G. McCormack, E. Jaffe, & M. Goodman-Lavey (Eds.), *The occupational therapy manager* (4th ed., pp. 177-192). Bethesda, MD: American Occupational Therapy Association.

Richmond, T. (2004). Marketing plan. In T. Richmond & D. Powers (Eds.), *Business fundamentals for the rehabilitation professional* (pp. 81-97). Thorofare, NJ: SLACK Incorporated.

Ryan, J. D., Ray, R., & Hiduke, G. (1999). *Small business: An entrepreneur's plan.* Fort Worth, TX: The Dryden Press.

Scott, L. (2013). *From passion to execution: How to start and grow an effective nonprofit organization.* Boston, MA: Cengage Learning.

Shoemaker, T., & Virden, C. (1992). Marketing. In J. Bair & M. Gray (Eds.), *The occupational therapy manager* (rev. ed., pp. 123-136). Bethesda, MD: American Occupational Therapy Association.

IV

Review and Evaluation Phase

Program Evaluation
Measuring Programming Goals, Objectives, Outcomes, and Impact

---

LEARNING OBJECTIVES

1. To understand the purpose of program evaluation in achieving and maintaining quality services

2. To identify various methods that may be used to measure program effectiveness

3. To appreciate the importance of the needs assessment to program evaluation

4. To understand the link between the goals and objectives of the program and the evaluation of outcomes and impact

5. To evaluate outcome measures in earlier researched evidence-based practices with similar goals and populations

6. To distinguish between the various levels of evaluation

7. To consider the summative measurement of individual progress to facilitate the assessment of program outcomes

8. To appreciate the function of formative measures to ensure program efficiency and effectiveness

9. To explore the rationale for selecting both quantitative and qualitative measures to evaluate program outcomes and to ensure quality

10. To appreciate the value of participatory action in the development and evaluation of community programs

11. To develop an evaluation plan for the program you are designing and developing

---

Fazio, L. S. *Developing Occupation-Centered Programs With the Community, Third Edition* (pp 257-276).
© 2017 Taylor & Francis Group.

KEY TERMS

1. Program evaluation

2. Stakeholders/participants/clients

3. Utilization-focused evaluation/participatory evaluation

4. Meta-evaluation/meta-analysis; evidence-based practice

5. Program effectiveness/outcome evaluation

6. Process evaluation

7. Formative evaluation/summative evaluation

8. Efficiency evaluation/effect evaluation

9. Community needs assessment

10. Impact evaluation

11. Program theory/process theory/effect theory/impact theory

12. Baseline measures

13. Quantitative and qualitative measures of outcome

14. Pretests/post-tests

15. Program logic model

16. Project level evaluation

17. Cluster evaluation

18. Participatory action research (PAR)

19. Community-based participatory research (CBPR)

What is program evaluation and why should it be done? Patton (1987) posits that evaluations, in a broad sense, are primarily concerned with the effectiveness of programs. Evaluation is part of an ongoing cycle of program planning, implementation, and improvement—it is beginning to end. MacDonell (1996) describes **program evaluation** first of all as a "system" that is put into place "to provide information that an organization can use to improve performance to an agreed-on level that meets desired outcomes" (p. 398). Ensminger, Scaffa, and Reitz (2014) say simply that program evaluation is used to make a judgment of merit, worth, or value of a program (p. 96). Therefore, we know that program evaluation is intended to improve programming performance and that it does so in the process of meeting our desired outcomes (our goals and the accompanying objectives). Brownson (2001) reminds us that an evaluation plan is a strategy and that it is developed as part of the overall program plan. Such a plan is effective only if it is done with the input of key **stakeholders** (partners, supporters) and of course present and potential **participants** or **clients** (Brownson, 2001, p. 113). The importance of program evaluation to stakeholders is also emphasized by Bryson, Patton, and Bowman (2011), as is the reliance of the programmer/evaluator on the various stakeholder groups to help develop the essential questions for the evaluation. The evaluation will be an evaluation of individual program participants or a population that is initiated through programming goals and objectives at a formative level ("forming" the foundation for our longer-term outcome and impact measurements). This formative measurement of programmatic effects is closely causally linked to outcomes and the impact of more temporally and causally distal programmatic effects.

Evaluation of the effects of the program provides data and information that can be used to alter the program intervention to more carefully and specifically ensure that we are doing the right things to achieve the objectives and goals we have established in order to ensure our longer-term outcomes and ultimate affects.

For occupational therapy practitioners and other health care providers, the impetus for scrutinizing the effectiveness of our services began some 30 years ago with the then newly developing social programs, but it has only been in the last 10 or 15 years that evaluation has become imperative for programs to remain viable. Through our unfolding history, we have placed the provision of quality patient care at the top of our priorities and, in providing that care, we have focused our attention on the process of therapy. In many ways, this attention to process at the exclusion of outcome has created inefficiency in our treatment styles and a tendency to trust in the effectiveness of our services rather than devise ways to effectively measure those outcomes. Clearly, we need both.

The field of physical rehabilitation was perhaps most effective in the 1970s and 1980s in the refinement of outcome measures, but effective measurement of outcomes did not quite happen for psychosocial practices, and we now see the results with shrinking service provision for the mentally ill. Since much of our work in the community considers the needs of those persons with severe and persistent mental illness, it is imperative that we work to refine outcome measures and determine the most efficient programming to obtain results. If our future is to include occupation-centered, community-based programs in the areas of prevention and health maintenance, we will have an even greater challenge as we design and implement outcome measures. It is our obligation not only to be aware of the evidence that exists to support positive results of practice models, but also to contribute to this work through the publication of our designs, methods, and outcomes.

HEALTH PROGRAM EVALUATION AND PLANNING: A BRIEF HISTORY

Health program planning and program evaluation have begun to overlap in recent history. Program planning has the longer history. Rosen (1993) argued that public health planning began approximately 4000 years ago with planned cities in the Indus Valley that had covered sewers. It is difficult to argue with that. However, it is likely that the development and use of the *Healthy People* goals, best known since the late 1970s (U.S. Department of Health, Education and Welfare, 1979) and continuing to the present (U.S. Department of Health and Human Services, 2010; 2020 *Goals*), has brought the importance of public health to our attention. These agendas reflect the accelerating rate of emphasis on nationwide coordination of health promotion and disease prevention efforts and a reliance on systematic planning to achieve this coordination.

The history of evaluation, from which the evaluation of health programs grew, is far shorter than the history of planning, beginning roughly in the early 1900s (Issel, 2014). The first evaluators were educators who were interested in evaluating student progress and teaching strategies (Patton, 2008). Through the late 1960s, evaluators became interested in using goals and objectives as the basis for evaluation; they were influenced by the managerial/business trend of management by objectives (Issel, 2014). With the introduction in the 1960s of broad innovation and initiation of federal social service programs (including Medicare, Medicaid, and Head Start), the focus of evaluations shifted to establishing the merit and value of these programs. Issel (2014) notes that, in the early days of evaluating education and social programs, the results were not used in that federal health policy was not driven by whether evaluations showed the programs to be successful (pp. 6-7).

Beginning in the 1980s, a new generation of evaluations emerged; what Guba and Lincoln (1987) referred to as the *third generation of evaluations*. During this generation, evaluators began to acknowledge that they were not autonomous and that their work needed to respond to the needs of those being evaluated, thus known as the "responsiveness generation" (Guba & Lincoln, 1987, p. 203). From the work of these evaluators, several lines or approaches to evaluation have emerged; **utilization-focused evaluation** and **participatory evaluation** are perhaps the most widely known. In utilization-focused evaluation, the evaluator's primary concern is with developing an evaluation that will be used by the stakeholders (Patton, 2008). These evaluations differ from those that are focused on outcomes alone. Participatory evaluations are typically guided by an "expert" but are actually generated and conducted by those most invested in the health problem (Whitmore, 1998). Sometimes referred to as an *empowerment approach*, participatory evaluation invites a wide range of stakeholders into the activity of planning and evaluation, providing those participants with the skills and knowledge to contribute substantively to the programming activities and fostering their sense of ownership in the program. It is this approach that best supports sustainable programs, and one we favor as occupation-centered programmers.

Worthy of mention is what is described as the fourth generation, which emerged in the mid-1990s; this is **meta-evaluation**, the evaluation of evaluations conducted across similar programs (Issel, 2014). This type of evaluation is consistent with the trend across the health professions toward the use of the **meta-analysis** of existing research for the development of **evidence-based practice**.

A culture of evaluation now pervades the health services, and huge data sets are being generated and are available for use in meta-evaluations. Funders are requiring outcome evaluations and are helping programmers gain this information and skill set. United Way, a major funder of community-based programs, offers assistance with evaluation in the form of a user-friendly manual (United Way of America, 1996) that can be used by professionals and nonprofessionals in the development of basic program evaluations. The W. K. Kellogg Foundation also offers similar assistance (W. K. Kellogg Foundation, 1998).

In general, we can say that the activities constituting program planning and program evaluation are cyclical and interdependent. The activities occur more or less in stages or in sets, much as we have described the full process of program planning and implementation in this text. In general, one flows into the next. We can say that they are interdependent in that the learning, insights, and ideas that result in one phase are likely to influence decision making and actions at the next phase/stage. Most programmers would agree, however, that the processes of program planning and evaluation are messy at best, so trying to separate the phases/stages is a pedagogical approach, not the reality. Planners must be flexible and creative.

TYPES OF EVALUATIONS USED BY COMMUNITY PROGRAMMERS

Let us investigate further the different ways to evaluate **program effectiveness.** Forer describes **outcome evaluation** as the method of evaluation that "concentrates on the *results* of services, programs, treatments, or intervention strategies" (Forer, 1996, introduction). Our primary goal in all of our programming efforts is, of course, the evaluation of the effectiveness of our program—not just outcomes, but the full component of services. Weiss (1972) emphasizes that program evaluation is a broader concept than outcome evaluation and suggests that the components of program evaluation be expanded beyond outcome evaluation to include the following: needs assessment, process evaluation, program efficiency, program effectiveness, impact of the program, and outcome evaluation.

Rossi, Lipsey, and Freeman (2004) suggest that program evaluation be conducted around five main foci to include the following:

1. The full process of the needs assessment

2. The program theory

3. Actual program implementation

4. The program impact

5. Program efficiency

Formative and Summative Evaluations

In general, evaluation can be said to fall into one of two broad categories: **formative evaluation** and **summative evaluation** (Centers for Disease Control [CDC], 2008; Issel, 2014). Formative evaluations are conducted during the program development and implementation process and are useful in providing direction on how best to achieve your objective and goals. They include measurements of your objective and inform you about how to improve your programming. These assessments occur as you are "forming" your program, during the initial stages of implementation, and they continue to provide a link to your summative evaluation. Issel (2014) suggests that formative evaluations can be diagnostic, identifying early problems that can be fixed. Summative evaluations should be completed once your programs are well established and you have generated some data. They will tell you to what extent the program is achieving its goals. Summative evaluations are done at the conclusion of a program to provide a statement regarding program effectiveness (Issel, 2014). Often, summative evaluation is used to refer to both outcome and impact evaluation. Outcome evaluations generally are measurements of short- and medium-term changes in program participants that result directly from the program, such as information/knowledge and awareness, attitude change, beliefs , behavior change, etc. These then relate to the objectives and goals you have established for your participants.

Evaluating Process

We have already mentioned process evaluations that begin when the program starts. These evaluations focus on the degree to which the program has been implemented as planned and often on the quality of the implementation. These can be considered formative evaluations as well. The framework for designing the **process evaluation** comes from the process theory component of the overall program theory selected during the planning phase. The theory or theories you have selected to guide your programming has provided you with general programming ideas, sometimes the actual programming activities and resources, and the interventions that are needed to achieve the health and/or behavior/knowledge change in the program participants or recipients. The selected theories may also have provided you with assessments that helped you establish programming goals and objectives and can be used to measure individual and, perhaps, group progress.

In addition, you may choose to do **efficiency evaluations** to examine the costs and benefits of a program in terms of quality of operations and the outcomes produced. Efficiency evaluations often include staffing and daily operations. In general, all information gleaned from the evaluation of process is used to plan, revise, and/or improve the program.

There is another type of evaluation that is intended to determine the effect of the program—to demonstrate or identify a program's effect on those who participated. According to Issel (2014), **effect evaluations** answer the basic question, "Did the program make a difference?" (p. 20). In this respect, and with some guiding theories that may be selected by the occupational therapy influenced programmer such as those supporting engagement in occupation, these may look much like process evaluations, and they are often used to revise the program as well. Effect evaluations, though, are more commonly used as outcome or impact evaluations than for ongoing process (Issel, 2014, p. 20).

It is timely to revisit the evidence you have gleaned to support the goals, objectives, structure, and content of your programming. In the evidence-based practices you reviewed, what outcome measures were used to determine effectiveness? Are these appropriate for your circumstances? Using similar measures of effectiveness and reaching similar results will strengthen your programming and options for continued or new funding. Karsh and Fox (2003, 2014) and Knowles (2002), in discussions of program evaluation for successful grant applications, consider two levels of evaluation. The first level is evaluation of program implementation, or process (i.e., carefully reviewing and evaluating what you have done). Issel (2014) also discusses the evaluation of "process" to determine the extent to which the program is being provided as planned, as mentioned previously. This process evaluation can be thought of as a formative evaluation, as you are fine-tuning what you have done thus far. The data and findings from the process evaluation are key feedback items in the planning and evaluation cycle; they can (and perhaps should) lead to revisions in the program delivery. As an example, the CDC (2008) offers a discussion of process evaluation in tobacco use prevention and control. The second level of evaluation, then, is that of program outcome and impact. What differences has the program made? This is a strong indication that you have reduced the "need."

Needs Assessment as Evaluation

Issel (2014) lists several types of activities classified as evaluations (pp. 19-22). A **community needs assessment** can be described as a type of evaluation that is intended to collect data about the health/social problems of a particular group. Programs cannot happen unless there is a clear, agreed-upon understanding and definition of "the problem" the program is to address. This is the purpose of needs assessments. In this text, you are encouraged to approach the community needs assessment as a way to further verify the need you often initially identified based on a review of pertinent literature. The on-site data you retrieve are then used to verify what you have learned from the development of your profiles and to include new information that is used to build a program specific to the needs and distinctive characteristics of the members of the selected community as well as the stakeholders to obtain the "just right fit" between the population and the programming. This text approaches the learning of programming in this way so that the classroom environment can support the process as you become accustomed to community programming; however, you should be keenly aware that approaching the needs assessment in this way, rather than beginning directly with the community, permits an opportunity for bias in that the programmer may make assumptions that are not appropriate to the needs of this particular community. A careful and unbiased assessment of need as reflected by your specific community members and stakeholders is always an important early phase and cannot be dismissed. Over the course of a program's life, additional needs assessments may be done to ensure currency in programming choices and the continuous matching between goals, objectives, and outcomes.

Summative Measures: Outcomes and Impact

Impact evaluation is a summative measure that determines the ultimate impact you wish to see when the outcomes are determined. Impact measures are community-level changes or longer-term results (i.e., changes in disease risk status, morbidity, and mortality) that have occurred as a result of the program/intervention. These impacts are the net effects on the entire school, community, city, organization, society, or environment. Although it is beyond the scope of this text, you will want to be aware of the field of health programming and evaluation study that attempts to chart the path between program outcomes and impacts. To serve this effort, **program theory** is advocated by a number of authors including Issel (2014), Rossi et al. (2004), and Potvin, Gendron, Bilodeau, and Chabot (2005). Program theory, like any theory, attempts to explain how something works. It is used to make sense of the relationship among variables; thus, a program theory is a conceptual plan with some details about what the program is and how it is expected to work (Issel, 2014, p. 182). We are selecting various theories (occupational therapy and others) to explain and predict the relationship between our programming objectives, our goals, and specific interventions. Think of this theory selection process as one of the building blocks toward the overall program theory. As mentioned earlier, the portion of program theory related to resources and actions is called the **process**

theory, and the theory about intervention and outcomes is called **effect theory**. You will recognize the similarity between program theory and the logic model; however, program theory as compared with a logic model offers a more explicit explanation of the relationship of the factors related to the health problem with the intervention (Issel, 2014, pp. 182-183). **Impact theory** is one element of effect theory and explains how the outcomes lead to impacts. Impact theory helps substantiate the sometimes wishful claims of program planners about the effects of their program by specifying the relationship between the immediate outcome of the program and the long-term, ultimate changes to the health problem (Issel, 2014, p. 200). Funding agencies commonly specify program impacts, and you will look for this when you review their requests for proposals. An example might be a reduction in infant mortality or a reduction in the incidence of juvenile diabetes. You can see that these problems are complex, so it is possible to have multiple impact theories for one long-range impact, especially if multiple intervention theories and interventions are used in one program. Sometimes, these impacts might be stated as program goals that the funded programs are to achieve. In these cases, the programmer works backward to determine programming. If you would like to learn more about program theory, the resources that Issel (2014) has referenced are recommended.

Outcome evaluations focus on the more immediate effects of the program, although this varies from months to years; impact evaluations have a more long-term focus over several years. As mentioned previously, these evaluations are often referred to as *summative evaluations*, indicating that they occur at the conclusion of a program. These are contrasted with formative evaluations, which are conducted earlier in the program's implementation. There is some confusion in the literature and the workplace over these terms and their meaning, so it is always a good idea to clarify with your stakeholders.

One final evaluation for discussion is the **meta-evaluation**. This evaluation is done by combining the findings from the previous outcome evaluations of various programs targeting the same health concern. The purpose is to gain insights into which of the various programmatic approaches has had the most effect. This type of evaluation relies on the use of a specific set of methodological and statistical procedures and is usually conducted by evaluation researchers, not programmers.

If you have worked with the guidelines of the Commission on Accreditation of Rehabilitation Facilities/Rehabilitation Accreditation Commission (CARF) or the Joint Commission on Accreditation of Healthcare Organizations, you know that these organizations place a great deal of emphasis on outcomes. CARF documents define program evaluation as "a systematic procedure for determining the effectiveness and efficiency with which results are achieved by persons served during the service delivery phase and following program completion as well as the individual's satisfaction with them" (CARF, 1995, p. 2). We have not discussed participant satisfaction as an evaluation measure, but we do measure it under what we are describing as marketing and our accompanying marketing surveys of satisfaction.

In these evaluations, the program's performance is always measured against the goals and objectives established by the planner or planning group. Therefore, the careful, accurate, and early expression of the goal and the objectives coupled with a well-articulated and comprehensive plan to achieve them will not only provide accurate guidelines for measurement of outcomes, but also ensure that those outcomes compare favorably with the intent of the planner and with other similar programs.

What Are Your Evaluation Options?

Evaluation plans are specific to the program and the kinds of evidence one needs to collect. There are many ways to collect data. The first approach, though, is to maintain records of the program. You will need to track participation, including the numbers of participants. In some cases, you may even track hits on the program website. The data you will track in your record keeping are based on the goals of the program, the objectives you have established to meet those goals, and the specific measurements required by the evaluation plan (Doll, 2010, p. 285). We may want to use surveys or questionnaires to record such things as reported behavior change (i.e., increases in exercise participation or changes in diet).

Ultimately, we would expect that our programs will have an effect on the health and well-being of the individual program participants. Certainly, one cannot design a program with accompanying goals and objectives without considering the needs of the client/participant. Those needs collectively provide the basis for the program. All of our programs deliver services to a client/participant group and, for most programs, monitoring individual process and progress provides us with incremental measures that ultimately contribute to our evaluation of the program's effectiveness. Thus, formative measures benefit the progress of the participants and the "process" of programming. Simply, these measures allow us to know how the group is responding to the objectives and goals of the program, and to the programming itself. These formative measures are then coupled with summative measures that occur at the end of a programming cycle. Beyond tracking attendance, numbers of participants, and additional record-keeping data, we will also want to consider other evaluation methods.

You may wish to consider such evaluation methods as (1) results of observations; (2) analyses of focus groups; (3) individual interviews; (4) participant and staff reflections/narratives and stories; (5) case analysis; (6) content analysis of agendas, training, and meeting minutes; and (7) video/ photography. Satisfaction surveys are sometimes recommended; however, as mentioned previously, these have more meaning as a marketing tool than as an evaluation measure. Certainly, you want your participants to like the program and to enjoy the interventions; we might assume that this will keep them attending; however, for our evaluation, we want to show achievement of goals and objectives.

You may wish to develop your own evaluation instruments based on the goal and objectives of your program. In some cases, you also may choose to purchase evaluation instruments for individual participants that are designed to accompany the theoretical orientation or model you have selected to guide your programming. You may need to research what is available for your population and your theory/model and what will meet the needs structured by your objectives and goal. Some assessments can be copied from texts or articles, while others are restricted. An excellent resource is Asher's (2007) *Occupational Therapy Assessment Tools: An Annotated Index.* You may wish to review this text and others should you consider individual evaluation of clients/patients as part of your formative and/or summative program evaluation process.

Your decision regarding individual assessments will be based on what the results of these will tell you about the effectiveness of your program. Your program evaluation is linked to the progress your individual clients make, so some consistent **baseline measure** of their performance must be made; the points where you will begin to monitor the impact of your programming or the outcomes. In some instances, that measure will be made by other agencies/practitioners and you will need to access the information.

For example, if we are providing day camp services for children who are currently being seen by other therapists, we might assume that these children have already been evaluated. There is no need for us to further evaluate each child (at least not in the same way). Certainly, we would collaborate with the therapist who is continuing to see the child or perhaps sees the child through a school year; we would have initiated this process with the needs assessment. The camp will provide intervention to enhance the treatment the child is receiving from the referring therapist and to assist in meeting the therapist's goals for the child. In addition, the camp experience might supplement the child's individual therapy with opportunities to learn socialization through structured group play.

In this example, you might wish to go further and consider establishing baseline measures and continuing formative and summative measures around the goal of socialization/ group play. Certainly, your marketing efforts for such a camp would be enhanced if you could demonstrate indicators of success in addition to what you expect the child's primary therapist might identify.

In some kinds of programs, a structured interview may also be used to establish a baseline assessment. You would likely establish the interview format yourself, which certainly would be based on your goal and on your chosen theory or model.

OTHER MEASURES TO CONSIDER

In many of the programs described in this text, there is no individual measurement of progress, as we may be accustomed to in our traditional occupational therapy models of evaluation and intervention, but we are always aware of the progress of individuals and that their goals and objectives are reflective of and companion to those of the program. For example, a program goal may target the development of moral judgment in adolescents as they transition to young adulthood. The goal may specifically target the development of skills to negate lawbreaking in the community. Accompanying objectives may focus on skills to find work and a residence or perhaps the provision of opportunity to explore and engage in alternative meaningful occupations. All of these objectives are measurable and all are related to outcomes. Not all of the adolescents participating in such a program may be successful in the attainment of each objective, and they may not all accomplish the goal; however, it is important to remember that a program may still be successful even if all of the participants are not. In some cases, we will establish a measure of objective attainment at 80% of the participants; in some cases, perhaps 100% can be realistic. We know that simple pre- and post-tests can begin to measure acquired information and perhaps skill acquisition. Frequently, though, we attach further measurement to information and skill acquisition through monitoring such things as employability, graduation from school, and perhaps reports of delinquency or lawbreaking. Intermediate measures to get at changes enroute to other outcomes such as the measurement of efficacy, locus of control, perceived well-being, and life satisfaction are helpful to see if our theoretical model supports anticipated outcomes.

Mandel, Jackson, Zemke, Nelson, and Clark (1999) utilized several measures of primary outcomes in the USC Well Elderly Research Study. Utilizing a pre-/post-test format with follow-up 6 months following completion of the programming, several instruments and measures were selected. The overall intent of programming was to improve health and slow aging-related declines in the elderly. Selected measures were the Functional Status Questionnaire (Jette & Cleary, 1987); Life Satisfaction Index-Z (Wood, Wylie, & Sheafor, 1969), Center for Epidemiologic Studies (CES) Depression Scale (Radloff, 1977), Medical Outcomes Study (MOS) Short Forms General Health Survey (Stewart, Hays, & Ware, 1988; Ware & Sherbourne, 1992), and RAND 36-Item Health Status Survey (Hays, Sherbourne, & Mazel, 1993). Collectively, these measures provided a comprehensive picture of the general health and well-being of the participants in the clinical trial before programming and following programming. The RAND SF-36 is particularly useful in measuring responses to much of our adult programming with populations seeking to maintain wellness and health. It is a self-report measure of health-related quality of life designed to measure health status efficiently from the consumer's perspective (Mandel et al., 1999, pp. 57-58; McHorney, Ware, & Raczek, 1993). The RAND SF-36 groups question items into eight domains: general health, mental health, physical functioning, social functioning, role limitations attributable to physical health problems, role limitations attributable to emotional problems, bodily pain, and vitality.

The best way to evaluate the objectives and, ultimately, the goal of your program is to ask yourself the following questions: How will I know if that actually happens, and when and how will I measure it when it does? All programs must be able to evaluate effectiveness in order to justify their continued existence. Such evaluation of process and outcome will not only justify their continuation, but also provide the information that is needed to continue to improve the match between the goal, objectives, and programming. This is the primary function of formative evaluation and provides the foundation for summative/outcome evaluation. The day-to-day program enables you to meet the program objectives and, ultimately, the goal. If objectives are not being met, then alterations, adjustments, and fine-tuning may be made in day-to-day programming. If the goal is not satisfied, then likely these adjustments are required in the objectives as well. As we have indicated, there are several dimensions or tiers of measurement needed to fully evaluate a program. We begin program evaluation by determining just what the dimensions are within which we will establish the measures of program success.

Measuring Outcomes in a Head Start Program for Children

To provide an example of outcome measurement in an occupation-centered, community-based program, we will highlight a program established to support the mission and goals of Head Start. As you may know, Head Start is a federally mandated program designed to aid preschool children in the attainment of skills that have been determined to be necessary for successful achievement when they enter school. Children who qualify for Head Start programs are those considered to be at risk with regard to lower economic status, some level of involvement with social services/child protective services, or physical and/or emotional disabilities.

The Head Start program was initiated with the community and population profiles followed by the needs assessments. The mission and philosophy of the Head Start program was discussed with the director and teaching staff of the selected site. In this first phase of needs assessment, which also included teachers in the district schools these children would attend, several unmet needs were identified that were appropriate for occupation-centered programming. The teachers expressed a strong desire to assist parents in assuming the role of prime educator of their child. Through this process, they would help to identify potential problems the child might be experiencing. They specifically identified the need for fine-motor/prewriting skill development and the additional need for early screening to determine which children might require more specific intervention before they entered school as opposed to those who might benefit from a little extra help in school or at home. In the focus group utilized for phase II (the later phase of the needs assessment) and performance skills deficits assessment, parents were concerned that they did not know what behaviors they should look for in their child that might present problems in school. If they did suspect problems, they did not know what to do about them. All parents concurred that they would like to help their child be ready for school if they knew what to do.

The goal of the program was essentially the same as that of the larger organization: to enhance the children's successful entry into school through parent-teacher-child teamwork. The ultimate impact would be a success measure perhaps of high school graduation and college admission.

The objectives to enable the accomplishment of the program goal mentioned previously were as follows:

1. The parents and teachers will be provided with information and activities to assist them in identifying deficits in the child's development that may indicate potential problems in school.

2. The parents and teachers will be provided with games and activities to engage in with children to encourage the development of fine-motor/prewriting skills.

3. Early developmental screening by occupational therapy practitioners will be conducted to assist in determining which children may require more extensive assessment and intervention.

The program provided a number of training sessions to parents and to teachers. Materials were developed to meet the needs of both groups in their efforts to help their children prepare for school. In addition, home and Head Start program visits and observations by occupational therapy practitioners and occupational therapy students assisted both parents and teachers in learning to identify potential problems. These visits were coupled with developmental screening of each child in the Head Start program. This program provided what might be considered both indirect and direct services. In community programming (perhaps in all occupation-centered programming), it is important to provide services that will empower the recipient and the family to share in meeting the responsibilities required to satisfy the program goal.

INITIATING PROGRAM EVALUATION

Now that we have our goal and objectives and we have conducted the program for a short period of time, we must ask ourselves the following process questions: Is the program effective? Does it do what we think it does? What about the mechanics of the programming, our methods? Is our staffing pattern effective? Are we utilizing our supplies and equipment effectively and efficiently? This is the point where changes can and often should be made. We may want to try a preliminary measure of the relationship between the objectives we have established and our goals. If our objectives are accurate in their expression of our goal and if they are measurable, we will have no problems in accomplishing this phase of evaluation.

To return to our example, there were three objectives for the Head Start occupation-centered program. All three objectives are measurable:

1. Parents and teachers *will be provided with information and activities* to assist them in identifying deficits in the child's development that may indicate potential problems in school.

2. The parents and teachers *will be provided with games and activities* to participate in with children to encourage the development of fine-motor/prewriting skills.

3. *Early developmental screening by occupational therapy practitioners will be conducted* to assist in determining which children may require more extensive assessment and intervention.

Regardless of the parameters of time established (such as 1 month, 6 months, 1 year, etc.), we should be able to measure these objectives. Did we provide the parents and teachers with information and activities to assist them in identifying deficits in the child's development that may indicate potential problems in school? Did we provide parents and teachers with games and activities to participate in with children to encourage the development of fine-motor/prewriting skills? Did we provide early developmental screening by occupational therapy practitioners to assist in determining which children may require more extensive assessment and intervention?

Even though we always begin formative evaluation by measuring the objectives established for our program, this alone is not enough. Even if we can clearly answer yes to all of the objectives, we really know nothing about the effectiveness or success of our program. We simply know that our program has provided the services that we promised. A positive evaluation of an objective that is designed to measure the dissemination of information and materials is only as meaningful as the quality of the materials and the mode of dissemination. Our professional knowledge, skills, and experience contribute to our clinical reasoning in helping us to provide the programming (the information and materials) that will be effective.

Recall our example of the Denver sanctuary program introduced in Chapter 7. The goal of encouraging self-efficacy was enabled through an objective of providing developmentally appropriate information and skills with which to make informed choices about practiced sexual behaviors. As was mentioned previously, this is very different than simply offering condoms. The success of this program is contingent on all of the embedded "clues" known to occupation-centered practitioners. By linking efficacy to cognitive and moral development and to the expression of sexuality as occupation, our clinical reasoning guides us to arrive at a program that is far more than providing information and skills; rather, we can provide information and skills that result in the program's success.

Exercise 16-1

The First Step in Formative Program Evaluation: Measuring Objectives

1. Considering the previous examples, discuss with your classmates or colleagues ideas for how you will measure the program you are designing. We are thinking now about the evaluation that occurs after or alongside formative measures of process. We can measure objectives as an early process measure to provide information about the effectiveness of our program, followed by program changes that may need to be made. Later, measures of objectives will be considered in summative data. Revisit your goal or goals and your objectives. In the space provided, write the goal or goals for your program, your objectives to support your goal, and the time you have established for measurement.

Your goal:

_____

_____

_____

_____

_____

Your objectives:

_____

_____

_____

_____

_____

Re-examine the evidence gleaned in your early literature reviews and the research that you used to support your programming model. What measures of outcome were used? Were individual assessments/measures utilized in gathering outcome data? Consider whether you will use individual assessments and, if so, what you will use. Will you be able to obtain baseline assessment data for your population from other sources?

For each of your objectives, determine the quantitative measures that you will utilize:

_____

_____

_____

_____

_____

Clearly, the first step in evaluating any program is to meet the objectives we have established as our first line of measurement. These first measures are **quantitative**; that is, we determine who received the services and how often. Without first knowing that everyone has received the services specified in our objectives, we cannot go further to determine additional quantitative measures and/or the **qualitative measures** necessary to evaluate whether our services met our expectations and were therefore effective.

However, the question of how we measure the outcomes to determine whether the program is effective still remains. Earlier, we listed several methods—both quantitative and qualitative—we can use to accomplish this task. One commonly used method to determine simple programming effectiveness is the pre- and post-test.

By carefully logging contact hours with parents and teachers and by videotaping the informational meetings, it was clear that the foundation (the quantitative measure) of the first two objectives for the Head Start program had been satisfied (27 parents and 4 teachers had received the information).

Over the course of 6 weeks, all of the children (23) had been screened to determine if any of them might require more extensive assessment and intervention. Following review of the screening results, six children were referred for further occupational therapy assessment.

Following review of the three objectives that were established, it was determined that the third objective required no further evaluation. There were no qualitative measures required to further assess this objective as it was written. In fact, it is arguable whether this objective relates to the goal for the program, which was "to enhance the children's successful entry into school through parent-teacher-child teamwork." Although nothing in this objective directly relates to parent-teacher-child teams, there is certainly an assumption that early screening and any resultant intervention will enhance the child's successful transition to school. In any further work with this program and to ensure funding for this objective, it would be necessary to evaluate this assumption through extensive literature review and by following each child's progress in school either by single case or compared to children who did not receive assessment and intervention.

THE USE OF PRETESTS AND POST-TESTS

When we use the term *outcome*, we are referring to the results that were obtained near the completion of our program and, perhaps, at intervals after programming has ceased for the participant. However, as we have indicated previously, one cannot measure the result of a program, or a treatment for that matter, without first obtaining some kind of base measurement. If we were to use this method in our Head Start example, at the first meeting of parents, teachers, and occupational therapy practitioners, a brief **pretest** or questionnaire would be developed and administered to determine how much the teachers (one group) and parents (one group) knew about the developing child generally, how much they knew about the identification of potential deficits, and how much they knew about the development of fine motor skills related to prewriting specifically.

For our example, the pretest would ask specific questions regarding the developmental markers for fine motor coordination in children between the ages of 3 and 4 years (the ages of the children in the program). A video might be used in conjunction with the questionnaire to provide examples of motor skills.

The same questionnaire/test (a **post-test**) would be given following the in-service or series of in-services. The comparison of responses to the pre- and post-tests provides a further marker for how successful the intervention (the in-service) was in meeting the objective of providing information, games, and activities. Our post-test will also provide us with information regarding how effective we were in developing materials that were appropriate to the needs of each group (parents and teachers). From this information, we could return to the materials and the way they were provided to make necessary changes to enhance their receptivity.

Since the first objective of our example suggests that the information we provide will assist the parent and teacher to identify any deficits in the child's development that may indicate potential problems in school, we would want to evaluate whether this happened or not in order to further ensure the effectiveness of our program. We might do so by asking the parents and teachers to note any deficits they observe on a chart or check sheet. This information might then be correlated with the results of the occupational therapy practitioner's screening. Positive correlations would add further strength to the results provided by this objective. If these correlations were not found, then we might wish to return to our programming to determine how our process might be more effective. Stronger and more definitive research designs might also be employed to measure the effectiveness of this program.

Meeting the second objective goes beyond the quantitative measure of providing games and activities and assumes participation by the parent-teacher-child to encourage the development of fine-motor prewriting skills. To provide a valid measurement of this objective, each child's fine-motor prewriting skills would need to be measured before the program (pretest) and again following the program (post-test). Although these tests would not provide enough information to definitively say that our program supported improvement in these skills, such test results could strongly suggest such a finding, particularly if we had measures of normative parent-child or teacher-child participation in our suggested games and activities.

Revisiting Programming Goals

It is wise to continue to revisit our goal to be sure that our evaluation of objectives has not caused us to become blind to our purpose. Although the objectives for our case example are sound and do relate clearly to the goal, it is likely that we will want to have one or two more. None of the objectives truly address the idea of teams mentioned in our goal and, as indicated in earlier chapters, teams can be empowering. Teamwork assumes a sharing of responsibility and equal distribution of rewards. Without a specific objective, we do not know whether we have established programming that will encourage the formation of teams or the philosophies and ideas that support teamwork. Without such an objective, the child appears to be the targeted "problem" in this program rather than a shareholder in the outcome. Although not formally tied to an objective, videotaping all aspects of the program offered a potential opportunity to qualitatively evaluate the formation of teams from the early stages of program design through actual programming, and the elements of teamwork did emerge. You might like to write an objective that would target the development of parent-child-teacher teams to help us more fully support our goal. Our goal also uses the subjective term *successful* to describe the desired transition from Head Start to school. Our objectives translate the results of our needs assessment into the skills we believe to be necessary for this transition to successfully occur. The results of the needs assessment also identified the need for children to be socialized to the school environment before actually entering it, although we did not develop an objective to meet this need. Can you suggest one?

Exercise 16-2

Going Beyond Quantitative Measures to Measure Quality

1. Again review your objectives and your goals. Are there further measures you will need to make in order to determine the effectiveness of your program? How will you measure the quality of your program? First, consider other quantitative measures and then more qualitative ones. Note what additional measures you will require here:

_____

_____

_____

_____

_____

2. Do you have a mode of measurement for every aspect of your objectives? Will the results of these measures determine whether you have met the goals for your program? Will they help you determine if changes in programming may be necessary? Make notations here for any alterations you may need to make now:

_____

_____

_____

_____

_____

3. What are some ideas for further process evaluation measures that you might use to determine if your program is operating efficiently and effectively? Note them here:

_____

_____

_____

_____

_____

Continuing program evaluation at whatever interval you've determined—3 months, 6 months, yearly, or all of these—will also be the time you re-evaluate your goals. Even a year is likely too soon to question the original goals (assuming your needs assessment was accurate), but it is not too soon to make changes in objectives and/or programming. This is what process evaluation is about and the time devoted to it varies by program. This will also be the time to evaluate staffing, costs, and the program environment. How do these factors impact the quantity and quality of your intervention? Most federal granting agencies expect at least yearly outcome reports and provide the program a 2- or 3-year running period before reapplying for continuation. This offers a reasonable time to measure outcomes and make minor alterations in programming. Consider, too, repeating your phases of needs assessment as a way of evaluating the connection between need, your goals, and your program design. You may wish to conduct a focus group as a qualitative measure of program effectiveness whether you used this technique in assessing need or not. Such a group can provide a strong measure of how you are doing. A focus group of parents and one of teachers would be extremely useful as a formative or a summative measure for our Head Start example. There may be other stakeholders to consider and others interested in our outcomes. In our example, the federal government is a significant participant/stakeholder. Let us take a moment to consider who may be interested in our program outcomes and impact.

WHO WILL USE PROGRAM EVALUATION RESULTS?

In our initial planning, it was suggested that the W. K. Kellogg Foundation logic model (or another of your choice) be used as an early planning instrument (W. K. Kellogg Foundation, 2001, 2004). This instrument permitted us to think broadly, and long-term about what difference we hoped to make (our impact), what outcomes we wished to have, and how to link all of the program planning phases to the proposed "impact" and the evaluation outcomes. As we are anticipating how we will measure outcomes, we will also think about exactly who will use our evaluation data and how. The usefulness of an evaluation depends on the extent to which questions that need to be answered are, in fact, answered. Evaluation results, for the most part, are used by our stakeholders. In defining and identifying our stakeholders, we will determine what they need and want to know, and for what purpose.

Issel (2014) suggests that one of our significant stakeholder groups is the funding organization. By using the W. K. Kellogg Foundation Model for early guidance, we can easily see that program evaluation is important to them and, by reviewing the programs they've funded, we can see their funding priorities. We can do the same by reviewing other funding sources, federal agencies, and private foundations.

Some funders use process evaluations to determine program accountability and longer-term evaluations for determining program effectiveness toward meeting broader initiatives and outcomes. Of course effectiveness is important to you, as a planner, and to your staff as a basis to seek further funding as well as for making improvements to your program.

Community action groups, community members, and program participants and recipients (and their families) form a significant group of stakeholders. This stakeholder group is most likely to advocate for a community health assessment and to use process evaluation results (including evaluation of community asset building) as a basis for seeking additional resources, or to hold the program accountable. There may be other stakeholders, such as policymakers and scholars and health professionals, but for much of our work (at least for novice planners), the first three stakeholder groups listed previously are likely most important.

OUTCOMES OVER TIME

It is often of interest and/or critical to determine if your program has lasting effectiveness—effectiveness after the program has been terminated for the participant. We have alluded to this in our Head Start case example with the recommendation that the children be followed through their school experience to effectively determine whether we have enhanced their progress and success. Evaluation over time is more difficult to achieve and will require more manpower and financial resources than formative and summative short- and mid-term evaluations. A long-term follow-up evaluation will require a system to track participants and a set of measures related to your original goals. If follow-up effectiveness seems critical to what you want to achieve, then your original goal(s) should state the follow-up outcomes as well as the immediate measures of success. If you initiated your planning with a logic model, you have already considered the impact you want your program results to achieve. Perhaps you have already included the specifics of evaluation on your timeline.

If you intend to manage numerous outcome measures, particularly over time, you will need an effective data management system to do so. Forer (1996) also offers a substantial reference section that provides a list of publications describing programming in a variety of disability areas as well as outcome evaluation techniques appropriate to differing kinds of programming. Review the discussion of sample programs in Part V for examples of program evaluation plans and instruments.

Exercise 16-3

Measuring Impact

1. Revisit your logic model. What is the impact you wish to make? Remember that impact is long-term and at the community level. Note the impact (large-scale change) you want to make here:

_____

_____

_____

_____

_____

2. What are some measures that might be used to determine this impact?

_____

_____

_____

_____

TRACKING PRESENT AND FUTURE TRENDS IN PROGRAM DEVELOPMENT AND EVALUATION

There is little doubt that our present emphasis on establishing programs that ensure successful outcomes will continue, and with more expectation of rigor than ever before. We have already devoted a substantial portion of this chapter to a discussion of outcome measurement and attention to program impact. Outcomes and funding will not likely ever be separated. The W. K. Kellogg Foundation has been a strong proponent of outcomes evaluation for some time. The Foundation identified their core mission in this way: "to help people help themselves through the practical application of knowledge and resources to improve their quality of life and that of future generations" (2001, 2004, introduction). In line with its core mission, the Foundation made evaluation a priority as early as 1998.

In Chapter 4, we introduced the use of a **program logic model** as a helpful planning instrument for the programmer. The W. K. Kellogg Foundation's recent guide to evaluation is designed to assist programmers in the use of this program logic model to facilitate evaluation. The program logic model is defined as "a picture of how your organization does its work…the theory and assumptions underlying the program…such a model links both short and long-term outcomes with program activities/processes and the theoretical assumptions/principles of the program" (W. K. Kellogg Foundation, 2001, 2004, introduction). The approach to programming described in this text (need, goal, objectives, theory) establishes a sound foundation to layer the language of a logic approach to evaluation.

As you may recall, in its simplest form, the logic model begins with a picture of your program (the multiple profiles, the structure, the programming). This picture includes your theoretical base and your rationale for why your approach, and what you put into the program (action-inputs), will result in an anticipated outcome (outputs). This is a sequence of "if-then" relationships and may be considered the core of planning and evaluation. Outputs, then, are a result of what we do (activities) and who we do it for (participation). Outcomes, according to the logic model, are what results for individual participants, for organizations, and, ultimately, for communities.

The foundation recommends evaluation at three levels. The **project level** is where we have focused in this text, measuring the effectiveness of our specific programming as efficiently as we can. The second level is **cluster evaluation**, or aggregating outcomes of projects with similar goals across the country to monitor change. The third is to use the levels of outcome measurement to influence policy making (W. K. Kellogg Foundation, 1998, p. 14).

The planner may choose differing approaches to utilization of the logic model. The theory approach models emphasize the theory of change that has influenced the design and plan for the program. The outcomes approach models focus on the early aspects of program planning and attempt to connect the resources and/or activities with the desired results in a program. These models likely measure change (outcomes prompted by a given set of activities) over time: short-term (1 to 3 years), long-term (4 to 6 years), and impact (7 to 10 years) (W. K. Kellogg Foundation, 2001, pp. 9-10). The activities approach models pay the most attention to the details and specifics of the implementation process. These models describe what a program intends to do and, as such, are most useful for the purpose of program monitoring and management. You are encouraged to visit the W. K. Kellogg Foundation website and others listed at the close of the chapter for current information on evaluation, particularly as it is linked to potential funding of programs.

Participatory Action Research

Participatory action research (PAR), in fact, informs several sections of this text. It is placed here because it can be extremely useful as a method/process to support program evaluation; however, as an extension of empowerment theory, it informs much of our goal development in community-based practices. PAR is particularly well suited to community intervention as it involves consumer participation, power, and leadership. It can inform the development, implementation, and evaluation of services (Reason & Bradbury, 2001; Suarez-Balcazar, Martinez, & Casa-Byots, 2005; Taylor, Braveman, & Hammel, 2004). This method of research grew out of community development work in developing countries (in particular, Latin America and Africa). PAR has been a central methodology to both rural and urban development in the third world for more than two decades. Huizer (1997) describes projects to enhance people's participation in development on their own behalf in Thailand, Sri Lanka, Zambia, and Sierra Leone.

PAR is an advocacy tool for a grassroots, bottom-up approach to community development that purposefully incorporates participation from disenfranchised or marginalized groups in society—the poor, minorities of all kinds, women, and children (Green & Haines, 2016; Huizer, 1997). Participation involves researchers, funders, and communities—both the people who are researched and the people whom the research is for. Action refers to the researcher's involvement in real projects with participants; working with people in their communities to create change. In this method of research, communities develop the goals, help collect the data, are involved in analyzing the data, and interpret the results (Green & Haines, 2016).

Community-based participatory research (CBPR) is intended to "create an effective translational process that will improve population health and increase connections with members of underserved communities" (Hacker, 2013, prospectus xi). Reason and Bradbury provide this definition: "Action research, as a method, may be described as a participatory, democratic process concerned with developing practical knowing in the pursuit of worthwhile human purposes" (Reason & Bradbury, 2001, introduction). Such a method seeks to bring together action and reflection and theory and practice in participation with others. It can be described as a practical method because it seeks solutions to practical problems (what people grapple with every day of their lives) and, in fact, practical problem solving is the venue of community practitioners. "Community" implies people mutually involved in identifying problems and seeking solutions to solve them. First identifying and then solving problems requires collective action—sharing strategies, information, and skills. Thus, participatory action is the crux, whether it contributes to the development of a community-based program and/or the evaluation as well as contributing to the research base for scaffolding further understanding and inquiry.

It is with somewhat these same interests that the programming descriptions shared by Kronenberg, Algado, and Pollard (2005) offer us examples of a kind of community practice driven exclusively by the expressed needs of the people involved. The practitioner is there to provide what is needed to help people (empower them) to solve their own problems and to provide guidance, encouragement, information, skills training, and effective ways to disassemble the bureaucracies. Is this not what all community practices should be?

Occupational therapy practitioners are also using participatory action methods in community programming, evaluation, and research. Taylor et al. (2004) describe their recent work utilizing this approach with two case examples: one with persons who have chronic fatigue syndrome, and the other with persons who have AIDS. As in other successful participatory action approaches, services and outcomes were consumer-driven and relevant. Participants in both projects were empowered to "recognize, use, and build upon their existing resources to accomplish their goals" (Taylor et al., 2004, p. 81).

Addressing the needs of an underserved Hispanic population in the Midwest represents the PAR of Suarez-Balcazar et al. (2005). Community residents participated in five public forums or focus groups intended to elicit needs, establish action agendas, and brainstorm solutions to address health and community needs that included the lack of affordable bilingual dentists and youth involvement in gangs, drugs, and alcohol (Suarez-Balcazar et al., 2005, p. 146).

Both of these examples emphasize the collaborative relationship between participant and practitioner. Both groups broadened their skills and knowledge through participation/action.

SUMMARY

This chapter has provided the rationale for program evaluation. The reader is reminded to always link the goal or goals of the program and the objectives to the evaluation of outcome. Program evaluation is not only necessary to determine the effectiveness of a program, but it can also provide a measure of the quality of the programming. Both measures of effectiveness and quality are necessary to enhance the successful future of a program and often are necessary to guarantee its continuation. These measures will also provide information with regard to the effectiveness of your staffing and the impact of your intervention environment and may also help you to re-evaluate costs. You have also been introduced to various tools and approaches for measuring outcomes as well as present and future trends in evaluation measures. A brief history of health-related program evaluation and planning is offered to provide you with a foundation for how this evaluation process fits the larger picture.

REFERENCES

Asher, E. (2007). *Occupational therapy assessment tools: An annotated index* (3rd ed.). Bethesda, MD: American Occupational Therapy Association.

Brownson, C. (2001). Program development for community health: Planning, implementation, and evaluation strategies. In M. Scaffa (Ed.), *Occupational therapy in community based practice settings* (pp. 95-118). Philadelphia, PA: Davis.

Bryson, J. M., Patton, M. Q., & Bowman, R. A. (2011). Working with evaluation stakeholders: A rationale, step-wise approach, and toolkit. *Evaluation and Program Planning, 34*(1), 1-12.

Centers for Disease Control and Prevention. (2008). *Introduction to process evaluation in tobacco use prevention and control.* Atlanta, GA: U.S. Department of Health and Human Services, Centers for Disease Control and Prevention, National Center for Chronic Disease Prevention and Health Promotion, Office on Smoking and Health.

Commission on Accreditation of Rehabilitation Facilities. (1995). *Survey standards for medical rehabilitation* (pp. 1-89). Tuscon, AZ: Author.

Doll, J. (2010). *Program development and grant writing in occupational therapy.* Boston, MA: Jones and Bartlett.

Ensminger, D., Scaffa, M., & Reitz, S. M. (2014). Program evaluation. In M. Scaffa & S. M. Reitz (Eds.), *Occupational therapy in community-based practice settings.* (2nd ed.). Philadelphia, PA: F. A. Davis.

Forer, S. (1996). *Outcome management and program evaluation made easy: A toolkit for occupational therapy practitioners.* Bethesda, MD: American Occupational Therapy Association.

Green, G. P., & Haines, A. (2016). *Asset building and community development* (4th ed.). Los Angeles, CA: Sage.

Guba, E. G., & Lincoln, Y. S. (1987). Fourth generation evaluation. In D. J. Palumbo (Ed.), *The politics of program evaluation.* Newbury Park, CA: Sage.

Hacker, K. (2013). *Community-based participatory research.* Los Angeles, CA: Sage.

Hays, R. D., Sherbourne, C.D., & Mazel, R.M. (1993). The RAND 36-item health survey 1.0. *Health Economy, 2,* 217-227.

Huizer, G. (1997). *Participatory action research and people's participation: Introduction and case studies.* Nijmegen, The Netherlands: Third World Centre, Catholic University of Nijmegen.

Issel, L. M. (2014). *Health program planning and evaluation: A practical, systematic approach for community health.* Burlington, MA: Jones and Bartlett.

Jette, A.M., & Cleary, P. D. (1987). Functional disability assessment. *Physical Therapy, 67,* 1854-1859.

Karsh, E., & Fox, A. (2003). *The only grant-writing book you'll ever need.* New York, NY: Carroll and Graf.

Karsh, E., & Fox, A. (2014). *The only grant-writing book you'll ever need* (2nd ed.). New York, NY: Carroll and Graf.

Knowles, C. (2002). *The first-time grantwriter's guide to success.* Thousand Oaks, CA: Corwin Press.

Kronenberg, F., Algado, S., & Pollard, N. (2005). *Occupational therapy without borders: Learning from the spirit of survivors.* London: Elsevier.

MacDonell, C. (1996). Program evaluation. In American Occupational Therapy Association (Eds.), *The occupational therapy manager* (pp. 398-410). Bethesda, MD: American Occupational Therapy Association.

Mandel, D., Jackson, J., Zemke, R., Nelson, L., & Clark, F. (1999). *Lifestyle redesign: Implementing the well elderly program.* Bethesda, MD: American Occupational Therapy Association.

McHorney, C. A., Ware, J. E., & Raczek, A. E. (1993). The MOS 36-item short form health survey (SF-36): II. Psychometric and clinical tests of validity in measuring physical and mental health constructs. *Medical Care, 31,* 247-263.

Patton, M. Q. (1987). *Qualitative research evaluation methods.* Thousand Oaks, CA: Sage.

Patton, M. Q. (2008). *Utilization-focused evaluation: The new century text* (4th ed.). Thousand Oaks, CA: Sage.

Potvin, L., Gendron, S., Bilodeau, A., & Chabot, P. (2005). Integrating social theory into public health practice. *American Journal of Public Health, 95,* 591-595.

Radloff, L. (1977). The CES-D scale: A self-report depression scale for research in the general population. *Applied Psychological Measures, 1,* 385-401.

Reason, P., & Bradbury, H. (2001). *Handbook of action research: Participative inquiry and practice.* London, UK: Sage.

Rosen, G. (1993). *A history of public health.* Baltimore, MD: Johns Hopkins University.

Rossi, P. H., Lipsey, M. W., & Freeman, H. E. (2004). *Evaluation: A systematic approach* (7th ed.). Thousand Oaks, CA: Sage.

Stewart, A. L., Hays, R. D., & Ware, J. E. (1988). The MOS short-form general health survey. *Medical Care, 26,* 724-735.

Suarez-Balcazar, Y., Martinez, L., & C. Casas-Byots. (2005). A participatory action research approach for identifying health service needs of Hispanic immigrants: Implications for occupational therapy. In P. Crist & G. Kielhofner (Eds.), *The scholarship of practice: Academic practice collaborations for promoting occupational therapy: Occupational therapy in health care* (Vol. 19, No. 2). Binghamton, NY: Haworth Press.

Taylor, R., Braveman, B., & Hammel, J. (2004). Developing and evaluating community based services through participatory action research: Two case examples. *American Journal of Occupational Therapy, 58*(1), 73-82.

United Way of America. (1996). *Measuring program outcomes: A practical approach.* Alexandria, VA: Author.

U.S. Department of Health and Human Services. (2010). Healthy People 2020 (ODPHP Publication No. B0132). Washington, DC: Author. Retrieved from https://www.healthypeople.gov/

U.S. Department of Health, Education, and Welfare. (1979). *Healthy people.* Washington, DC: Author.

Ware, J. E., & Sherbourne, C. D. (1992). The MOS 36-item short-form health survey (SF-36): I. *Medical Care, 30,* 473-481.

Weiss. C. (1972). *Evaluation research: Methods for assessing program effectiveness.* Englewood Cliffs, NJ: Prentice Hall.

Whitmore, E. (Ed). (1998). *Understanding and practicing participatory evaluation: New directions for evaluation.* San Francisco, CA: Jossey-Bass.

W. K. Kellogg Foundation. (1998). *The Evaluation Handbook.* Battle Creek, MI: W. K. Kellogg Foundation.

W. K. Kellogg Foundation. (2001, 2004). *Logic model development guide.* Battle Creek, MI: W. K. Kellogg Foundation.

Wood, V., Wylie, M. L. & Sheafor, B. (1969). An analysis of a short self-reported measure of life satisfaction. *Journal of Gerontology, 24,* 465-469.

Related Websites

Joint Commission on Accreditation of Healthcare Organizations (JCAHO): http://www.jcaho.org

Logic Models Information and Examples: University of Nevada, Reno Western CAPT: http://www.unr.edu/colleges/educ/captta/prev/evaluate.html

Rehabilitation Accreditation Commission (CARF): http://www.carf.org

United Way of America's Outcome Models: http://www.unitedway.org/outcomes/contents

W.K. Kellogg Foundation: http://www.wkkf.org

V

Programming Stories
Program Examples for Children, Adolescents, Adults, and Older Adults

Programming to Support Engagement in Meaningful Occupation and Balance for the Disenfranchised and Homeless

The Development of a Community Programming Proposal

LEARNING OBJECTIVES

1. To appreciate the condition of homelessness
2. To understand the impact of homelessness on the program participants' choices and on their participation in occupation
3. To appreciate the impact of severe and persistent mental illness on the occupations of homeless persons
4. To identify how a shelter may be utilized as a site for occupation-centered programs
5. To follow the development of a programming proposal from identification of need to outcomes

---

KEY TERMS

1. Disenfranchised
2. Chronically homeless/homelessness
3. Severe and persistent mental illness (in homelessness)

Fazio, L. S. *Developing Occupation-Centered Programs With the Community, Third Edition* (pp 279-295).
© 2017 Taylor & Francis Group.

INTRODUCTION AND BACKGROUND

The Homeless Population Is Complicated

According to *The International Webster New Encyclopedia Dictionary* (1975), the definition of **disenfranchised** is "to deprive of the right to vote or some other right of citizenship." Therefore, the use of the word in connection to the homeless population is not entirely accurate, although it does carry with it an assumption about the rights of a citizen. If the citizen has obligations to the community, does not the community have obligations to the citizen? Having access to shelter is the foundation for any attention to meaningful occupation and must be attended to for the achievement of purpose. The **chronically homeless** are defined as "individuals or families who have been continuously homeless for a year or more or have had at least four episodes of homelessness in the past three years" (U.S. Department of Housing and Urban Development, 2014). Although accurate figures are extremely hard to obtain, according to numbers recently released by the U.S. Department of Housing and Urban Development (2015), the City and County of Los Angeles, CA, have the most chronically homeless people in the country, and nearly all of them sleep on the streets. The chronically homeless population in Los Angeles has grown to 12,536, since 2013, with total numbers of homeless reported as high as 54,000 (U.S. Department of Housing and Urban Development, 2015). The chronically homeless account for about 15% of all people in that category. New York City has experienced the second largest spike in chronically homeless people and families, with the rest of the country remaining basically flat with a 1% increase.

When this program was in the original stages of development, it was reported that there were approximately 7 million people (men, women, and children) experiencing **homelessness** during the latter half of the 1990s (CalWorks: Homeless Families, 2005; National Coalition for the Homeless, 1997). Moreover, at any one time and complicating these numbers, approximately 20% to 25% of the single, adult homeless population were considered to be experiencing some form of **severe and persistent mental illness** (Koegel, 1996). In a 2005 fact sheet, the National Coalition for the Homeless (2006) reported similar numbers (approximately 20% to 25%) of the single, adult homeless population suffering from some form of severe and persistent mental illness. However, this is actually a fairly small percentage of the 44 million people living with mental illness in the United States (National Institute of Mental Health, 2005). The general deinstitutionalization of the mentally ill during the 1950s and 1960s may have initiated some of the developing increase in the homeless mentally ill; however, the vast increases in these numbers did not occur until the 1980s (Federal Task Force on Homelessness and Severe Mental Illness, 1992). Why did this occur? Koegel (1996), Kaufman (1997), and the report of the Federal Task Force on Homelessness and Severe Mental Illness (1992) attribute the cause, among other things, to the general decrease in incomes and the loss of housing options for marginalized populations. These factors remain current among the homeless today (National Law Center on Homelessness and Poverty, 2014). The mentally ill experience these causes as do those associated with debilitating illness; frequently, they are also unable to access or receive medication and other therapy services. They are likely to remain homeless (without shelter) for longer periods of time and to have less contact with family and friends than others who are homeless. Their opportunities for employment are fewer, and they tend to be in poorer physical health than their homeless peers (Federal Task Force on Homelessness and Severe Mental Illness, 1992; National Law Center on Homelessness and Poverty, 2014). Although it has been a widely accepted belief that the homeless mentally ill refuse rehabilitative services, it would appear that those individuals with serious mental illness are willing to use services that are easily accessible and that meet their perceived needs. Of course, there are others who are homeless and have debilitating illness, such as drug and alcohol abuse and HIV infection. These persons require similar access to services as do the mentally ill. A related problem is experienced by homeless adolescents, who often engage in sex in exchange for food, clothing, and shelter; they are at great risk for contracting HIV-related illnesses as well as various other STDs. Robertson (1996) has reported on the results of a series of studies performed in four cities across the United States in which a median HIV-positive rate of 2.3% for homeless persons under age 25 years was found. Naranbhai, Abdool, and Meyer-Weitz (2011) have conducted research on risky sexual behaviors for youth who are homeless and determined they are at extremely high risk for HIV infection. Their research has resulted in the development of interventions to modify sexual risk behaviors in this population. These populations are discussed in more detail in Chapters 20 and 21, and specifically in our Denver Shelter Program case example introduced in Chapter 7.

We have identified some of the problems of the homeless who are ill, but who are the homeless who are not ill? Do they share common characteristics whether they are found in urban areas or in rural ones? Do the homeless populations in the East, Midwest, South, or West have common characteristics? What about the growing numbers of homeless around the world who are a migratory population pushed from their countries of origin by famine and conditions of conflict? Homelessness resulting from conditions of conflict occurs in our own country. In the United States, during the 12-month period from October 2011 to September 2012, homeless veterans from both Vietnam and more recent wars and conflicts accounted for 1 in 156 veterans. On a single night in January 2014, veterans accounted for about 11.3% of all homeless adults (National Law Center, 2015). Even though we are able to make estimates of the numbers of homeless persons based on the numbers of people in shelters and on the street, those estimates are undoubtedly below the actual numbers. Many people who lack a stable, permanent residence and, for example, are living from friend to friend or in a car, have few shelter options and remain uncounted. In fact, in a 1996 study of homelessness in 50 U.S. cities, the estimated number of homeless people greatly exceeded the number of emergency shelter and transitional housing spaces (National Law Center on Homelessness and Poverty, 1996). Today, the numbers of homeless have increased far beyond the slight increase in emergency shelters (National Law Center on Homeless and Poverty, 2014). In addition, Aron and Fitchen (1996) reported that, although there are significant numbers of homeless in rural areas of the United States, there are virtually no shelters; where there are few shelters, it is also likely that there are fewer support programs.

Women and Children Who Are Homeless

According to a study conducted by the Thurston County Homeless Point-in-Time Census Report (2005), the leading cause of homelessness among women and children within half of the examined cities was domestic violence. As of 2013, more than 90% of homeless women were victims of physical or sexual abuse, and they were in shelters if they could find them. Female-headed families made up 84% of homeless families in 2014 (Green Doors, 2014). The average homeless family is made up of a mother in her late 20s with two children; they comprise 34% of the total homeless population and are considered the fastest-growing segment within this population (Green Doors, 2014). Most of the adults who are homeless (both men and women), particularly in families, have experienced loss of employment and resultant loss of housing. This loss, coupled with little formal education or vocational training, often prompts moves across the country in search of opportunities—a search that often leads to homelessness in a strange city. Loss of employment is certainly not the only contributor to homelessness, but it is a significant one.

Programming for homeless or near homeless women and families can take many forms, ranging from interventions that are offered within shelters, providing the basics of comfort and safety, to day-shelter programs that provide temporary housing for at least the waking hours. Dear (1996) noted that the homeless are sometimes referred to as the *service-dependent*. By intention or neglect, those services that are accessed by the homeless—including health care, social welfare, emergency shelter, and job training—are most often localized to areas of the city known as "skid row" or something similar. This area, which becomes the community of the homeless, is where they live, eat, talk to friends, and often work. According to Dear (1996), it is a well-defined time-space prism, and living there is a coping mechanism for the homeless (p. 109). Perhaps this community is a sanctuary, just as your home may be after a long week at work. Most likely, any occupation-centered programming, as an extension of this service network, will also be part of this community. Partners and stakeholders will also be here. Any effort to move programming outside of the location where homeless people are congregated is often met with resistance from those living in the outside neighborhood or community. Whether this resistance is merited or not, if programming is to occur outside and a new community is to be created, there would probably be related goals that would make this the most desirable circumstance. Good or bad, this is often a reality of so-called urban renewal that is occurring everywhere in the larger U.S. cities. If this is the case, we must consider accessibility and motivation, and a transitional program might be the best way to initiate services.

Programs can be provided for children and adolescents within various educational formats (formal or shelter schools), but attention must be focused on the needs and concerns of these children who have lived without homes and the safety of a stable shelter. Neville-Jan and associates (1997) described one such program that included some foster-care children who had experienced homelessness (pp. 144-157). Although this program included a broad range of children with varying needs, during the course of the programming, it was noted that the children who had experienced what might be described as the culture of homelessness were more likely to engage in protective negative social behaviors such as hoarding of supplies, lying, and petty theft—attributes that were likely extremely adaptive on the street. Certainly, these characteristics challenge the practitioner beyond what might be expected when programming focuses on the development of social skills and behaviors that enhance and support learning.

The following example is a description of a student-designed program for a homeless women's shelter in South-Central Los Angeles, CA. This example will provide you with a step-by-step discussion from the first examination of the site and the population to the final steps of evaluation. The programming described may give you ideas you can use for programming with similar populations where you live.

Programming for a Homeless Women's Shelter

The History of the Sunshine Mission Program

This particular program is the oldest running community program designed and operated by a community programming occupational therapy class at the University of Southern California. Although there have been many permutations, the goals of the varied programming have always been about strengthening the communities that surround the university's campuses and to do so through the knowledge and skill building brought by student volunteers. It has sustained through many changes in the neighborhoods and stakeholders making up this community. The original programming was initiated well before the first edition of this text was written and continued to thrive when the second edition was published (Fazio 2001, 2008). At the time of the second edition, the program had evolved to newer interests and needs, and the culture of the homeless women was a bit different in terms of the experiences that had led to their homelessness. Human trafficking was present in the lives of some of these women, but the term was not then in general use and little was known about it. As of this writing, the site of the Sunshine Mission is closed for refurbishing, but it remains a historical landmark for the city of Los Angeles. Its future as a service site is currently unknown.

The students in the occupational therapy student residence (O.T. House) have now turned their volunteer programming attention to neighborhood children who are at substantial risk for unsuccessful school experiences and who also feel pressure from surrounding gangs that recruit from these neighborhoods. This program, too, evolved from a student-designed project into a popular and thriving venture. Project ENGAGE has a student resident coordinator who organizes programming with the volunteer help of other residents and student volunteers from other campus organizations. They meet weekly in the shared common space for activities, events and field trips (Project ENGAGE, 2008).

The Original Site

Founded by radio evangelist Sister Essie Binkey West, the Sunshine Mission began to offer shelter to homeless women in downtown Los Angeles in 1941. In later years, the city condemned the downtown facility and another was purchased just north of the University of Southern California campus. Functioning first as a school, followed by a hotel, and then a United Service Organizations facility, this building, Casa de Rosas, enjoyed a colorful history. In 1951, Sister West moved her entire Old Time Faith programs—including her radio broadcasts, publications, and services to the homeless and needy—to this site, and she remained there until her death in 1976. The Old Time Faith operated with donations from Sister West's followers, and they continued to support the Sunshine Mission with donations through its history.

In 1989, the organization ended its religious affiliation and reorganized itself into Casa de Rosas, Inc., a tax-exempt California corporation. The volunteer board of directors and management team initiated numerous programs to restore the agency both physically and financially. Support included a range of government contracts, corporate charitable grants, fundraising events, and regular individual donations. The physical structure was renovated by the city and state as a historic residential project. The building is now part of the community's architectural history and, for a time, was an example of modern safe housing for its homeless and low-income residents.

When the Sunshine Mission Program was initiated by students, the mission provided housing, food, and life necessities to adult single women for periods of 30 to 60 days. The structure could comfortably house 20 women per night, and each woman was expected to work with the shelter manager to develop and implement a plan to assist her in returning to independent living.

Adjoining the Sunshine Mission was the Casa de Rosas Hotel, which provided single-occupancy accommodations for the near homeless. Residents included senior citizens, the disabled, people in recovery, and working people of low income. The hotel could house 45 tenants who paid low monthly rents.

This information was incorporated in the mission statement of Sunshine Mission/Casa de Rosas, Inc. (1996), portions of the Agency Effectiveness Report, selected literature to support the development of the profiles , and a phase I needs assessment interview provided by the manager.

The Community Profile

When this program was first developed, the Sunshine Mission was one of several connected buildings surrounding a central plaza, and it was secured from outside entry. It is located in South Central Los Angeles, approximately 7 miles from downtown. The area is bordered by the 110 Freeway, the 10 Freeway, Vermont Street to the North, and the USC University Park Campus to the South (approximately three-quarters of a mile). The area is diverse, with a mixed population of African American, Hispanic, East Indian, Middle Eastern, and Caucasian (mixed origin) middle- and low-income families. Housing remains as remnant of the downtown Los Angeles early affluent Victorian style, with most converted to small apartments (many occupied by students). There are also apartment structures built in the 1970s and in more recent years and an assortment of small older homes. The area is also dotted with university-owned housing occupied by students and faculty. There are several gangs occupying territory in the adjacent neighborhoods and, although the mission is secured, it is situated within a high crime area. According to 2004–2005 Los Angeles Police Department (LAPD) statistics, nearly 50% of all crimes committed in Los Angeles County were perpetuated in the South Central area where the mission is located. Although still considered a high crime area today, the statistics indicate a substantial drop in violent crimes (LAPD, 1996, 2004, 2005, 2015).

The Target Population

From our earlier discussion, it would appear that there are multiple factors that contribute to and sustain the problem of homelessness. Many of these are no different in Southern California than in the larger United States. According to Jaffery and Linderstorm (2015), a state of emergency was recently declared in Los Angeles to address the growing issue of homelessness. According to these authors, since 2013 in the city alone, there has been a 12% increase in homelessness, totaling 26,000 homeless individuals and families, 18,000 of whom are unsheltered. In September 2015, Los Angeles Mayor Eric Garcetti pledged $100 million to housing services (stating that the issue is lack of affordable and sustainable resources) (Jaffery & Linderstorm, 2005). According to the 1993 Report of the Glendale, CA Task Force on Homelessness, some of these factors include illiteracy, lack of competitive job skills, substance abuse, emotional trauma from histories of child abuse, extensive employment layoffs, deinstitutionalization of the mentally ill, working poverty, and lack of affordable housing. Much of the reported information remains current and deals primarily with the male homeless population, but it is not difficult to draw the conclusion that women fare far less well overall. A more recent report from CalWorks Homeless Families (2005) demonstrates that African American and Hispanic females head most homeless families in Los Angeles County and that females were more likely to seek shelter services than males.

Initial statistics provided by the mission show that 60% of the women in residence were African American, 20% were Caucasian, and 20% were from various other cultural groups. The typical age range was 26 to 45 years. Fifteen percent of the women reported a background of domestic violence, and 12% had a history of alcohol and/or drug abuse. The average educational level was completion of elementary school, and some had differing amounts of vocational training. Most of the women had held previous jobs.

The Needs Assessment

> *Note:* In this early example, we arbitrarily divided the needs assessment process into two phases. As our work continued over the years and other programming evolved, we began to realize how important it was to conduct a thorough literature review, gather evidence, locate stakeholders, and talk to experts before and alongside what we had earlier termed the *phase I needs assessment;* thus, we began to think of the assessment of need as simply a process rather than two distinct phases. What we had earlier described as phases I and II of the needs assessment began to be referred to as the *early phase of the needs assessment;* the *community/on-the-ground portion* was the later phase.

The shelter manager was contacted by student representatives to gain a perspective on what programs were currently being offered and what needs the residents might continue to have that could be considered in designing a useful and meaningful occupation-centered program. The manager was also questioned regarding past, present, and future trends concerning homeless women at the mission.

The students then did further research to develop the service profile and determined that in 1995, the homeless population in Los Angeles was estimated to be approximately 83,900. The Shelter Partnership of Los Angeles (1995) estimated this population to be even larger. Statistics for the same area in 2004 demonstrated a slight increase. This information coupled with a review of national as well as local community statistics over time seemed to support a trend that the numbers of homeless would only increase and that their needs would become greater. This is demonstrated by the current statistics, which are not showing any decreases. In addition, women were becoming more proactive in seeking services and were advocates for other women. All of this information pointed to an increased demand for information and services tailored to the needs of women and was useful when resources were required.

A search for evidence to support the direction of successful programming for women or women with families who were homeless resulted in a review of programs currently in place at that time, including Solutions at Work, Cambridge, MA; homeless shelter programs in Maryland, including Baltimore, Capital Heights, Frederick, Hagerstown, and Westminster; and personal contact with programs in Los Angeles County. A search of the occupational therapy literature resulted in descriptions of programming with similar populations reported by Tryssenaar, Jones, and Lee (1999).

According to the manager, during the phase I assessment of need, the mission and the residents would be most interested in programs to prepare the residents for the job-search process. A review of shelter programs and the report of CalWorks (2005) supported the need for programs with a work or return-to-work emphasis. Following this comprehensive review of the needs of shelter populations in general and of women in particular, brainstorming to generate ideas for programming that might be useful adjuncts to the present programs and considering the manager's perspectives, a phase II needs assessment was developed for distribution to the current residents. (See Figure 17-1 for the phase II needs assessment.)

Following a trial distribution, it was soon discovered that the phase II assessment instrument was too broad and open-ended; residents requested services that the students were not prepared to provide or were beyond the scope of the program being considered. Thus, a second version of the phase II needs assessment survey instrument was designed and distributed to residents in the dining hall. The students distributed the assessment personally, answered questions, and collected the assessments before leaving the site. Distributing the needs assessment at a time when the majority of residents were available, answering questions, and collecting the completed assessments before leaving the site were all ways to ensure a maximum number of responses.

This second assessment instrument was aimed at identifying what realistically could be provided in a mission environment with very little financial support, but still meeting the needs identified in phase I. This instrument incorporated the ideas of the students and the concerns of the manager. The students wanted to ensure that the programs could be utilized and were also cognizant of the need to design programs that could be conducted by volunteers from the community and perhaps by occupational therapy students without loss of the goal structure.

Results of this second questionnaire indicated that the largest percentage of residents identified employment skills and money management as being of greatest concern to them. Coping skills, followed by life skills, completed the ranking of the results.

Selection of a Theoretical Orientation to Support Goals and Programming

At the time, a collection of theories derived from occupational behavior perspectives were thought to most likely be of use in helping to understand and structure the selection of a rationale to guide programming for the women at the Sunshine Mission. Two are of particular importance: the Model of Human Occupation (MOHO) and Occupational Adaptation. MOHO is useful in that it helps to structure our thinking as we approach our participants in those processes of occupational adaptation described as volition (personal causation, values, and interests); and the volitional processes incorporated under the broader category of habituation (habits and roles) (Kielhofner, 2002; Kielhofner, Forsyth, & Barrett, 2003). MOHO addresses motivation for engagement in occupation, the routine patterning of occupations, the nature of skilled performance, and the influence of environment on occupation (Kielhofner et al., 2003, p. 212). All of these features are of significance for the women at the mission as they engage in a normalizing round of daily activities in preparation for finding employment and living independently. Programming to encourage personal initiative, engagement in activities of interest, and awareness of the multiple contexts of performance, as well as the development of skills seems on target to meet the women's needs and ensure positive outcomes.

Sunshine Mission Survey

We are interested in providing programming that will assist you in preparing for your return to the community. To do this, we would like to know what activities you would find most useful. Please fill out this survey to help us identify your needs and interests. **Check all that apply:** (Rate 1 through 6, with 1 being the area you are most interested in and 6 the area you are least interested in)

I am most interested in activities that will help me:

_____ learn how to get a new or better job

_____ meet people I can do things with

_____ learn about free or low-cost services in Los Angeles

_____ take better care of myself

_____ relax and enjoy life more

_____ develop new interests and/or skills

Things I would be interested in trying:

_____ arts and crafts

anything in particular _____

_____ home skills

    _____ apartment hunting: how and what to expect

    _____ cooking/baking

    _____ nutrition/healthy meal planning

    _____ shopping/how to find coupons and discounts

    _____ small plot (or) community gardening

    _____ budget decorating

    _____ sewing

    _____ other (please describe): _____

_____ learning about the community

    _____ seeing Los Angeles on a budget

    _____ the Los Angeles library services

    _____ riding public transportation

    _____ activities of "singles" organizations

    _____ assisting others in need of help

    _____ Los Angeles community social services

    _____ religious outings

    _____ other (please describe): _____

_____ pre-employment skills

    _____ how to "job search"

    _____ developing a resume

    _____ how to fill out a job application

    _____ how to interview well

    _____ other (please describe): _____

_____ self-care

    _____ exercise classes

    _____ how to relax and manage stress

    _____ safety education/women's self-defense

    _____ grooming and hygiene

    _____ other (please describe): _____

Thanks for your time; you will be seeing programs posted by the end of the month. See you there!

Figure 17-1. Needs assessment survey.

The second model, the model of Occupational Adaptation, comes from the work of Schultz and Schkade (2003) and complements our interpretation of the MOHO. Occupational adaptation considers the person (the interaction) and the occupational environment. The authors' emphasis on the desire for mastery, the press for mastery, and the demand for mastery as translated through these interactions is appropriate for our understanding as we design programming that will present an occupational challenge, and a resulting occupational response. It will be our task to provide mediating opportunity and assistance for adaptive response formation (through the design of programming) that will help our participants reach their goals and achieve successful long-range outcomes.

> *Note:* Over time, we have come to realize how significant change theory is to understanding this population; particularly, the resistivity that often occurs. Motivational interviewing and the recognition of ambivalence regarding change is also helpful (Miller & Rollnick, 2013).

Drafting Goals and Objectives

Following careful review of the results of the needs assessment, the mission statement, characteristics of the facility, and the characteristics of the population, two goals for the program were drafted and were followed by measurable objectives, as shown by the following examples. Goals and objectives are intended to support programming that will result in employment and in independent living.

> *Note:* Although we did not use the term *outcome* in the description of this early project, it is implicit in the foregoing statement regarding employment and independent living. Neither were we talking about impact at that point in time, but ultimate impact would be measured by an increase in employment that produced a wage that would support independent living and a reduction in the numbers of homeless women over a specified period of time, first in this shelter population and then in the city of Los Angeles.

Program Focus: Attention to Healthy and Balanced Independent Living

Goals

1. To be healthy and balanced by increasing awareness of healthy living strategies to include nutrition, personal care, exercise, relaxation, stress management, job and apartment search, self-defense, and safety.

2. To control one's destiny by increasing the individual's sense of personal causation, self-esteem, and self-efficacy, resulting in sustained employment and independent living.

Objectives

1. (a) Fifty percent of the residents at the Sunshine Mission will attend four out of the six sessions (nutrition, personal care, exercise, stress management, job and apartment search, self-defense, and safety).

   (b) Of the women attending each session, 80% will demonstrate knowledge of information and techniques provided in that session.

2. (a) Of those women attending all of the sessions, 80% will demonstrate increased self-efficacy, self-esteem, and personal causation by the time they leave the mission programming.

   (b) Of those women attending all sessions, 80% will find employment.

   (c) Of those women finding employment, 80% will sustain such employment for 6 months.

The Program

Single-session workshops that each lasted approximately 1.5 to 2 hours were developed in each of the identified areas (nutrition, personal care, exercise, stress management, job and apartment search, self-defense, and safety). These areas were selected from the four broader areas of the needs assessment: employment skills, money management, life skills, and coping skills. Nutrition was added by the planners when it became evident that concerns regarding appearance, healthy activities, and self-esteem could be somewhat alleviated with attention to nutrition.

Nutrition

The session on nutrition was initiated with a verbal survey of how and what the residents preferred to eat and what, if any, problems they were experiencing that they thought might have a relationship to their nutritional likes and dislikes. Most of the residents preferred less expensive "fast food" when they were not receiving mission meals, and many were either under or over their preferred weight.

From earlier discussion with the manager and some of the residents, the students were prepared with materials gleaned from the fast-food restaurants regarding their own statistics for calorie, fat, and salt content.

> *Note:* This kind of information has now become commonplace and nutritional tracking can be easily done.

This information was coupled with some suggestions for balancing fast-food meals and some hints for ways to reduce cholesterol and calories. Meeting the residents' basic needs was important to the success of this session and provided a good foundation from which other nutritional sessions such as healthy meal planning and cooking could develop.

Personal Care, Exercise, and Stress Management

Personal care in the forms of personal hygiene and makeup were important as an adjunct to job searches. Enthusiastic volunteers were solicited from neighborhood shops to provide demonstrations of manicure and pedicure techniques and application of makeup. A local beauty school provided no-cost haircuts and styling techniques.

> *Note:* We would now find these neighborhood volunteers and stakeholders early on through an identification of population and community assets (see Chapter 9).

A group walking program was established both for exercise and stress management, and an aerobics dance class was initiated. Both quickly came under the direction of residents. Relaxation techniques and guided imagery sessions rounded out the program.

> *Note:* Over time, we began to introduce "mindfulness" meditation and yoga to enhance relaxation.

Job and Apartment Search

Job-search skills consisted of exercises in learning how to read the classified section of the newspaper, how and where to access other job announcements, how to develop a skills-based resume that would not negatively highlight periods of unemployment, and how to write a cover letter. Videotaped role-playing provided practice in interviewing.

> *Note:* This was considered to be innovative at the time, and continued to be extremely useful in building confidence. A similar format was used in finding and evaluating apartments for location (near public transportation, shopping) and cost.

Self-Defense and Safety

A community martial arts studio volunteered the time and expertise of a female instructor to provide instruction in physical self-defense techniques. Small-group discussions followed the self-defense instruction to assist in the emotional buffering necessary for some women who had histories of physical abuse.

Representatives of the LAPD and the University Crime Prevention and Rape Awareness Group provided information verbally and in the form of handouts to assist the residents in being safe on the street and in the neighborhood, including safety precautions to follow if they were living on the street.

Since the residents frequently rotate, a set of programs can be repeated. This is positive in that the students have time to develop and enhance existing materials, but it can be something of a disadvantage when relying on volunteers from local shops and agencies.

Staffing

As noted previously, staffing for the sessions/workshops was provided by neighborhood volunteers in the form of representatives from local shops and agencies. Residents were trained to become facilitators whenever possible—not only to assist in providing "womanpower," but, more importantly, to provide as many residents as possible with leadership opportunities.

> *Note:* This speaks to sustainable skills, knowledge, and resulting efficacy.

Another important source of assistance for the ongoing success of the program was the linkage to the Student Occupational Therapy Association and the O.T. House, as well as the university housing residential advisors and coordinators. All of these organizations "adopted" the mission as an ongoing service project. Occupational therapy graduate students also obtained service-learning credit for participation in and expansion of the programs and activities. The on-site manager supports student involvement and acts as a liaison between the occupational therapy student programs and the needs of the residents. All activities are supervised by a department faculty member, as well as the resident advisors who live in all university student residences.

> *Note:* This has continued although programming has now moved to other neighborhood populations.

Space

When the students first went on site to conduct the tentative needs assessment, they explored the space (including storage) and materials/supplies that would be available to them. Two rooms provided the space and work tables necessary for the planned programming—the existing dining room and a conference room. In addition, the outside courtyard and kitchen could be used for some activities.

All space was used for multiple purposes and had to be scheduled at the convenience of the Mission. For the convenience of all concerned, it was determined that following the evening meal was the preferred time for activities (although it was a competitive time with television). Weekend times offered additional possibilities.

Tables could be moved aside for activities that required floor space. There was one file cabinet where some space could be provided, but secured storage was limited and could not be relied upon. The rooms contained electrical outlets that could accommodate a radio, VCR, and/or CD player, and the adjoining kitchen was well supplied with utensils. A small storage area contained rulers, pencils, and paper, and a typewriter and personal computer were available for the residents' use (donations). Secured parking for volunteers was limited.

Supplies and Equipment

Efforts were made to design activities requiring minimal equipment and supplies and minimal requirement for storage. Equipment was available through the mission facilities. All activities utilized the existing tables and chairs in the dining area and/or conference room, the kitchen, and the floor space in the dining area.

Cost

Even though most of the activities relied on donated supplies, a cost breakdown of supplies and equipment was done in order to anticipate replacement costs (if required) and to assist those who wished to donate by establishing a cost/value for items.

Funding

Since residents of the mission were provided with services and information free of charge to assist them as they prepared for independent living, this was clearly a service program. The program required the mission to absorb minimal cost, if any, for supplies, and these costs were incorporated into the existing budget.

The occupational therapy students explored the processes of fundraising, including those activities already in existence through the mission. Successful efforts were made to build collaborative bridges with local shops and agencies for ongoing relationships to provide volunteer staff and donated supplies. A sense of community and community responsibility was created between the university, the local residents, and the local businesses and agencies; all were partners in encouraging success for the residents.

> Note: The term *stakeholder* was not popular at the time, but that was the nature of this effort, alongside ensuring that the program would become sustainable.

In addition to the efforts already mentioned, the creation and maintenance of community was of equal importance to the occupational science and occupational therapy academic programs that assumed some fiscal responsibility for the student-related mission activities as part of their Occupational Therapy-Los Angeles (OT-LA) community service and community service-learning programs and projects.

Marketing

There is some marketing to be done, even with community service programs. The first marketing, of course, was to the mission manager, who, in turn, brought the ideas to the board of directors. This first effort was accomplished in the initial on-site meeting. The students were prepared with appropriate and relevant questions and could offer a brief scenario of their interests in working with the residents. This was also an excellent opportunity for the students to market some of the basic tenets of occupation, meaningful engagement in activity, and occupational therapy. In addition, they were able to link their interest in occupation with the work of the mission.

Second, the residents needed to be informed of the program's activities. This was done initially through the needs assessment and the verbal/visual introduction to the students who would be involved. When plans for programming were finalized, the students prepared colorful flyers advertising the full program and giving information about the activities as well as how residents could benefit. These were supplemented by weekly flyers highlighting the "program of the week." Programming was offered whether there was one participant or 20 participants. There was also marketing to the potential students and residents who might wish to become involved in programming. Flyers were posted in dormitories, and program planners/coordinators attended floor meetings at the beginning of the semester to explain the program.

The next phase of marketing required some substantial networking as well as leg work. The purpose of the mission's activities and the goals and objectives of the students' programming was taken to the shops and agencies that the students' had targeted as providing services that would benefit the residents of the mission. The idea of volunteering time and, in some cases, services and supplies had to be "sold" to the shop owners and employees. The students found this to be the most disconcerting aspect of marketing the program, but in many ways, it turned out to be the easiest.

It should not be lost that this third phase of marketing strongly involved the encouragement of responsibility—and perhaps obligation—to the community. This was made even stronger through the residence of the programmers within the neighborhood where the mission existed. Certainly, students are transients, but the responsibility that is created by an investment in the shared premise of community can become a legacy handed from one student group to another through the investment of the institution (the university) and the academic department.

Outcomes

Taking time to work and rework program goals and objectives is worthwhile when it comes to determining how effective the program has been and continues to be. Of course, to really know long-term effectiveness, it is necessary to follow the residents' progress in obtaining employment and acquiring suitable housing. This follow-up was attempted by the mission, but for numerous reasons, it was difficult to accomplish. Record of first employment following completion of the program can be attained and 6-month follow-up can be accomplished; however, if the participant leaves employment or is fired (and does not return to the mission), it is not likely that she would be identified for follow-up. As the occupational therapy students' programming continues to attract residents and if that programming is effective, we would expect to see this reflected in any data the mission is able to obtain.

The goals and objectives of the students' programming can be measured for short-term effectiveness in the following ways:

Goal

1. To be healthy by increasing awareness of healthy living strategies to include nutrition, personal care, exercise, stress management, job and apartment search, self-defense, and safety.

Objective

1. (a)   Fifty percent of the residents at the Sunshine Mission will attend four out of six sessions.

Measurement

This objective is measured simply by an organized system of attendance marking and is compared to the number of women who are in residency during the programming. The relationship of the objective to the goal carries the assumption that being present during the session does, in fact, increase awareness. Since awareness is a fairly superficial goal, the objective is likely being measured adequately. Measurement of this objective could be strengthened with the use of an observer/ participation checklist similar to the one shown in Figure 17-2, which can be used to note the level of each participant's engagement in the session.

Objective

1. (b)   Of the women attending each session, 80% will demonstrate knowledge of information and techniques provided in that session.

Measurement

This objective is best measured in two ways. A brief questionnaire can be distributed following each session to focus on the information that the facilitator wishes to convey, or a brief structured interview can be utilized for participants in a small group. It is important that the facilitators think carefully about the content and reflect the main ideas in their questionnaire/interview. Always ask the following question: What is really important to assist the participants in meeting the goal?

CLIENT ATTENDANCE AND PERFORMANCE RATING FORM

Name	Session 1	Session 2	Session 3	Session 4	Session 5

KEY:

Rating	Performance
0	Did not attend
1	Attended session but did not participate in activity
2	Quietly participated but not interactive with others
3	Engaged, active participation, interaction with others

Figure 17-2. Observer check sheet for participation level.

If there are demonstrated techniques, as there were with the sessions on personal care, exercise, job search, and self-defense, then an observer checklist is again appropriate. The facilitator must determine the level of competency that is desired to assess achievement of the objective and measure at that level. An actual resume was required as part of the session(s) on job search—either this was accomplished or it was not. If a particular level of quality is expected when something is actually produced, then this must be reflected in the checklist.

SAFETY SELF-ASSESSMENT

Please read the following statements carefully. Rate each statement using the following scale:

1 = strongly agree
2 = agree
3 = doesn't apply/don't care
4 = disagree
5 = strongly disagree

  1) I feel that I can protect myself. _____

  2) I feel that I DON'T give up easily when faced with problems. _____

  3) I feel safe when walking to the store. _____

  4) I feel comfortable saying "No." _____

  5) I understand the difference between verbal abuse and physical abuse. _____

  6) I feel comfortable when a stranger approaches me. _____

  7) I feel that I know how to deal with confrontation. _____

  8) I feel that I can rely on myself. _____

  9) I feel confident that I would survive an attack. _____

10) I know when to use my words and when to use my fists to protect myself. _____

11) I feel that I have control over my life. _____

12) When I want something, I work hard to get it. _____

Figure 17-3. Safety self-assessment pre- and post-test.

Pre- and post-tests could be utilized to get a truer measure of information the participants bring to a session as opposed to new information they acquire in a session. For the purposes of this program, it was thought that a pretest was most useful to determine at what level to introduce information. (See Figure 17-3 for an example of a pre- and post-test.)

Goal

2. To control one's destiny by increasing the individual's sense of personal causation, self-esteem, and self-efficacy.

Objective

2. (a) Of those women attending all of the sessions, 80% will demonstrate increased self-efficacy, self-esteem, and personal causation.

Measurement and Supporting Rationale

An important aspect of this objective is the requisite that all of the sessions be attended. The selection of content, or enabling activities, was made with the belief that mastery would, in fact, increase the participant's self-esteem, self-efficacy, and sense of control over her environment or personal causation. Further, it was assumed that the participants were deficient in these characteristics (validated through pretest measures) and that this could be the area that would make a difference in their future successes in seeking employment and living independently.

In this case, pre- and post-test measurements were selected. The Generalized Expectancy for Success Scale (GESS; Asher, 1996; Fibel & Hale, 1978), and the Self-Efficacy Scale (SES; Asher, 1996; Sherer et al., 1982), were given to all participants at the first session in the series, and individual scores were calculated. The measures again were given to all participants (those who had attended all of the sessions) at the last session of the series. It is doubtful that improvement in these measures would be sustained over time with such a short programming window; however, if all mission programming was considered as contributing to efficacy, then a post-test prior to leaving the mission might be more valid.

Differences in individual scores were calculated for participants. Although the numbers attending all sessions were small, there was improvement in each set of scores. Of course, there may have been many factors affecting the increased scores. Some formative questions we could consider were: Why did some residents attend one session and not another? How did the women who attended all sessions differ from those who did not? How did their initial scores compare? Did the content of some sessions affect the scores more than others (e.g., self-defense or personal care)? These are all legitimate questions that would strengthen the measures, both formative and summative.

Time Frame

The programs were prepared over the course of an academic semester (15 weeks), with student groups meeting once each week for 2-hour periods. The initial program, healthy living, was conducted in 2-hour sessions, once per week, over a 6-week period.

Minimal supplies were required and there was no substantial lag time for acquisition. The most difficult aspect of the timeline was the substantial marketing effort to those organizations that would provide volunteer time and the scheduling of sessions for their convenience and for the convenience of the residents.

SUMMARY

The disenfranchised and homeless include children, adolescents, and adults, and their numbers are growing daily. Homelessness is sometimes by choice, but most often, it is a product of the individual's loss of control over his or her life. Matters of economics and loss of income are integrated with loss of meaningful occupations and hope. One program has been described to provide an example of services for the homeless and/or those in shelter environments. This was an in-depth description of a program provided for homeless women living in a shelter. The goals for this program included the pursuit of "health" and the development of knowledge and skills to "control one's destiny." To support the goals and to meet the objectives, programming focused on self-care, community awareness, holiday arts and crafts, home skills, and pre-employment skills.

This chapter offered the information as it developed when this program was little more than a vague idea. It was one of the earliest programs developed and conducted by community programming students and, during its operation (before the mission was closed by the city), the programs remained amazingly current; this is perhaps not so surprising because the problems of homelessness and the factors that contributed to that condition for women in particular have not disappeared. Boxed "notes" are offered in the preceding text to show where more current thinking and information may influence the program design and/or evaluation.

REFERENCES

Aron, L. Y., & Fitchen, J. (1996). Rural homelessness: A synopsis. *Homelessness in America* (The "series" of pamphlets/reports). Washington, DC: Oryx Press/National Coalition for the Homeless.

Asher, E. (1996) *Occupational therapy assessment tools: an annotated index* (2nd ed.). Bethesda, MD: American Occupational Therapy Association.

CalWorks: Homeless Families. (2005). *Report to the County of Los Angeles Board of Supervisors.* Los Angeles, CA: County of Los Angeles, Department of Public Social Services.

Dear, M. (1996). Time, space, and the geography of everyday life of people who are homeless. In R. Zemke & F. Clark (Eds.), *Occupational science: The evolving discipline* (pp. 107-114). Philadelphia, PA: F. A. Davis.

Fazio, L. S. (2001). *Developing occupation-centered programs for the community.* Upper Saddle River, NJ: Prentice Hall.

Fazio, L. S. (2008). *Developing occupation-centered programs for the community* (2nd ed.). Upper Saddle River, NJ: Prentice Hall.

Federal Task Force on Homelessness and Severe Mental Illness. (1992). *Report: Homelessness and severe mental illness.* Washington, DC: Author.

Fibel, B., & Hale, W. D. (1978). The generalized expectancy for success scale—A new measure. *Journal of Consulting and Clinical Psychology, 46,* 924–931.

Green Doors. (2014). *Statistics about the female demographic within the homeless community.* Author. Retrieved from GreenDoors.org

The International Webster New Encyclopedia Dictionary of the English Language. (1975). Chicago, IL: The English Language Institute of America.

Jaffery, S., & Linderstorm, D. (2005). *Letter to editor. Daily Trojan.* Los Angeles, CA: University of Southern California.

Kaufman, T. (1997). *Out of reach: Rental housing at what cost?* Washington, DC: National Low Income Housing Coalition.

Kielhofner, G. (2002). *Model of human occupation* (3rd ed.). Philadelphia, PA: Lippincott, Williams and Wilkins.

Kielhofner, G., Forsyth, K., & Barrett, L. (2003). The model of human occupation. In E. Crepeau, E. Cohn, & B. Schell (Eds.), *Willard and Spackman's occupational therapy* (10th ed., pp. 212-219). Philadelphia, PA: Lippincott, Williams and Wilkins.

Koegel, P. (1996). The causes of homelessness. In *Homelessness in America.* Washington, DC: Oryx Press, National Coalition for the Homeless.

Los Angeles Police Department. (1996, 2004, 2005, 2015). *Los Angeles county crime report.* Los Angeles, CA: Author. Retrieved from http://www.lapdonline.com

Miller, R., & Rollnick, S. (2013). *Motivational interviewing* (3rd ed.). New York, NY: Guilford Press.

Naranbhai, V., Abdool, K. Q., & Meyer-Weitz, A. (2011). Interventions to modify sexual risk behaviors for preventing HIV in homeless youth. *Cochrane Database System Review, (1),* CD007501.

National Coalition for the Homeless. (1997). *Homelessness in America: Unabated and increasing.* Washington, DC: National Coalition for the Homeless. Author.

National Coalition for the Homeless. (2006). *Mental Illness and Homelessness.* Washington, DC: National Coalition for the Homeless. Author.

National Institute of Mental Health. (2005). The numbers count. Bethesda, MD: Author. Retrieved from www.nimh.nih.gov

National Law Center on Homelessness and Poverty. (1996). *Mean sweeps: A report on anti-homelessness laws, litigation and alternatives in 50 United States cities.* Washington, DC: National Law Center on Homelessness and Poverty.

National Law Center on Homelessness and Poverty. (2014). *Homelessness in America.* Washington, DC: Author.

National Law Center on Homelessness and Poverty. (2015). *Homeless veterans in America.* Washington, DC: Author.

Neville-Jan, A., Fazio, L. S., Kennedy, B., & Snyder, C. (1997). Elementary to middle school transition: Using multi-cultural play activities to develop life skills. In L. D. Parham & L. S. Fazio (Eds.), *Play in occupational therapy for children* (pp. 144-157). St. Louis, MO: Mosby.

Project ENGAGE. (2008). Unpublished community programming proposal. Los Angeles, CA: Chan Division of Occupational Science and Occupational Therapy, University of Southern California.

Report of the Glendale, California Task Force on Homelessness. (1993). Glendale, CA: City of Glendale, California.

Robertson, M. (1996). *Homeless youth on their own.* Berkeley, CA: Alcohol Research Group.

Schultz, S., & Schkade, J. (2003). Occupational adaptation. In E. Crepeau, E. Cohn, & B. Schell (Eds.), *Willard and Spackman's occupational therapy* (10th ed., pp. 220-223). Philadelphia, PA: Lippincott, Williams and Wilkins.

Shelter Partnership of Los Angeles. (1995). *Annual Report.* Los Angeles, CA: Author.

Sherer, M., Maddox, J. E., Mercandante, B., Prentice-Dunn, S., Jacobs, B., & Rogers, R. W. (1982). The self-efficacy scale: Construction and validation. *Psychological Reports, 51,* 663–671.

Sunshine Mission/Casa de Rosas, Inc. (1996). *Mission statement: Agency effectiveness report.* Los Angeles, CA: Author.

Thurston County Homeless Point-in-Time Census Report. (2005). *What are some statistics about homeless women?* Author. Retrieved from https://www.reference.com/world-view/statistics-homeless-women-d04271ef7404737a?qo=cdpArticles

Tryssenaar, J., Jones, E., & Lee, D. (1999). Occupational performance needs of a shelter population. *Canadian Journal of Occupational Therapy, 66(104),* 18-23.

U.S. Department of Housing and Urban Development. (2014). The 2014 Annual Homeless Assessment Report (AHAR) to Congress. Retrieved from https://www.hudexchange.info/resources/documents/2014-AHAR-Part1.pdf

U.S. Department of Housing and Urban Development. (2015). *Los Angeles chronically homeless.* Retrieved from http://documents.lahsa.org/planning/homelesscount/2015/HC2015CommissionPresentation.pdf

18

Intervention and Support Programming in Day Camps, Sleep-Away Camps, and "Adventures"

Fazio, L. S. *Developing Occupation-Centered Programs With the Community, Third Edition* (pp 297-310).
© 2017 Taylor & Francis Group.

This chapter offers some examples of what might be described as programming that showcases environment/context-centered occupations that provide significant meaning for all ages. Although certainly not restricted to one season, this type of programming does carry with it the flavor of summer with its games, crafts, fun, being outdoors, and being with friends, and perhaps even nursing a sunburned nose, a few bug bites, and a bruised knee. Adults hold these moments of play/leisure in pockets of pleasurable memory, and children relish the time spent at play.

The selected environments for programming provide a comfort zone for children and adults with or without significant disability. They are user-friendly environments that offer all participants equal access and the opportunity for the development of competency, autonomy, and relatedness rather than dependency; what Ryan and Deci (2000) describe as *self-determination.* In other words, they are **normalizing environments.** Day camps are probably the simplest to develop and program. Sleep-away camps, on the other hand, are more challenging and more costly but provide significant opportunities for building positive experiences, self-esteem, and efficacy for both the young and those who are older.

What is meant by "adventures," the third category of programming included in this chapter? Coming from the word *advent,* which means "to begin or to commence," adventure is the undertaking of doing so (Random House, 1984). When they are participating in an adventure-oriented intervention program, it is not unusual for clients to exclaim, "I'm alive again!" or, "This is living!" The adventures of Christopher Robin at Pooh Corner, Alice in Wonderland, Robin Hood and his Merry Band, Luke Skywalker in Star Wars, Zorro, or Batman conjure up exciting images of new places, new events, mysteries, and maybe a little danger. These are the attributes that put the keen edge on "meaningful occupations" for many.

Yerxa (1999) has described the need for people to become "effective managers of their own environments" and noted that, through this process, there is undoubtedly an accompanying need to "search for novelty," perhaps the core of intrinsic motivation. Yerxa (1999) refers to *homo occupacio* to describe the human link with occupation: "Occupation helps construct who I am" (lecture). What better way to initiate this construction than through the novelty imbedded in an adventure? Whether these adventures come in the form of horseback riding, spending the night on a hiking trail high in the mountains, diving in the ocean, driving with the top down, spying an unseen species of bird, or another activity of equal challenge, they are all adventures.

Throughout this text, we have discussed that the prerequisite to programming for any population is to "know" that population on all levels. A thorough investigation of the developmental expectations, along with the parameters of any disability or differing ability, is of absolute necessity to provide programming that will be formative or preventative. Since day camps, sleep-away camps, and adventures are typically adjunct to other programming the clients are receiving, communications with other providers is important to maintain and support the goals for intervention that are already in place.

THE DAY CAMP

Day camps can be developed for clients of any age. They can be developed for the child alone, the child and a sibling, or the child and a parent; or they can be developed for the adult alone or the adult and a caregiver, depending on the goals of the program. Although not discussed at length here, day programs for adults, particularly those with cognitive dysfunction, are actually day camps. If you think of them in that way and incorporate many of the activities of a typical children's day camp (scaled to adult needs and interests) in the adult treatment environment, goals can be attained while supporting the pleasurable attributes and nostalgia of "camp." Most adult programs for clients with Alzheimer's disease in fact do this by combining a routine of indoor and outdoor activity, rest, snacks, and celebration of life events (holidays, birthdays, and so on). Since the day programming offers some respite for the caregiver, much of the programming is for the client; however, selected shared adventures such as trips away from the treatment environment and the immediate community can provide an opportunity for the client and caregiver to enjoy positive experiences together. These shared experiences can assist in alleviating some of the daily stressors and often the accompanying guilt that may overpower the caregiver.

Supportive programming for children can occur anywhere; many after-school and Saturday day camp models are in the practice settings common to pediatrics. If at all possible, however, this kind of programming, particularly a day camp that occurs for a period of time (e.g., daily for 2 weeks), should be held at a camp site. This dissociation from the treatment environment provides a new arena for children to experience new challenges and opportunities to meet these challenges in different ways. Of course, some day camp programming can be for children who have no apparent cognitive, emotional, or physical disabilities. These day camps for children who may be considered to be at risk for losing out on what we might describe as "life's rewards" are excellent ways to provide supportive and preventative programming. The "club" models described in Chapter 19 highlight programming examples of this kind.

An Example of Programming for a Children's Day Camp

The Needs Assessment

The program we will examine in this section came to fruition when the City of Los Angeles Department of Recreation and Parks experienced numerous requests from parents and teachers to add children with emotional, cognitive, and physical disabilities to their summer camp programming. These requests were not new and efforts had been made previously to mainstream these children into the existing structures, but with limited success.

The mission of the City of Los Angeles Department of Recreation and Parks included the following sentence: "To unify Los Angeles by providing diverse recreational opportunities, beautiful facilities, and innovative leadership for the universal enjoyment of our residents and visitors by providing a broad range of recreational opportunities at various facilities to the general population, especially youth, and to *all special need segments of the population* [italics added]" (City of Los Angeles, 2015). Thus, providing such a camp was well within the scope and interests of this department.

The department employed a recreation therapist (RT) and several adolescent assistants from the surrounding community to operate the summer day camp programs. The adolescents were thought to be at risk (for gang affiliation, drugs, and engagement in criminality) and had been selected to participate in an "opportunity for success" employment program operated under the auspices of the Los Angeles Police Department, a significant stakeholder. The RT recognized that the potential campers identified with special needs were of sufficient number and variability to require several small groups with different programming for any meaningful outcomes to occur.

Since occupational therapy, an added partner and collaborator, became involved late in the process and the time frame was fairly short, an occupational therapist, along with other therapists who were or had been seeing some of the children for varying kinds of therapeutic programming, volunteered time to further develop the needs assessment. The children ranged in age from 5 to 8 years old. Some were no longer receiving therapy, and some continued to receive therapy on a weekly basis; others had never received therapy services. All available information regarding individual therapeutic goals for the children was gleaned from a variety of services, and individual objectives were developed for each of the 15 children who were expected to attend. The children were then grouped according to their objectives rather than by age or disability status.

A goal was developed for the camp and was shared by all of the children. "Camp for Friends" was designed to help each child increase his or her interpersonal and general social skills. The collective responses to the assessment of need provided assurance that the goal and objectives for the program were on target for all of the participants.

Thus, this example actually was initiated with the first expressed need. It would appear that the initial planning steps outlined in Parts I and II of this text were bypassed; however, it is important to note that an enterprising and experienced programmer carries all of the process in his or her head. The therapist involved in this example recognized the trends toward inclusion of differently abled children but also recognized that inclusion requires cognizance of appropriate and meaningful goals. In addition, this therapist knew how to expand the needs assessment to include community assets and capacities so that programming ensures that the goal or goals are satisfied as well as the needs of stakeholders, and resources are not wasted.

The programmer should also know that, with skillful activity analysis and appropriate adaptations and modifications, a full round of camp activities can be enjoyed by every child in the program. This programmer will also be able to successfully market the uniqueness of occupation-centered intervention coupled with program evaluation methods so that a future for occupational therapy practitioners is assured in this particular community-based practice environment. When the programmer works cooperatively with the RT and other staff as well as community organizations and services, a full round of therapeutic and supportive activities can be developed by this team and the concept of community can be strengthened and maintained.

Programming

Daily programming for the campers in our example was not unlike what other summer day camps were utilizing. Programming was held Monday through Thursday from 10 a.m. to 4 p.m. and lasted for 1 month. Transportation to and from camp was provided by vehicles from the parks and recreation department, which also accommodated the two children in wheelchairs.

Daily programming consisted of arts and crafts, field trips, swimming, games, and pet care combined with snacks/lunch and a short rest period. Arts and crafts were similar to those enjoyed by all summer campers (including T-shirts sponge-painted with the camp logo, lanyards for ID badges, leathercraft, and an assortment of other ideas all analyzed and adapted to ensure full participation and successful outcomes).

Cooking was also a favored activity, which was tailored to the out-of-doors camp environment (such as chocolate, graham crackers, and marshmallow S'mores, hot dogs on sticks, toasted marshmallows, etc.). Field trips included an amusement park, the local children's museum, the beach, and the zoo. The children collected an assortment of objects from the beach for a collage to be constructed later, and the wet sand provided an interesting tactile challenge for bare feet and bodies. Swimming also offered opportunities to practice dressing—getting in and out of swimsuits—grooming wet hair, and toweling dry.

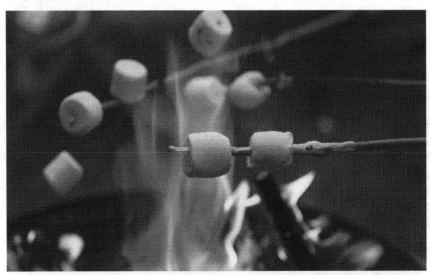

Toasting marshmallows over a campfire, is there anything more fun?

An activity-analysis previsit by the therapist and/or students to all of the field trip sites paved the way for successful access and the "just-right" challenge with regard to managing the terrain and crowds and avoidance of potential exhaustion with resulting temper tantrums. Bathrooms and lunch areas were also mapped so that children would not experience any potentially embarrassing accidents or unintentionally be the brunt of discrimination.

Most games were played outdoors, with the favored ones involving the parachute and variations of the parachute with foam balls that were large enough for all to grasp and throw. Pet care was actually serendipitous with the discovery of a frog, which was later joined by a duck that happened to enjoy the swimming pool and rabbits that were adopted. One of the premises supporting pet care by children is that of offering the opportunity to experience responsibility—relentless as it is when it comes to feeding and taking care of an animal. More important to our community was the normalizing process of caring for a pet that most children can access and many take for granted. The campers had more often been the recipients of caretaking rather than the providers of care.

You will find a number of resources at the close of this chapter to help you with camp programming. One of these resources, *Backyards and Butterflies: Ways to Include Children With Disabilities in Outdoor Activities,* includes descriptions of several adaptations to assist with pet care (Greenstein, Miner, Kudela, & Bloom, 1993).

Space, Staffing, and Cost

Space for this camp was in a city park with an adjoining secured building and was shared with other programs. The building provided some office space, a large gymnasium, a kitchen, and rooms for small-group activities. A playground with newly designed equipment, a swimming pool, and child-sized picnic tables and benches was adjacent to the building.

Since there were other camp activities scheduled at the same time as these camps, it was necessary to coordinate not only these groups through daily programming, but also with other groups as well for the use of the swimming pool, vehicles for field trips, and the gymnasium. Several times each month, there were opportunities for some shared activities, and many of the children had siblings in the other camps.

Since the budget had already been established before the camps were conceptualized and developed, the first summer of the program, the occupational therapy personnel were largely volunteer or minimum-wage employees. There were also four paid adolescent assistants assigned through a separate agency. Following the first summer, an occupational therapist, an occupational therapy assistant, additional adolescent assistants, and two level II occupational therapy and/or occupational therapy assistant students were expected to be added to the programming. It was also anticipated that there would be additional campers following further marketing efforts.

Costs for the activities were subsumed under the regular camp costs. The cost of supplies for 1 month of programming was approximately $120 per child. These were budgeted items for craft and activity supplies and did not include transportation, field trip admissions, or lunch, nor did they include the cost of salaries or use of space. These items were part of the larger budget of the parks and recreation department obtained from individual fees, city funds, and donations. Some of the per-child tuition was funded through tuition assistance in the form of gifts from businesses, individuals, and the police and fire departments.

Keep in mind that many day camp sites make use of community assets in the form of donated or minimal-cost lease sites with summer availability, including school buildings and grounds and community buildings. Having access to a swimming pool or beach is ideal, but if either of these are not available, wading pools can be substituted to satisfy some of the water-related programming. It must be remembered that some or all staff must be responsible for the appropriate credentials to ensure safety and liability (such as water safety and instruction).

Because normalizing environments can be dangerous, programming efforts must provide a median or safe zone between risk and safety. A sufficient number of personnel is critical, and one staff member per child is not excessive. Never permit yourself to be maneuvered into enrolling too many children for your available staff; if you have a greater need than you can safely manage, then run more and shorter-duration camps (e.g., 1- or 2-week rotations).

Marketing

Because the need and requests for services initiated the programming in this example, marketing was an afterthought. However, a brochure describing the occupational therapy services was sent to all recipients of parks and recreation department mailings, and these services were also highlighted in that organization's newsletter. Keeping occupation, occupation-centered intervention, and, in this case, therapy strongly linked to the camp was a critical part of continued involvement in this setting.

Summer day camps or Saturday camp programming are excellent private practices or extensions of existing therapy practices. These may be specialty camps utilizing specific theoretical orientations or frames of reference such as sensory-integration or behavioral models for a number of differently abled children, or they might be specific to a diagnosis/condition such as asthma, muscular dystrophy, eating disorders, spinal injury, or autism spectrum.

As in this day camp example, camps may be mixed, without particular attention to diagnosis. In all of these cases, marketing and the other processes of program development will be followed by conceiving (as a first step) and then developing a program. Marketing will be to parents, other professionals, stakeholders, and community members (perhaps to the owner of a building and to potential donors of a tuition scholarship).

In general, most of the supply costs can be covered by tuition and some donations. Tuition can be paid out of pocket by consumers or can be partially covered by therapy payment services (for those continuing therapy goals) and/or tuition donations. For such a freestanding camp, corporate giving can be an important contributor depending on the mission of the program and the clientele.

Evaluation

Initial evaluation is, of course, directly tied to the goal or goals and to the objectives of the program. If campers bring with them individual therapy goals established by another practitioner or by "individualized education plan" goals, then these must be integrated into the goals of the programming; if they are not integrated directly, then the program goals must complement individual goals. For these children, progress will be measured by the programmer or, in some cases, by the occupational therapy practitioner who is seeing the client external to the camp. Camp experiences are excellent venues to maintain the goals and objectives of school-based therapies because these goals otherwise may be abandoned over the course of a summer without continued programming. For goals supporting social skills development (appropriate for most participants regardless of diagnosis or functional abilities), an observer checklist provides a marker for daily observations of those behaviors determined to be appropriate to social skills goals and objectives.

For instance, for some children making eye contact with a therapist or another child is indicative of an objective at least partially achieved; for another, giving up a toy or receiving one would merit a mark. The person recording the observer checklist can be someone who is not directly involved in programming, such as a volunteer. You could also consider the employment of a minimally cognitively impaired adult, which would be an excellent way to utilize the skills of therapy "alumni" who may be transitioning to a work environment. With some assistance and practice, they can make a significant contribution to this task that cannot be done by someone who is directly involved in activities with the children. There are other measures of social skills, but for the limited exposure of a summer camp, we are assuming that individual evaluations will occur at the primary therapy site and that our programming will enhance goal performance or at least assist in maintaining stability.

SLEEP-AWAY CAMPS

Anyone who has ever participated in a **sleep-away camp** knows what a life-changing experience being away from daily support systems can be for a child. There is probably no experience more frightening or more freeing for a child—abled or differently abled. Unfortunately, the differently abled child is most often restricted from such experiences. First of all, few opportunities exist for them, and for those that do, marketing such a camp to protective and concerned parents can be daunting. The cost of the additional and professional personnel can be high, and ensuring accessibility and comfort in existing away-camp structures can be difficult, although both of these factors can be managed by an enterprising programmer.

Although not carried to fruition (more because of time constraints than anything else), a pilot plan for a sleep-away camp was developed as a programming proposal by graduate students. This camp was designed to accommodate 8- to 10-year-old children with mild to moderate cognitive and physical disabilities, but of such significance that they would not likely be permitted to join most sleep-away camp groups. Programming was developed for the pilot group of 10 children to be at the camp for a period of 1 week. The reader may wish to explore the *Hole in the Wall Gang* system (www.HITWGCAMPS.org) of sleep-away camps for children who are terminally ill. This organization, sponsored initially by Paul Newman and Joanne Woodward, is an excellent example of what can be accomplished with such a model and with effective and persuasive fundraising efforts.

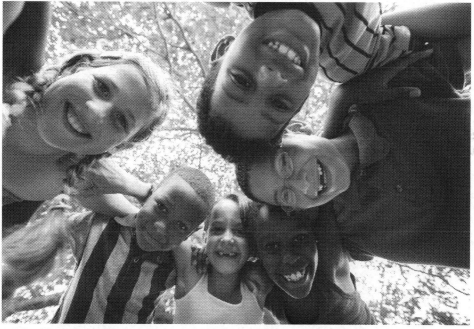

Just hanging out together.

Goals

The broad goals for this occupation-centered program included (1) team building, (2) positive interaction with others, (3) exploration of new interests, (4) development of new skills, (5) accepting and meeting responsibilities, and (6) having fun.

Programming

Programming would provide a set of activities that would be as normalizing as possible. A typical daily routine might include the following:

- Wake-up call at group tents (three children and a counselor)
- Get ready for the day (morning routines and dressing)
- Breakfast in the dining tent
- Animal care/pet therapy
- Morning exercise according to individual abilities and needs
- Activities to include hiking (also wheelchair hiking trails), water sports, paddle boating, and burro trail riding
- Lunch in the dining tent
- Kitchen cleanup and help routines
- Rest, sleep, and/or story telling
- Preparation for Family Day skits/mini plays
- Camp craft, vegetable gardening, pet care, and games
- Dinner in dining tent
- Campfire stories and activities
- Preparation for bed and "good night"

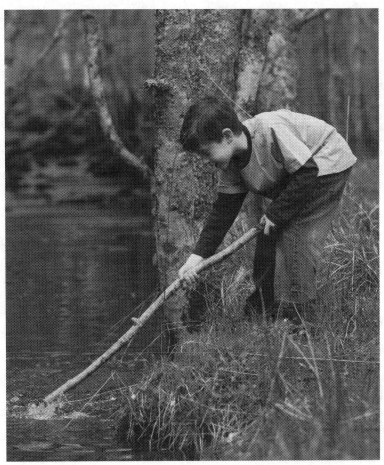

For a child who has grown up in the city, a pond is a potential "adventure."

Staffing

Staffing for a program such as this is best when overlaid on an existing camp structure with staff such as employed cooks, kitchen help, horse/burro wranglers, and lifeguards. In fact, many organizations such as the YMCA and the 4-H Clubs have such camp facilities. There are also similar camp facilities located in national parks and forests and in some state and city parks and recreation facilities.

Overlaying occupation-centered programming on such existing structures is far easier than trying to do the whole thing yourself. If you would like to develop a pilot camp such as this, first do an assessment of assets in the community to help identify partners, collaborators, and stakeholders. Then, do a thorough two-phase needs assessment including other care providers in the community as well as potential parents/caregivers, then locate a suitable existing camp facility and market your proposed program there.

The facility's administrators may be able to offer you funding or at least support funding for their services if you can obtain tuition for your attendees and perhaps some matching funding from the community for the programming you are suggesting and for the additional specialized personnel you will require.

You will likely need one-to-one counselors (preferably high school or college students) under the supervision of an occupational therapist or an occupational therapy assistant. In addition, prerequisites include any specialized staff to ensure safety and personnel with the therapeutic skills to be sure that each child is meeting the goals and objectives of the camp experience. The credentials and experience of your professional staff will be of extreme importance in your marketing efforts to parents.

Supplies and Cost

Assuming you are able to get the support services to offer the sleep-away experience, supplies and materials will not be unlike those described for day camp programming. Many parents would pay tuition out of pocket for such a camp experience for their child; for those who could not, corporate sponsorship could probably be obtained through your marketing and fundraising efforts.

For an ongoing camp such as the one described here, the primary cost would be in the professional personnel and perhaps for some initial physical alterations in camp structures that may be required to ensure accessibility (e.g., ramps, bathrooms, and wheelchair-accessible trails). Volunteer groups, parents, and patient advocacy groups are generally more than willing to assist with meeting these requirements, and Wilderness Adventure organizations and conservation groups can assist with cutting wheelchair-accessible trails and trails adapted for others (such as emphasis on scents and sounds for the vision-impaired camper).

A camp such as this offers excellent fieldwork opportunities for student involvement at all levels of development and marketing as well as in actual programming. Students from the University of Pittsburgh engage in a level I pediatric fieldwork experience that targets health promotion and prevention during a 1-week sleepover camping experience for children ages 4 through 16 years (Toto et al., 2012). Camp Watakamini in the Laurel Ridge Mountains of southwestern Pennsylvania is sponsored by a nonprofit organization that provides programs and activities for promoting self-esteem and responsibility. The occupational therapy program at the University of Pittsburgh works with this organization to offer the fieldwork experience and other fieldwork/camp experiences as well, all targeting children who come from families of low socioeconomic status who may be at risk for experiencing health problems, occupational performance limitations, and/or behavioral problems.

ADVENTURES

Of course, camps are adventures in the making, but we will also explore ideas for **adventures** programming geared toward young adults and "not so young" adults. Most likely the adventure is identified and defined by the participants themselves. As mentioned earlier, the client and the client's family are the best advocates for services. In these circumstances, the occupational therapy practitioner is the "coach" who provides information, access, and strategies for success. It is the practitioner who orchestrates the "just right challenge," or that set of circumstances where challenge and skills are exquisitely matched (Csikszentmihalyi, 1982).

Disabled Divers

Disabled Divers is a program that, in our example, combines the services and expertise of the Office of University Disability Services and Programs, the Handicapped Scuba Association, associated fundraising organizations and programs for university handicapped athletes, and the occupational therapy student organizations. Strongly motivated by the athletes with disabilities themselves, the purpose of this program was to encourage and develop students with disabilities who have an interest in water sports to become certified scuba divers. Occupational therapy students first contacted Denise Dowd, OTR/L, in Carpinteria, CA, to seek out her guidance and expertise regarding the Disabled Divers International programs (http://www.zoominfo.com/p/Denise-Dowd/398385674). Disabled Divers International is a nonprofit organization, with the aim of promoting, developing, and conducting disabled scuba diving training programs for professional and nonprofessional students (https://www.ddivers.org/about). Denise is a key member of this organization and organizes local kayaking trips for disabled paddlers as well as dive trips for disabled divers. She is an instructor with the Handicapped Scuba Association and also runs an instructor training course, teaching instructors how to work with the disabled in diving. Although strongly supported by spinal-injury participants in her California coastal occupational therapy practice, Dowd has also reported scuba diving interest from not only paraplegics and quadriplegics, but also amputees and the vision impaired. Water, at least for those who can swim, is truly a normalizing and equalizing environment. Dowd represents a common link among occupational therapy practitioners to mobilize the meaningful occupations they have selected in their own lives

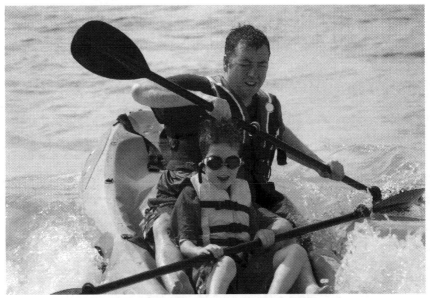

A paddler with a spinal injury enjoying an adventure with his son.

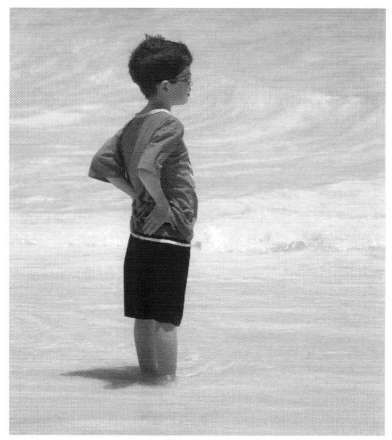

Sometimes, "adventures" are best enjoyed in small steps.

to motivate and encourage their clients. Occupational therapists who engage in "extreme" sports adventures were interviewed for an article in *OT Practice* (Waite, 2015). A common theme for these therapists was not just how occupational therapy knowledge helped the therapists complete these activities, but also how these activities helped them become better at their jobs; some have incorporated extreme sports into their practices (i.e., marathon training).

In many universities, colleges, and YMCAs, there is strong participant support for the differently abled to access sports such as wheelchair basketball, rugby, skiing, and snowboarding. Recent interest on a national and international level in the Paralympic Games has offered further support for the model of adventures through sports and, in many cases, competitive sports.

The Disabled Divers program has provided an incentive to many men and women with disabilities whose opportunities for engagement in their choice of meaningful occupations seemingly have been obliterated or at least threatened. Remember that you may have to occasionally exceed your own occupational boundaries in considering the world of your clients. Do not limit their engagement in adventure and their pursuit of meaningful occupations by not being aware of the opportunities that exist for them. For example, although you may not want to go near the water, if your clients do, you should find the best avenues possible to assist them in reaching that goal. Of course, safety must be a primary consideration, and for programs such as the one just described, every precaution is taken to protect the participants. Certified and quality instruction is critical; your task and that of your clients may be to educate the instructor with regard to the disability so that he or she can be prepared for the additional precautions that may be required. First, though, consult organizations like Disabled Divers and the Handicapped Scuba Association and ask for their advice.

Healing Through Surfing and Ocean Activities

A program that has come to fruition through the hard initial work realized in a student project is sponsored by the Jimmy Miller Memorial Foundation (www.jimmymillerfoundation.org). The mission statement for the foundation is as follows:

> The Jimmy Miller Memorial Foundation is a non-profit 501(c)(3) Foundation dedicated to honoring the life of our inspiration, Jim Miller, by supporting the healing of mental and physical illness through surfing and ocean related activities. Through recreational, educational and mentoring programs, the Jimmy Miller Foundation will bring together surfers, educators, therapists, lifeguards and friends to help people affected by mental and physical illness feel the joy and healing power of the ocean and surfing. The Foundation also supports other charities that support the protection, preservation, appreciation and safe enjoyment of the oceans, beaches and marine environment. Our mission is to carry on the legacy of Jim's pure love of surfing by showing the ocean's power to heal.

The final proposal for this ocean therapy program was designed and developed by an occupational therapist, Carly Rogers, OTD, OTR/L. It was initiated while she was a student in the author's programming class in the Chan Division of Occupational Science and Occupational Therapy at the University of Southern California. Knowing that she was an ocean lifeguard, a surfer, and an occupational therapist, the Jimmy Miller Foundation approached her for programming ideas and accepted her proposal for an ocean/surfing therapy program. Although now changed somewhat from the initial idea, the "story" of the early development of this program is described in some detail in a chapter by Fazio (2010, pp. 195-206). Since its beginnings as primarily a program for children, it now includes a very successful Wounded Warrior Program for veterans of Operation Enduring Freedom and Operation Iraqi Freedom (Rogers, Mallinson, & Peppers, 2014).

Another program that seats "adventure" in the ocean environment is Therapy in Ocean, owned and operated by Bethany Brown, OTR/L, in Florida. In this program provision of occupational therapy services include children and adults with a variety of special needs in a safe and therapeutic ocean environment (Brown, 2015). Mentioned in an earlier chapter is Israel "Izzy" Paskovitz's nonprofit surfing program called Surfers Healing. Motivated by the calming effect the ocean had on his son who has autism ("I had a feeling that maybe, just maybe, surfing might help other kids with autism like it had helped Isaiah"), Paskovitz founded Surfers Healing, the original surf camp for children with autism, in 1996 (Paskovitz, 2016). Today, the organization offers free camps during the summer months for autistic children from San Diego to Rhode Island as well as in Mexico and Puerto Rico. As of 2016, new camps opened in Sydney and in Perth, Australia.

In your investigation of potential adventures with your patient or client, also consider such venues as wilderness outings, kayaking, sailing, or boating. Look to align yourself with organizations that offer such programming to the general public in your community. Also consider the activities of organizations such as the Sierra Club or Elderhostel for those still seeking adventure but perhaps less gregariously. Although Elderhostel and Sierra Club activities are not specifically designed for populations with disability, careful choice of programming can help your clients achieve goals directed toward the accomplishment of a camera safari, wildflower viewings, and numerous other activities with these organizations. Adventure, after all, is in the eye of the beholder!

SUMMARY

The opportunity for a child, adolescent, or adult to participate in what has been described as normalizing experiences is considered to be significant in providing meaningful engagement in occupation. These experiences may consist of the conventional model for day camp that might include weekly, after-school, or weekend programming. The day camp example provided demonstrates the relationship between the assessment of need; the programming; space, staffing, and cost; marketing; and evaluation. Although sleep-away camps are more challenging for the planner, they are recommended as a way to provide opportunities for the achievement of autonomy and skill-building for the camper.

"Adventures" are novel, challenging experiences and are defined as such by the participant. For some, adventures might involve diving in the ocean as our "Disabled Divers" program describes, surfing, or perhaps it is kayaking or a camera safari. For others, it may be viewing wildflowers from a wheelchair-adapted hiking trail.

The opportunity to play, have fun, and find challenges and freedom in the outdoors defines the occupations highlighted in this chapter; in this regard, they are those experiences that promote "normal" engagement in life—experiences that are of importance for the abled and the differently abled child, adolescent, and adult.

REFERENCES

Brown, B. (2015). Therapy in ocean. Retrieved from http://sheldonbrown.com/org/ocean

City of Los Angeles. (2015). *Mission Statement*. Los Angeles, CA: Department of Recreation and Parks.

Csikszentmihalyi, M. (1982). Toward a psychology of optimal experience. In L. Wheeler (Ed.), *Review of personality and social psychology* (Vol. 2). Beverly Hills, CA: Sage.

Fazio, L. (2010). Health promotion program development. In M. Scaffa, S. M. Reitz, & M. Pizzi (Eds.), *Occupational therapy in the promotion of health and wellness* (pp. 195-206). Philadelphia, PA: F. A. Davis.

Greenstein, D., Miner, N., Kudela, E., & Bloom, S. (1993). *Backyards and butterflies: Ways to include children with disabilities in outdoor activities*. Ithaca, NY: New York State Rural Health and Safety Council.

Paskovitz, I. (2016). Surfers healing. Retrieved from http://www.surfershealing.org/

Random House Thesaurus (college edition). (1984). New York, NY: Random House.

Rogers, C., Mallinson, T., & Peppers, D. (2014). High-intensity sports for posttraumatic stress disorder and depression: Feasibility study of ocean therapy with veterans of Operation Enduring Freedom and Operation Iraqi Freedom. *American Journal of Occupational Therapy, 68*(4), 395-404.

Ryan, R. and Deci, E. (2000). Self-determination theory and the facilitation of intrinsic motivation, social development, and well-being. *American Psychologist, 55*(1), 68-78.

Toto, P., Leibold, M. L., Boardman, S., Corcoran, M., Heichel, K., . . . Simon, R. (2012). Camp Watakamini: Promoting health and wellness for children and youth at sleepover camp. *OT Practice, 17*(14), 19-21.

Waite, A. (2015). Off-hour adventures: What happens when OTs go to extremes. *OT Practice, 20*(7), 15-17.

Yerxa, E. (1999, April 9). Confessions of an occupational therapist who became a detective. Lecture. Los Angeles, CA: University of Southern California.

You will find the following references helpful in designing and implementing camp programming for all ages:

Ashton, M., & Varga, L. (1995). *101 games for groups*. Tucson, AZ: Communication Skill Builders.

Brown, O. (1983). *The metropolitan museum of art activity book*. New York, NY: The Metropolitan Museum of Art and Harry N. Abrams.

Campbell, J. (1993) *Creative art in groupwork*. Bicester, Oxford, UK: Winslow Press.

Carlson, L. (1993). *EcoArt: Earth-friendly art and craft experiences for 3- to 9-year olds*. Charlotte, VT: Williamson.

Cohen, J. G., & Wannamaker, M. (1996). *Expressive arts for the very disabled and handicapped for all ages*. Springfield, IL: Charles C Thomas.

Complete book of arts and crafts, Grades K-4 (2009). Columbus, OH: School Specialty Publishing.

Dikengil, A. T., & Kaye, M. E. (1992). *Building functional social skills: Group activities for adults*. Tucson, AZ: Therapy Skill Builders.

Furrer, P. J. (1982). *Art therapy activities and lesson plans for individuals and groups*. Springfield, IL: Charles C Thomas.

Goldschadt, S. (2012). *Craft-a-day: 365 simple handmade projects*. Philadelphia, PA: Quick Books.

Gomez, A. (1992). *Crafts of many cultures*. New York, NY: Scholastic.

Gray, L. (1990). *Something special: Seasonal and festive art and craft for children*. Twickenham, UK: Belair Publishers. (Distributed by Incentive Publications, Nashville, TN.)

Henkes, R., & Smith, D. (1991). *Art projects around the calendar*. Portland, ME: J. Weston Walch.

Homer, H., & Miller, R. (2014). *101 kids activities*. Salem, MA: Page Street Publishers.

Kamiya, A. (1985). *Elementary teacher's handbook of indoor and outdoor games*. West Nyack, NY: Parker.

Kay, J. G. (1977). *Crafts for the very disabled and handicapped for all ages*. Springfield, IL: Charles C Thomas.

Kingloff, A. (2014). *Project kid: 100 ingenious crafts for family fun*. New York, NY: Artisan Publishers.

Knoth, M. (1995). *Activity planning at your fingertips*. Lafayette, IN: Valley Press.

Korb-Khalsa, K., Azok, S., & Leutenberg, E. (1995). *Self-esteem and life skills (S.E.A.L.S. +PLUS)*. Beachwood, OH: Wellness Reproductions.

Korb-Khalsa, K., Azok, S., & Leutenberg, E. (1996). *Self-esteem and life skills, too! (S.E.A.L.S. II)*. Beachwood, OH: Wellness Reproductions.

Martha Stewart's favorite crafts for kids .(2013). New York, NY: Editors of Martha Stewart Living.

Montano, M. (2008). *The big-ass book of crafts*. New York, NY: Simon and Schuster.

Moore, K. (2015). *DIY crafts*. artscraftsandmore.com

Morris, L. R., & Schulz, L. (1989). *Creative play activities for children with disabilities: A resource book for teachers and parents*. Champaign, IL: Human Kinetics Books.

Official duck tape craft book. (2012). New York, NY: LLC Shur Tech Brands, Design Originals.

Orlick, T. (1982). *The cooperative sports and games book: Challenge without competition*. New York, NY: Pantheon Books.

Rider, B. B., & Gramblin, J. (1987). *The activity card file*. Kansas City, KS: Rider and Rider.

Rider, B. B., & Scharfenberg, C. (1999). *The book of activity cards for D D adults: Designed for groups*. Kansas City, KS: Rider and Rider.

Rodriguez, A. (1984). *The special artist's handbook: Art activities and adaptive aids for handicapped students*. Palo Alto, CA: Dale Seymour.

Rohnke, K. (1984). *Silver bullets: A guide to initiative problems, adventure games and trust activities*. Dubuque, IA: Kendall/Hunt.

Rowland, A. (1995). *How I learned to make friends: A workbook of activities to help children make friends*. King of Prussia, PA: The Center for Applied Psychology.

Sattler, H. R. (1987). *Recipes for art and craft materials*. Beech Tree Productions. New York, NY: William Morrow and Company.

Sayne, J. T. (1996). Ability awareness day: Summer day camp disability-education program. *Parks and Recreation, 31*, 24.

Schwake, S., & Schwake R. (2012). *Art lab for kids: 52 creative adventures*. www.quarybooks.com

Sher, B. (1995). *Popular games for positive play: Activities for self-awareness*. Tucson, AZ: Therapy Skill Builders.

Smead, R. (1995). *Skills and techniques for group work with children and adolescents*. Champaign, IL: Research Press.

Sobel, J. (1983). *Everybody wins: 393 Non-competitive games for young children*. New York, NY: Walker.

Tedrick, T., & Green, E. (1995). *Activity experiences and programming within long-term care*. State College, PA: Venture.

Terzian, A. M. (1993). *The kids' multicultural art book: Art and craft experiences from around the world*. Charlotte, VT: Williamson.

The World's Best Mandala coloring book. (2015). New York, NY: Adult Coloring Books and Penny Farthing Graphics. Shutterstock.com

Wankelman, W. F., & Wigg, P. (2006). *A handbook of arts and crafts*. Dubuque, IA: William C. Brown.

Witoski, M. L. (1992). *It's not just a parachute: Integrative activities for children of all abilities*. Tucson, AZ: Therapy Skill Builders.

Wnek, B. (1992). *Holiday games and activities*. Champaign, IL: Human Kinetics Books.

Internet Sites

The Association of Hole in the Wall Gang Camps, Inc.: www.HITWGCAMPS.org

Disabled Divers International/Denise Dowd: https://www.ddivers.org

Elderhostel, United States and Internationally: www.elderhostel.org

Ocean Therapy/Carly Rogers, OTD, OTR/L: www.jimmymillerfoundation.org

Sierra Club: www.sierraclub.org

Surfers Healing/Israel "Izzy" Paskovitz: www.surfershealing.org

Therapy in Ocean/Bethany Brown: http://sheldonbrown.org/ocean/

19

Prevention and Wellness Programming Within Existing or Newly Formed Clubs
Collaboration and Partnering With Stakeholders

LEARNING OBJECTIVES

1. To understand the significance of the "club" as a structure within which to place occupation-centered programs

2. To appreciate how the structure of a club is defined by the developmental age and resulting needs of the child or adolescent

3. To appreciate the opportunities for collaboration and partnering with existing community organizations and stakeholders

4. To identify examples of existing clubs and associations whose mission and goals are compatible with occupation-centered programs

5. To consider the importance of gender in developing the goals and structure of club-based programs

6. To explore program examples housed in existing club structures and associations

7. To examine the design and development of free-standing club structures to meet the occupation-centered program needs of children, adolescents, and adults

Fazio, L. S. *Developing Occupation-Centered Programs With the Community, Third Edition* (pp 311-328).
© 2017 Taylor & Francis Group.

KEY TERMS

1. Clubs
2. Middle childhood
3. Adolescence
4. Gender-specific clubs
5. 4-H Club
6. Roots and Shoots
7. Boys and Girls' Clubs of America
8. YMCA/YWCA
9. Freestanding club

This chapter focuses on the concept of the **club** as a community within a community; it describes new and existing structures appropriate for the placement of occupation-centered programs. Included are program examples that offer a combination of preventative and restorative goals appropriate to the children and adults involved, and one—the Jazz/Blues Club—demonstrates the specific intention of strengthening and reaffirming community for the members.

A foundation for understanding why the context of *club* is appropriate for occupation-centered programming is established and examples are provided to describe the characteristics and goals of several organizational structures based on the concept of *club*. To highlight the importance of collaboration and partnering with other community organizations, stakeholder structures and examples of programs for children, adolescents, and adults are offered that have been incorporated into existing clubs with missions and goals compatible with our own occupation-based views of effective programming. Two examples are provided where a new, freestanding club was established to support the proposed programming.

The first example for children and adolescents is an occupation-centered program that utilizes the Roots and Shoots project sponsored by Jane Goodall, which is then placed within an urban 4-H Club. Second, a program that exists within the structure of a Boys and Girls Club is described, followed by two brief examples of programming under the umbrella structures of the Young Men's Christian Association (YMCA) and the Young Women's Christian Association (YWCA). The first is a program for adult client/members with Parkinson's disease and their spouses, and the second is a "Mommy and Me" program for adolescent mothers. The last two examples are of clubs created for the purposes of enhancing the goals and objectives of the developing occupation-centered programming. One is the middle-school Ice Cream Cart Club, and the second is the Jazz/Blues Club intended to create or establish community in a group of older adults disenfranchised by the gentrification of the inner city, with resulting changes in urban culture.

WHY CLUBS?

Think back to when you were a child. You most likely sought membership in both formal and informal clubs. Why are clubs so appealing to children? Perhaps some of the answers to this question can be found by exploring what is known of the social, behavioral, and cognitive development of children and adolescents that for each group would permit the club to be such a powerful motivator and, in that regard, a powerful agent for positive change. Florey (1998, 2003) and Florey and Greene (1997, 2008) discuss the occupation of play in middle childhood (ages 6 to 12 years) and the transition in social groups toward increasing structure and elaboration of membership requirements. Citing Boy Scouts and Girl Scouts as examples, Florey (2003) recommends that occupational therapy programming for children—particularly for children in middle childhood—include an emphasis on clubs to meet the inclusion needs of this age group.

Middle Childhood

In most cultures, the earlier years of **middle childhood** (ages 6 to 7 years) appear to be the time when both adults (parents and caregivers) and peer groups place fairly stringent demands on children for new and more sophisticated social behaviors. This is particularly so in societies where formal schooling is a central occupation for this age group. Even more than the often stringent parental expectations for more grownup behaviors, the peer group moves into position as perhaps the major context for continued development—particularly in the social and behavioral domain—during these years. Although adult control may appear to be absent in these peer groups, covert parental/adult sanctions are realized through the rules attached to games and, perhaps more specifically for our examples, through memberships in clubs or organizations. These club/organizational selections are often more formal in nature and are supported by the parent or adult caregiver. The peer-selected and peer-organized clubs are of a more informal nature but nevertheless have a tremendous impact on the child's social development.

Why do the child and adult parent both gravitate toward the idea of a club? The work of Jean Piaget (1960) would suggest that cognitive changes—particularly those that serve to mediate social and behavioral learning—are occurring in middle childhood. These changes permit children to appreciate actions and views of others that may be in disagreement with their own and, through this awareness, they may learn to mediate their actions to get along with adults and peers. The demands of this developmental "window" can best be realized through play, most likely through such forms of organized play as soccer, hockey, and baseball and the clubs organized around these sports. Membership and participation in such clubs have a set of prescribed rules/expected behaviors accompanying membership, and the rules for sports clubs might support cooperation, fairness, participation, spirit, and team building.

Adolescence

Many foundational developmental theorists, including Piaget (1960), Inhelder and Piaget (1958), Erikson (1968), Havighurst (1972), Kohlberg (1984), Keating (1980), Siegler (1981), Siegler and Eisenberg (2014), Gilligan (1982, 1993), and Sigelman and Shaffer (1995), have proposed numerous ways to define and understand development from childhood to older adulthood, of course including **adolescence.** Their varying theoretical perspectives describe development from an organismic view (biological, psychoanalytic, or cognitive-developmental) or an environmental view (sociological-anthropological or social learning–behavioral). Although agreeing on the general parameters, the developmental theorists differ in the emphasis they place on the influences that biology, cognition, social factors, environment, and culture have on the phases of development and on the psychological characteristics attached to it. As you review these theorists and others, you will likely find that you will be more influenced by some views than by others, and your programming goals and objectives will reflect this.

If middle childhood seems to hold the most opportunity and challenge for social behavior/rule development and seems to offer the strongest support for clubs, then the period of later childhood or adolescence, which begins at around age 12 years and continues to age 20 years or so and is accompanied by expectations for adult responsibility, is likely one of even greater potential social change. Numerous theorists, including those mentioned previously, have applied their knowledge to the period following middle childhood. This is the period that we have come to know as adolescence, which is derived from the Latin verb *adolescere* and means "to grow to maturity." Most agree that it is a developmental passage of fairly dramatic changes in all of the domains (physical, cognitive, psychological, and social). Expanding cognitive abilities often invite the adolescent to think about worlds he or she does not yet have the physical and social development to master. The adolescent is not quite an adult but also is no longer a child. The potential frustration and impatience prompted by this discrepancy coupled with the adult desire for independence and the child's need to self-validate through belonging offer support of carefully structured club programming for the adolescent as well as for the child.

According to Keating (1980), adolescents are developing ways of thinking that are different than those of middle childhood, and these ways of thinking must be considered and encouraged as we write programming. Adolescents are capable of (1) thinking about possibilities; (2) thinking ahead; (3) thinking about hypotheses; (4) thinking about thought (i.e., thinking about their own thought processes, or meta-cognitive thinking and second-order thinking, such as developing rules about rules); and (5) thinking beyond conventional limits (Keating, 1980, p. 609; Piaget, 1960)—all characteristics that must be considered by programmers.

These characteristics are in contrast to the middle childhood years, when much thought in response to choices and circumstances may be spontaneous and more self-centered. This is not to say that all adolescents have achieved the same level of thought or social/behavioral responsiveness, nor does it suggest that all younger children have not. Rather, it is always necessary to know the child regardless of chronological age expectations as there may be broad ranges of variation between developmental and chronological expressions of age.

Another developmental factor that may influence programming for adolescents is their generalized ability to consider questions regarding the social order, values, and ethics (Kohlberg, 1984). For example, a club membership may have an entirely different meaning for an adolescent than it might for a younger child. The opportunity to meet with peers in a club format for projects and discussions dealing with issues of moral responsibility and global concerns might not only engage the adolescent in positive peer interactions, but it also might assist in the achievement of the underpinnings necessary for choosing all present and future occupations holding meaning and personal fulfillment. For example, the Roots and Shoots Club may be equally appealing for younger children and for adolescents, but programming within the goals of the club would take on quite different features to hold the interest of the two age groups. Csikszentmihalyi and Larson (1984) have researched the lives of adolescents in order to provide a picture from the "inside out," or the adolescent's internal dimensions of experience. They explore many areas that can assist us in organizing programming for this age group, but much of the adolescent experiences appear to be ones of conflict between instinctual choices (perhaps more similar to middle childhood) and emerging values. This transition reinforces the use of activity experiences to assist in clarifying thinking with regard to daily and long-term occupational choices and to value systems that may be in the process of development.

Whether one supports the view of adolescence as a generally unpleasant and stormy period of transition, it is surely recognized as one of considerable potential stress and responsibility as the child prepares for new roles requiring independence. This is a time when intervention in the form of education, information, skill building, and supportive coaching/mentoring is needed to encourage self-efficacy and a smooth transition toward positive choices. You may wish to review the developmental theories of childhood and adolescence in depth as you prepare to work with these groups and as you select the conceptual framework or "window" through which to view your community group. When we consider the ideas for community programming with adolescent populations—whether these populations are thought to be at risk (note that some theorists believe this is such a difficult period that all adolescents may be "at risk") or whether we are working with adolescents who have recognized psychopathology—we must utilize what is known developmentally about these children to build our service profiles as well as to establish the goals for our programs.

If you are designing programming for children with known psychosocial dysfunction or children with delayed cognitive and social development, then you must be familiar with the literature on the seriously emotionally disturbed (a school system classification), autistic spectrum disorders, attention deficit disorder, and cognitive disabilities. Although it will not tell us much about the individual child's problems, the *Diagnostic and Statistical Manual for Mental Disorders* (American Psychiatric Association, 2013) is widely used to describe the clinical manifestations of these disorders. Florey (1998, 2003) and Florey and Greene (1997), however, caution us that there is confusion in identifying children with emotional problems. The reasons for this dilemma may include such factors as fear of stigma, financial constraints, and general lack of identification, which often results in children being inappropriately labeled collectively as "learning disabled" and/or "troubled."

The school system, which is where the child's primary occupation is enacted, is likely the community where much of your child-adolescent programming will take place (if not directly in the school, then in environments adjacent to the school). Alternative schools and detention centers are also excellent sites for programming; these are sites where children and adolescents may be placed following engagement in risk factors (such as substance abuse, delinquent behavior, and youth pregnancies) that may accompany seriously emotionally disturbed or learning disability diagnoses.

Gender-Specific Clubs

In thinking about the structure of a club or "community within a community," one must consider how much the structure/organization should mirror the "real world" or expected environment of the child and how much it should be adapted to provide opportunities for learning and preparation for a reality not yet attained. Young (1992) and Batsleer (1996) support the idea of community programming as a way to support young girls' and women's concerns separate from those of young men, and they offer an agenda to challenge what they describe as sexism in community work—at least from a social service perspective. Although their particular examples are from England, there is likely cross-cultural validity in their findings. Hooks (1984) proposes the use of the forum of community programming to assist in advocating for women and their emancipation and to assist in obtaining justice. In her view, community programming can support feminism in its effort to end oppression. In fact, community work with young women who have been abused, are pregnant in childhood, are young single mothers, or have been accustomed to becoming sexually and emotionally support to or codependent with young male gang members may have such an awareness and intention as an obvious or more likely covert agenda.

Women and men as "communities" may share some but not all social experiences. Mixing the same sex but different ages and cultures may offer new interpretations of experience and new identities. Taking risks and acknowledging differences and similarities may result in creativity in problem solving and resultant strength (Batsleer, 1996). Batsleer goes on to support offering young women relevant information in an environment where they feel comfortable and secure. The comfortable and secure environment may be the strongest support for **gender-specific clubs.** Beetham (1991) and Arendt (1986) refer to these community groups as "empowering," which is triggered by acting in concert. Arendt notes that "power is never the property of an individual; it belongs to a group and remains in existence only so long as the group keeps together" (1986, p. 64). Arendt goes on to say that same-sex groups (women in her examples) can exercise power by rules of exclusion. This exclusion of not only the opposite sex but also members of the same sex by arbitrarily changing "passwords" for entry or other such exclusionary rules is, in fact, part of the appeal of informal clubs in middle childhood. Unfortunately, exclusionary rules are factors in bullying behaviors as well.

Safe houses and other examples of community programming for abused women and their children are examples of what Arendt (1986, p. 64) might describe as "empowering practice." These are intended to be safe places to teach and support strategies for resisting or avoiding violence, but, more importantly, to establish links to the legal and social systems and to other women.

With any community, group empowerment seems to be a desirable agenda even if it is not the primary or even visible one. Programming that includes informed choices, self-reflection through the telling of life stories, and survival techniques offers empowering opportunities. The "Mommy and Me" Story Quilt Club program is an example. One should also note that empowerment is certainly not only for the young; older adults are often disenfranchised when it comes to issues of power and efficacy as well. An important feature of the study on aging performed by Clark and associates (1997) was that wellness was supported in part by knowing how to access the occupations in which one wanted to engage. In this way, the occupational therapists offered information and opportunity with regard to access not only to such things as public transportation, but, more importantly, to power and efficacy.

If these arguments seem too political for you, consider the work of several developmental theorists concerning gender and minority-group development. A number of researchers have studied identity formation as a critical stage of adolescent development, and several of these studies have focused specifically on gender differences (Abraham, Feldman, & Nash, 1978; Markstrom-Adams, 1992; Markus & Kitayama, 1991). Others have focused on minority differences where there appears to be much stronger evidence than for gender-based differences. Spencer and Markstrom-Adams (1990), for example, have researched identity formation among minority-group children in the United States. For these children, the progression through childhood and adolescence is further complicated by negative social stereotyping by their majority peers and often by lower incomes that push them to a social status lower than their majority peers. If you consider these factors alongside Marcia's (1966) stages of identity formation, then the children in this group may be at risk for altering their development through what he describes as foreclosure, or adopting an externally based identity and prematurely committing to roles rather than goals and values (p. 556).

Earlier theorists, including Freud (1935/1953) and Erikson (1968), believed there were significant sex differences in the process of forming an identity. More recent research offers mixed support for this earlier contention. In their work on identity development, role-taking skills, occupational knowledge, and career development in adolescence, Grotevant, Cooper, and Kramer (1986) and Grotevant and Durrett (1980) reported that adolescent girls scored higher levels of identity achievement than boys with regard to friendship. Their work was supported by Archer (1982, 1992), who found that girls score higher in areas of choice with regard to combining career and family. Based on this somewhat limited research, support for gender-based clubs is not as compelling as support might be for minority-based programming. If one considers other measurements of development in addition to identity formation, however, then perhaps a stronger case can be made. Certainly, gender- and minority-based programming will likely have a different mission, goals, and objectives than those where the population is more diverse. Neville-Jan and colleagues (1997) offer a description of a middle school program that focuses on transition. The programming interweaves the developmentally related needs of these children, along with minority-based concerns that extend into the family and the community.

THE CLUBS

Although this is certainly not an exclusive listing, there are many opportunities for programming across the country offered in conjunction with the following five organizations or clubs: the 4-H Club, the Jane Goodall Roots and Shoots Program, the Boys and Girls Clubs of America, the YMCA, and the YWCA. These organizations have been selected specifically because of the compatibility of their missions with our interests as occupation-centered practitioners. The following descriptions will provide you with some general background information on these groups; as you read about the organizations, think about compatible occupation-centered programming that you might develop.

The 4-H Club

I pledge my HEAD to clearer thinking, my HEART to greater loyalty, my HANDS to larger service and my HEALTH to better living.

Perhaps you recognize this as the motto, or pledge, of the **4-H Club** (www.4h-usa.org). The beginnings of the twentieth century also witnessed the beginnings of what might be described as the demise of the rural American lifestyle, which was represented through a sense of "rugged individualism" coupled with a concern and kindness translated as "neighborliness." The young people of rural America were rapidly leaving for the cities and perceived brighter futures in industry. Beginning as early as the late 1800s, several factors brought about the beginnings of the 4-H Club. These included a growing concern for the quality of rural education and the relevance of the public schools to country life and a concern for advancing agricultural technology that was being developed by land-grant universities but was not gaining rapid favor in most agricultural communities.

4-H appears not to be the idea of any one person; rather, it was developed as a widespread grassroots movement to encourage rural youth to "stay on the farm," but to do so while embracing new ideas for productivity as well as sound values and behaviors. By 1904, clubs were formed to teach life skills and learning-by-doing projects. Community service projects were developed to capture the joint efforts of adults and youth, first by appealing to boys through activities such as rewarding the best corn crop and then to girls by fostering sewing, canning of vegetables, and baking projects. Interest spread throughout the Midwest and Texas and, in 1906, Thomas M. Campbell, an assistant to George Washington Carver, organized clubs with similar goals for Black farmers and their children in the south. These so-called "corn" and "sewing" clubs came under the sponsorship of the Cooperative Extension System established by the Smith-Lever Act in 1914, and 4-H Clubs soon were started in nearly every state. The clubs for boys and girls tended to be organized separately. While boys were being encouraged to adopt new agricultural techniques and methods to increase production, the girls' groups were evolving to examine the roles of women in the rural home and community. Self-confidence and a commitment to community became shared goals.

Clubs were not only in rural areas, but in cities as well. Many of the city-based clubs were organized to encourage activities between rural and city youth and, by 1948, the exchanges were matched by those between American and European club members through the International Farm Youth Exchange.

Today, the 4-H Club movement continues to be strong and is more centered on the personal growth of the child. It is the nation's largest positive youth development and youth mentoring organization, empowering 6 million young people in the United States (www.4h-usa.org). 4-H partners with 110 universities to develop life-changing, well-researched programs. 4-H boys and girls clubs are most often combined under similar interests. Projects continue to be utilized in the development of lifelong skills, and efforts are rewarded. It is intended that participants become contributing, productive, self-directed members of society. Making decisions, learning to communicate, learning the characteristics of leadership, and learning how to cope with change are goals of today's clubs.

The 4-H Club remains a largely federally organized group with county and states retaining control over its programs. International programs are presently active in more than 80 countries. A wide and diverse range of interests was represented in the listing of the National Training and Events Activities of Clubs in 1997–1998; these included such topics as Partnerships for Preventing Violence; Habitat Evaluation; Engineering, Science, and Leadership; Dairy Conference; Safety Council Congress and Exposition; and the Poultry and Egg Conference (www.4H-usa.org).

Today's clubs, which have expanded to become some of the most successful youth clubs in existence, range from the community club model to urban interest groups, community resource development, special interest groups, school enrichment, camping, and interagency learning experiences. One of the more recent 4-H initiatives, in 2002, was the 4-H Afterschool (www.4hafterschool.

org), a volunteer-driven program designed to help kids find something fun, constructive, and safe to do in the hours after school. It is not difficult to recognize the similarities between the purposes and goals of 4-H and those of occupational therapy. An occupation-centered program focused on health promotion, social skills enhancement, and emotional risk reduction can be comfortably placed within the existing structures of 4-H Club programming while retaining the vitality of both. Opportunities for creative programming based on the principles of occupation are boundless.

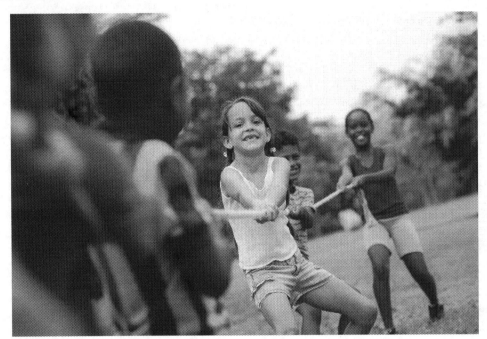

Enjoying an after-school 4-H Club activity.

Roots and Shoots

Roots and Shoots was established in the summer of 1991 with 12 students in Tanzania, and it now has 150,000 members in 130 countries. It is the Jane Goodall Institute's global, youth-led, community action program. Goodall is best known for her research on chimpanzee behavior in Tanzania, but she has become equally recognized for her substantial interests in sustainability, conservation, education, and animal welfare. Roots and Shoots is an international environmental education and humanitarian program for young people. It encourages and empowers children and young adults to coordinate constructive activities that promote care and concern for the environment, for animals, and for the human community. Roots and Shoots was the name selected to recognize that "children are the fertile ground in which seeds are planted" (Jane Goodall Institute for Wildlife Research, Education, and Conservation, 1995).

Once seeds germinate, of course, their roots spread in all directions and establish a firm foundation. Important work can be accomplished when each child is recognized as important to the future of all children. The fundamental concepts and philosophy of Roots and Shoots include "care and concern for the environment; care and concern for animals; and community enrichment through constructive service projects" (Jane Goodall Institute for Wildlife Research, Education, and Conservation, 2015, p. 1).

The example we will explore a bit later in this chapter is one of a club within a club, that is, Roots and Shoots within the structure of a 4-H Club. Although the interests of the occupational therapy providers/occupation-centered practitioners were in the enrichment of and concern for the individual child, all of the concepts and philosophies of both the 4-H Club and the Roots and Shoots organization were utilized as tools in the development of programming.

Boys and Girls Clubs of America

The Boys and Girls Club movement is a nationwide affiliation of local autonomous nonprofit organizations. The mission of the Boys and Girls Clubs of America is to "enable all young people, especially those who need us most, to reach their full potential as productive, caring, responsible citizens" (Boys & Girls Clubs of America, 2017b).

It is important to note that the Boys and Girls Club has a physical location, usually a neighborhood-based building where local community youth may congregate to participate in organized programs and activities. This is an important concept because the intention is to keep children off the street and preferably not at home when adult supervision is absent. The clubs are open every day after school and on weekends. Every club has paid, full-time, trained youth-development professionals who are selected to be mentors and positive role models. Volunteers are relied on for key supplementary support. Children pay a small amount of dues per year, but supportive moneys are provided through campaigned gift donations based on the club's proven delinquency-prevention programs.

There are currently nearly 4 million members in over 4,100 clubs including domestic and international military bases (Boys & Girls Clubs of America, 2017a). Of these members, 71% lived in urban/inner-city areas, 53% were from single-parent families, 51% were from families of three or more children, 56% were from minority families, and 42% were from families with annual incomes below $22,000. Ages of members range from 7 years and younger (16%) up to 18 years of age (21% are between the ages of 14 and 18), with the largest group (34%) between 8 and 10 years of age. Boys make up 62% of the children and girls the remaining 38%.

Boys and Girls Clubs are another excellent site for occupation-centered programming with general goals supportive of the prevention of behaviors leading to patterns of crime and delinquency.

A Programming Example of Multiple Collaborations: A Club Within a Club Within a Club

This example of the Jane Goodall Roots and Shoots programming was developed at two sites—in the 4-H Club after-school enrichment program established through the partial support of the Los Angeles Housing Authority and the County Parks and Recreation Department, and at an East Los Angeles Boys and Girls Club. There is likely no better example of layered and embedded collaborations and partnering. These programs were the result of the shared efforts of the Jane Goodall Institute's Roots and Shoots programming, the 4-H Clubs of America, the Los Angeles Housing Authority, the Los Angeles County Department of Parks and Recreation, the Los Angeles Zoo, the University of Southern California's Chan Division of Occupational Science and Occupational Therapy, and the Boys and Girls Clubs of America—Los Angeles.

The two sites selected serviced similar populations, which included Hispanic boys and girls between the ages of 7 and 11 years who were from low-income families. The community profiles presented similar pictures of apparent neighborhood neglect as evidenced by graffiti, numerous gang signs, and garbage. More optimistically, it was noted that two parks were in the process of being repaired and landscaped by the city.

The two occupation-centered programs were identical in their after-school structure and in their affiliation with existing clubs. The early needs assessment at both sites demonstrated an interest in programming that would support the existing goals of both the 4-H Club and the Boys and Girls Club. Both groups expressed interest in improving their community and suggested several ways they might do so that ranged from picking up trash, to planting gardens, to helping older residents run errands in the neighborhood. Because of its supportive structure for under-standing and building community through attention to one's habitat (in our case, neighborhood) and its already-developed programming ideas along these lines, the Jane Goodall Roots and Shoots structure was selected as a vehicle for the occupation-centered intervention. The success of the existing after-school 4-H Club at the Housing Authority site and the Boys and Girls Club as well as the chronological and developmental ages of the children involved supported the choice of a club format embedded within the existing programming.

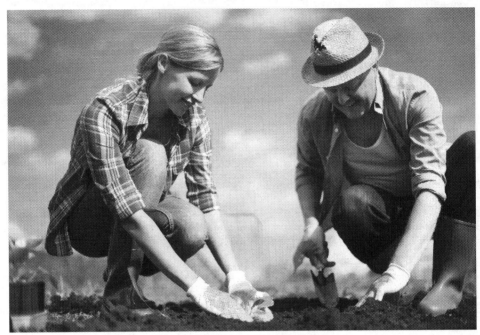

Planting community gardens encourages caring for the environment.

Although not necessarily articulated, the combined message of all of the clubs was empower-ment to effect change, first in one's community and secondly in oneself. In addition, building a community of caring and concerned children whose example would encourage those around them to also build rather than destroy was equally important. A review of the purposes of both organiza-tions demonstrates that the goal of "empowerment through positive change" and the objectives to demonstrate care and concern for the community through such enabling activities as conducting a community celebration of Earth Day are appropriate. The specific activities of exploring the habitats and migrations of butterflies and birds through research and field surveys, planting but-terfly gardens on windowsills of nursing care facilities and in backyards of public housing, trash patrols, and "acts of kindness" patrols all targeted care for the community and were visible enough to encourage the participation of other children and adults in the activities.

The Jane Goodall Roots and Shoots Clubs frequently form a liaison with local zoos, which offers additional programming opportunities. In this example, the Los Angeles Zoo provided an opportunity to study and assist with the design of a chimpanzee habitat for the zoo and to attend the official opening. What does that have to do with an inner-city Los Angeles community? It is very applicable if the programmer makes good use of the opportunity to demonstrate community as a common and global concern. In addition, if the club can be visited by Jane Goodall or by the local media news team or has the opportunity to join in world-wide conservation-environmental activities with children from other cultures and countries, then our goal of empowerment is enhanced through recognition and group consensus. These clubs also developed programming slogans around the ideas that human life—or at least the quality of life many enjoy or would like to enjoy—may be endangered. The similarities in the way that other endangered or extinct species used or abused their habitats was impetus for research and for planning.

For both programs, the low-budget activities were subsumed under existing resources in bimonthly programming. Existing space was utilized with all regular after-school club participants who were also participating in the Roots and Shoots activities. The personnel consisted of high school students who received service learning course credit for their contributions. At the Boys and Girls Club, older participants (teens) were paid by the club to assist with programming. At the 4-H Club, paid staff also was involved with programming. In both of these cases, the consistency in programming was maintained by the paid staff when students were not available. This is a critical adjunct whenever students are involved in community-based programming so that continuity is maintained when students are not enrolled. Having volunteers or paid staff who are members of the community where programming occurs also encourages participation and investment over time and takes advantage of local assets while building capacity. Equally important is the presence of a consistent faculty or clinical advisor/supervisor to provide direction as goals, objectives, and programming is turned over to others less invested. It is also an important feature when there are many partners sharing in the goals for programming, and in the outcomes.

In order to accurately evaluate the effectiveness of the program, it would likely need a more consistent format and perhaps some way to distinguish it from the value of the 4-H programming. A measure of the effectiveness of the combined programming, however, might be acceptable since the goals and objectives are so compatible. Evaluation of these two programs consisted of two levels: (1) information and skill building in protecting and building community (immediate) and (2) personal empowerment (long-term outcome). For the first level of evaluation, pre- and post-tests of questions to determine what the children knew before and after each programming session were used to obtain immediate factual information. For example, an activity named "Take a Closer Look" was designed to sharpen their observation skills and to serve as a reminder of individual differences (1998, p. 26). The pretest asked the children to carefully view color photos of the chimpanzees at the zoo (also identified by name), and the post-test consisted of matching the distinguishing characteristics of each and the names to the actual chimps in their habitat on a field trip to the zoo. This lesson was coupled with other activities supporting the importance of distinguishing ourselves as individuals while supporting the functions and roles of a group/community.

Teasing out the meaning associated with "empowerment" is much more complicated and takes much longer. In these instances, the Nowicki-Strickland Locus of Control Scale for Children, originally developed in 1973, was used at the beginning and end of the programming cycle and was recommended as follow-up 6 months to 1 year later. The scale was used in an attempt to distinguish each students' sense of internal personal control over his or her life and actions. This link between perceived control and empowerment is supported by the research of Gibson (1993) and by Chamberlin (1997), who broadened the link to include community involvement and group participation. The use of the instrument appeared to produce positive outcomes, but the population was too small and the programming too inconsistent in the earlier phases to provide a sound measure. However, continued work with the instrument seems advantageous as a potentially effective measure of the program's goal. In work on self-concept formation, Harter (1982, 1985, 1990a, 1990b) developed the Perceived Competence Scale for Children, which also would be an appropriate measure of the goals for the children in these programs, as would the work of Battle (1981), Battle and Blowers (1982), Bruininks (1978), and Bryan and Pearl (1979). As an additional measure to further define the factors that contribute to community building, empowerment, and personal control, one of the programs was videotaped to be qualitatively coded for further investigation. The programmer must always take into consideration the length of time children (or adults) are exposed to programming and the realistic time span to measure anticipated outcomes. How long before "change" will occur, and how long will it last? Although positive changes were noted with all of the instruments, they are not generally reliable for lasting results over time without continued programming to reinforce the gains.

Another consideration to keep in mind is that whenever you select a group as recipients of your programming (in the examples here, children), you must be very aware of the meaningful occupations those recipients (children) engage in during their normal round of activities. These children were primarily engaged in a combination of schoolwork and play during their week—not an uncommon combination for any child in early and middle childhood. The task of these programs was to support the goals of schoolwork and the developmental need for play through activities that supported and enhanced community. All of the selected programming did this, although not without some trial and error. If you would like to learn more about the use of play in occupational therapy, review Parham (2008), Parham and Primeau's (1997) discussions of play and Florey and Greene's (1997) discussion of play in middle childhood.

At the Boys and Girls Club site, continued programming for older participants that is external to the 4-H Club structure included the development of a newsletter project as well as other similar group projects to produce one shared outcome. These projects were designed to meet the goals of developing skills in the realm of leadership, communication, vocational choice, and writing and organization—all within and in support of the basic parameters of community.

As you develop your own programming, if you elect to support occupation-centered goals for children to encourage the enhancement of normal development, support of school-room performance, or as a deterrent to negative-outcomes ("clubs" in the form of gangs), you may wish to more carefully examine the goals of 4-H, Boys and Girls Clubs, and, specifically, Roots and Shoots. As the Roots and Shoots programming was developed, planners discovered a number of conservation-concerned groups that provided volunteers and dollars to enhance programming. These groups included Wildlife on Wheels; Seeds of Simplicity; Heal the Bay; Tree People; The Audobon Society; and numerous parks, gardens, zoos, and museums. You will likely find similar organizations in your area.

THE YOUNG MEN'S CHRISTIAN ASSOCIATION (YMCA)

The **YMCA** was founded in London in 1844 by Sir George Williams (knighted in 1894 for his lifelong service to boys). Impetus for the establishment of the organization was the unhealthy social conditions of the times apparent in the large urban cities at the end of the Industrial Revolution. The founding young businessmen wished to help young workers avoid the social "dangers" of idleness (such as gambling and drinking) through Bible studies and prayer meetings. The organization quickly gained popularity and spread to the industrial centers of North America and throughout Europe. The first YMCA to be established in America was in Boston in 1851, and by 1854, there were 26 associations in the United States and Canada (YMCA, 2017).

In 1862, the attention of the association was turned to the welfare of American Civil War prisoners. This was the first civilian volunteer organization dedicated to the welfare of war prisoners and other servicemen, and this work continued through World War I and World War II. The YMCA continued to work not only with prisoners of war, but also with displaced persons, refugees, and soldiers. In 1941, the YMCA joined with five other organizations to form the United Service Organizations.

The post-war YMCA continued to evolve by incorporating libraries, gymnasiums, summer camps, colleges, night schools, swimming pools, mass swimming instruction, and hotel-type rooms. It is of interest that to meet the need for a "vigorous recreation suitable for indoor winter play," an instructor at the Springfield, MA, YMCA, Mr. James Naismith, invented basketball in 1891 (Naismith & Baker, 1996). At this YMCA, which is now Springfield College, volleyball was invented in 1895 by William G. Morgan, the physical education director of the YMCA in Holyoke, Massachusetts. The YMCA also assisted in the development of other groups such as the Red Cross, Boy Scouts, the Student Christian Movement, World Council of Churches, and CampFire. The years between the 1930s and the 1960s were marked by diminished interest in the activities of the YMCA and difficult financial times. In the late 1970s, however, there was renewed public interest in health and fitness, and child care was added to the organization's programs to meet the demands and needs of young mothers.

Currently the YMCA serves upward of 14 million people per year. Local YMCAs are independent and autonomous and are dedicated to local community needs and service and have as their goal the provision of values-based experiences that nurture the healthy development of children and teens, support families, and strengthen communities. Their mission is "to put Christian principles into practice through programs that build healthy spirit, mind, and body for all" (YMCA, 2017). Each YMCA is a charitable, nonprofit organization. The YMCA provides many opportunities to occupation-centered programmers for knowledge and skills development in small group venues and in a structured class format. You may find it useful to review two resources provided to occupational therapy practitioners for understanding and conducting the high functioning *groups* found in many of these organizational structures: Schwartzberg, Howe, and Barnes' (2008) *Groups: Applying the Functional Group Model* and Cole's (2012) *Group Dynamics in Occupational Therapy.*

THE YOUNG WOMEN'S CHRISTIAN ASSOCIATION (YWCA)

The **YWCA** is the largest and oldest women's organization in the United States (YWCA, 2017). Its mission is to eliminate racism; empower women; and promote peace, justice, freedom, and dignity for all. This mission was adapted by the General Assembly in 2009. The YWCA opened the first day nursery in the United States in 1864 and today continues to train child care providers and babysitters. Other child-related services are found in the forms of resource and referral agencies, child care for homeless children, services to family day care homes, and parenting education. Services for women include basic life skills training, GED courses, adult education, welfare-to-work programs, nontraditional employment, and other related services. It should be noted that women worked in the YMCA military canteens in World War I, but it was not until after World War II that they were admitted to full YMCA membership. The YWCA, however, establishes specific goals to meet the general needs of women.

Globally, the YWCA represents more than 25 million women worldwide in 120 countries. The YWCA provides shelter, child care, employment training, racial justice, physical fitness, youth development, leadership training, and world relations. Each year, more than 535,000 women come to the YWCA for safety services and support to overcome violence (YWCA, 2017).

Programs in Collaboration With the YMCA and the YWCA

Programs can be developed within the mission of an umbrella organization but can also be very different in their goals and objectives and in the population that they serve. There is no "recipe" for programs within the 4-H Club, the Boys and Girls Club, or the YMCA/YWCA. The ability to see opportunities for creative expression of an organization's mission through the exercise of occupation is entirely at the pleasure of the programmer. We will now briefly contrast two programs, each carefully articulated with the mission and goals of the YMCA/YWCA.

A Shared Exercise Program for Client/Members With Parkinson's Disease and Their Spouses

An exercise program for client/members of the YMCA with Parkinson's disease and their spouses was initiated in a fairly common way—at the request of a participant in an outpatient occupational therapy program. This participant was also a member of a YMCA in an affluent neighborhood where he had long been a strong advocate for his community in many ways. He expressed to his occupational therapist a concern that he would like to return to his YMCA for an exercise group. At the time, there was no such group that took into consideration the specific needs of people with Parkinson's disease, but there was another agenda as well: "meaning" for this patient was not only a wish to resume what for him had been a fairly normalizing activity ("adult play at the YMCA"), but also there was a need to continue or perhaps to encourage the expression of bonding and support by including his spouse. As a skillful and intuitive occupational therapist elicited this patient's story, she recognized other meanings being expressed as well. Perhaps the patient wanted to not only engage in exercise and spend time with his spouse but also, and more importantly, wanted to return to a more proactive role in his own life and his community (to be an advocate and someone who could still get things done). Perhaps he also wanted to return to a more normalizaing spousal role in which he could engage in an activity with his spouse where she was not the caregiver, but the partner. Oftentimes, personal collaborations are as worthy of encouragement as are the larger, professional shared ventures.

With some guidance, the client/member (or, simply, the community-member) developed an advocacy plan to encourage the initiation of a couples' exercise/dance program for himself, his spouse, and others with similar needs. The program was developed much like what has been described in this text. When a needs assessment demonstrated that there was enough interest to start with several classes a week, the YMCA added the classes for a fee in a similar structure to other programming and took care of the promotion and marketing. The occupational therapist, who was also an aerobics instructor and an avid "line-dancer," was hired to develop the programming along with the assistance of the participants. This program demonstrates a nice bridge between the treatment setting (one of the arenas of occupational therapy) and the community (one of the arenas of the occupation-centered practitioner). It also demonstrates the true art of the practitioner—that of recognizing and enabling the strengths of the participant to once again put them in control of their own lives.

The "Mommy and Me" Story Quilt Club

Another example appropriate to our discussion is that of a "Mommy and Me" program established in a YWCA in a far less affluent neighborhood than the one described previously. Affluence does not have much to do with these two stories except that it does seem to go hand-in-hand with one's perceived sense of control over one's destiny, which makes for some difference in the selection of goals and objectives for a successful program. Following its own somewhat informal needs assessment, this program was initiated at the request of the YWCA. The YWCA was interested in two programs—one for young mothers (13 to 16 years old) and another for these mothers and the fathers. The program for the mothers was designed to also actively include the babies. The format consisted of classes, which was similar to other programming at this facility, but fees were not charged directly to the participants. The mother and baby classes involved the shared and enmeshed occupations surrounding the physical care of the baby and also the "learning how to play together" emotional care of both mother (an adolescent) and baby.

Perhaps the most successful activity associated with this program (as reported by the mothers) was one that focused on meaningful occupation and self-advocacy, which was a theme in the previous example as well. The activity consisted of making an oversized quilt block that was large enough to function as a baby coverlet. The design of the block was developed as the mother's "story" that she wished to give her baby as her legacy or gift. The story was an expression of the mother's meaningful occupations, her values, her interests, and the things about life she most wanted her baby to know and remember. An important piece of the block also carried the theme of what the mother still wished to do with her life. Although the blocks were constructed individually, the activity was carried out as a group—the "quilting club"—and this community of young storytellers shared and validated their experiences and came away with a tangible record. This class was conducted by student volunteers as a university-related campus residential life community service project and later became the full responsibility of the YWCA.

FREESTANDING CLUBS

The last two examples are again quite different from each other in terms of population, intention, and geography and are both examples of **freestanding clubs**; although, collaboration and partnering with other service providers, organizations, and stakeholders in the community were strong factors in both. The Ice Cream Cart Club was a rural, midwestern venture, while the Jazz/ Blues Club was an inner-city urban experiment.

The Ice Cream Cart Club

The Ice Cream Cart Club was developed in response to a need, which was expressed primarily by teachers in the beginning to better integrate children with learning disabilities and autistic spectrum disorders into the student life activities of the middle school environment. All of the students identified first by the teachers were described as "socially isolated." The program was developed as a club in consideration of the developmental needs of this group (chronologically aged 11 to 14 years), and this idea was also strongly supported in the second level of needs assessment accomplished with the children who wished to be involved. All of the children first identified by the teachers were invited to be members but none were required to be. By consensus the children elected to start a lunchtime ice cream cart business. The programming involved multiple skill development in sales, marketing/promotion, accounting, and personnel management. Although significant in helping students to focus on future goals and staying in school (long-range outcomes), foundational goals were centered again around empowerment, advocacy, and self-esteem—a theme that continues to resurface in much of our programming, particularly with children and adolescents. Weekly club meetings were facilitated by a school-based occupational therapist who helped develop individual goals for each child as well as goals for the collective club. The club meetings were often indistinguishable from the goal-directed adolescent psychosocial group model (the goal being the business to be accomplished for the week). Continued programming has included the addition of several high school mentors for the group to assist in the transition from middle school as well as mentors from local businesses.

The Dunbar Hotel Jazz/Blues Club

The second example of the development of a club model—in this case to create community—is that of the Jazz Club. The Dunbar Hotel is located in downtown Los Angeles and is part of the Dunbar Economic Development Corporation. In 1975, the Dunbar Hotel Black Cultural Historical Museum was established to save the Dunbar Hotel. Through these efforts, the Hotel was designated as a city and national historical landmark (Dunbar Economic Development Corporation, 1996). Today, the hotel is newly renovated and available for tourist lodging; it is also the site of the Central Avenue Jazz Festival and other jazz-related festivals and events.

In recognition of low-income housing needs, in 1988, the hotel was financed for mixed use to include housing (73 units of low-income senior housing), commercial facilities, and cultural facilities. The intent of the occupation-centered programming that was developed in the early 1990s was to create a sense of shared community for these residents. In order to identify the characteristics of community and the meaning these residents assigned to their lives and their history, it seemed appropriate to investigate the history of the hotel. Oftentimes, a building or neighborhood has forgotten history that, when resurrected, can structure the goals and objectives of a program. In this case, the history was that of the jazz music tradition. In its original 1920s state, the hotel was a first-class hotel for Blacks. It was surrounded by jazz clubs and became the hub of the Los Angeles Black night life. As integration grew into the 1950s and Black entertainers and clubgoers were no longer restricted to downtown, the hotel and the neighborhood drifted into decay. One of the occupational therapy students, an amateur jazz historian, took an interest in the hotel and in the present residents. Upon closer investigation and a cursory needs assessment accomplished with the assistance of the social service coordinator, it was determined that the general health and well-being of the residents could likely be enhanced if they could be encouraged to become less isolated and share in some kind of activity programming. Although there was a space designed for shared activities, no one frequented the room and attempts at programming by volunteer groups had not been successful.

Upon further investigation it was discovered that many of the aging residents had been participants in the vibrant neighborhood of the jazz era, and a number were musicians themselves. Although we cannot assume that everyone continues to assign meaning to their own histories, with the kind of shared interests evident at the Dunbar, it was a fair guess that jazz and blues, in some way, continued to have meaning for many of the residents. With the resources of the museum, the Jazz/Blues Club was organized first to plan and celebrate birthdays of Black jazz and blues performers, and then to organize jam sessions and miniconcerts. Residents were first involved as the audience, but those who were able to quickly became more active participants and/or contributors.

Again, this example includes the theme of "meaning" as the significant indicator of well-being and therapy. In this example, the meaning is assessed through linkages with history, and those linkages weave the fabric of community.

SUMMARY

Clubs are examples of communities within communities. They offer the child, the adolescent, and the adult structures that support and encourage their cognitive and social development. In this way they provide the potential for powerful interventions. The cognitive and social development of middle-childhood and adolescence has been discussed to provide a foundation for understanding how the structure of clubs can be utilized to support a program that is developmentally sensitive. Whether the program planner wishes to encourage gender-specific clubs or to mix participants has also been considered. Understanding the developmental period of the participant will assist the planner who wishes to place a program within a club in selecting an appropriate club structure from existing ones or in the creation of rules and structures for a new club.

Existing club structures have been described, such as the 4-H Clubs, Jane Goodall's Roots and Shoots Clubs, Boys and Girls Clubs of America, and the YMCA/YWCA. Examples have been provided for occupation-centered clubs within the aforementioned existing club structures. In addition, the development of two freestanding clubs, the Ice Cream Cart Club and the Jazz/Blues Club, have been briefly described. All of the examples involve collaborations and partnering with the community and local stakeholders. In all of these examples, efforts were made to identify assets and strengthen capacity not only in the larger communities, but in the individuals who occupy them. The concept of "club" within developmentally appropriate contexts and rule-bound structures can provide a frame for the placement of successful occupation-centered programs for all ages.

REFERENCES

Abraham, B., Feldman, S. S., & Nash, S. C. (1978). Sex role self-concept and sex role attitudes: Enduring personality characteristics or adaptations to changing life situations? *Developmental Psychology, 14*, 393-400.

American Psychiatric Association. (2013). *Diagnostic and statistical manual of mental disorders* (5th ed.). Washington, DC: Author.

Archer, S. L. (1982). The lower age boundaries of identity development. *Child Development, 53*, 1551-1556.

Archer, S. L. (1992). A feminist's approach to identity research. In G. R. Adams, T. P. Gulotta, & R. Montemayor (Eds.), *Adolescent identity formation* (Advances in Adolescent Development, Vol. 4, pp. 32-37). Newbury Park, CA: Sage.

Arendt, H. (1986). Communicative power. In S. Lukes (Ed.), *Power* (pp. 64-71). Oxford, UK: Basil Blackwell.

Batsleer, J. (1996). *Working with girls and young women in community settings.* London, UK: Arena.

Battle, J. (1981). *Culture free self esteem inventory, self esteem inventory for children and adults.* Seattle, WA: Special Child Publications.

Battle, J., & Blowers, T. (1982). A longitudinal comparative study of the self-esteem of students in regular and special education classes. *Journal of Learning Disabilities, 15,* 100-102.

Beetham, D. (1991). *The legitimation of power.* London, UK: MacMillan.

Boys & Girls Clubs of America. (2017a). Facts and figures. Retrieved from http://bgca.org/whoweare/Pages/FactsFigures.aspx

Boys & Girls Clubs of America. (2017b). Who we are. Retrieved from http://bgca.org/whoweare/Pages/WhoWeAre.aspx

Bruininks, V. L. (1978). Actual and perceived peer status of learning disabled students in mainstream programs. *Journal of Special Education, 12,* 51-58.

Bryan, T. H., & Pearl, R. (1979). Self-concept and locus of control of learning disabled children. *Journal of Clinical Child Psychology, 8,* 223-226

Chamberlin, J. (1997). A working definition of empowerment. *Psychiatric Rehabilitation Journal, 20 (4), 43-46.*

Clark, F., Azen, S., Zemke, R., Jackson, J., Carlson, M., Mandel, D., Hay, J., . . .Lipson, L. (1997). Occupational therapy for independent-living older adults. *Journal of the American Medical Association, 278*(16), 1321-1326.

Cole, M. B. (2012). *Group dynamics in occupational therapy.* Thorofare, NJ: SLACK Incorporated.

Csikszentmihalyi, M., & Larson, R. (1984). *Being adolescent.* New York, NY: Basic Books, Harper and Row.

Dunbar Economic Development Corporation. (1996). *Organizational history.* Los Angeles, CA: Author.

Erikson, E. (1968). *Identity: Youth in crisis.* New York, NY: Norton.

Florey, L. (1998). Psychosocial dysfunction in childhood and adolescence. In M. Neistadt & E. Crepeau (Eds.), *Willard and Spackman's occupational therapy* (9th ed., pp. 622-635). Philadelphia, PA: Lippincott, Williams and Wilkins.

Florey, L. (2003). Psychosocial dysfunction in childhood and adolescence. In E. Crepeau, E. Cohn, & B. Schell (Eds.), *Willard and Spackman's occupational therapy* (10th ed., pp. 731-744). Philadelphia, PA: Lippincott, Williams and Wilkins.

Florey, L., & Greene, S. (1997). Play in middle childhood: A focus on children with behavior and emotional disorders. In L. D. Parham & L. S. Fazio (Eds.), *Play in occupational therapy for children* (pp. 126-143). St. Louis, MO: Mosby.

Florey, L. & Greene, S. (2008). Play in middle childhood: A focus on children with behavior and emotional disorders. In L. D. Parham & L. S. Fazio (Eds.), *Play in occupational therapy for children* (2nd ed., pp. 279-299). St. Louis, MO: Mosby.

Freud, S. (1935/1953). *A general introduction to psychoanalysis.* (J. Riviere, Translator). New York, NY: Permabooks.

Gibson, C. M. (1993). Empowerment theory and practice with adolescents of color in the child welfare system. *Families in Society, 74*(7), 387-396.

Gilligan, C. (1982). *In a different voice: Psychological theory and women's development.* Cambridge, MA: Harvard University Press.

Gilligan, C. (1993). *In a different voice: Psychological theory and women's development* (Rev. ed.). Cambridge, MA: Harvard University Press.

Grotevant, H. D., Cooper, C. R., & Kramer, K. (1986). Exploration as a predictor of congruence in adolescents' career choices. *Journal of Vocational Behavior, 29,* 201-215.

Grotevant, H. D., & Durrett, M. (1980). Occupational knowledge and career development in adolescence. *Journal of Vocational Behavior, 17,* 171-182.

Harter, S. (1982). The perceived competence scale for children. *Child Development, 53,* 87-97

Harter, S. (1985). *Manual for the self-perception profile for children.* Denver, CO: University of Denver Press.

Harter, S. (1990a). Issues in the assessment of the self-concept of children and adolescents. In A. M. LaGreca (Ed.), *Through the eyes of the child: Obtaining self-reports from children and adolescents.* Boston, MA: Allyn and Bacon.

Harter, S. (1990b). Processes underlying adolescent self-concept formation. In R. Montemayor, G. R. Adams, & T. P. Gullotta (Eds.), *From childhood to adolescence: A transitional period?* Newbury Park, CA: Sage.

Havighurst, R. (1972). *Developmental tasks of education* (3rd ed.). New York, NY: David McKay.

Hooks, B. (1984). *Feminist theory: From margin to center.* Boston, MA: South End Press.

Inhelder, B., & Piaget, J. (1958). *The growth of logical thinking from childhood to adolescence.* New York, NY: Basic Books.

Jane Goodall Institute for Wildlife Research, Education and Conservation. (1995). *Roots and Shoots Fact Sheet.* Ridgefield, CT: Author.

Jane Goodall Institute for Wildlife Research, Education and Conservation. (2015). *Roots and Shoots Fact Sheet.* Ridgefield, CT: Author.

Keating, D. P. (1980). Thinking processes in adolescence. In J. Adelson (Ed.), *Handbook of adolescent psychology.* New York, NY: Wiley.

Kohlberg, L. (1984). *The psychology of moral development: The nature and validity of moral stages.* New York, NY: Harper and Row.

Marcia, J. (1966). Development and validation of ego identity status. *Journal of Personality and Social Psychology, 3,* 551-558.

Markstrom-Adams, C. (1992). A consideration of intervening factors in adolescent identity formation. In G. R. Adams, T. P. Gullotta, & R. Montemayor (Eds.), *Adolescent identity formation. Advances in adolescent development* (Vol. 4). Newbury Park, CA: Sage.

Markus, H. R., & Kitayama, S. (1991). Culture and the self: Implications for cognition, emotion, and motivation. *Psychological Review, 98,* 224-253.

Naismith, J., & Baker, W. (1996). Basketball: Its origin and development (2nd ed.). Omaha, NE: University of Nebraska Press, Bison Books.

Neville-Jan, A., Fazio, L. S., Kennedy, B., & Snyder, C. (1997). Elementary to middle school transition: Using multicultural play activities to develop life skills. In L. D. Parham & L. S. Fazio (Eds.), *Play in occupational therapy for children* (pp. 144-157). St. Louis, MO: Mosby.

Nowicki, S., & Strickland, B. R. (1973). A locus of control scale for children. *Journal of Consulting and Clinical Psychology, 40,* 148-154.

Parham, L. D. (2008). Play. In L. D. Parham & L. S. Fazio (Eds.), *Play in occupational therapy for children* (Introduction). St. Louis, MO: Mosby.

Parham, L. D., & Primeau, L. (1997). Introduction to play and occupational therapy. In L. D. Parham & L. S. Fazio (Eds.), *Play in occupational therapy for children* (pp. 2-21). St. Louis, MO: Mosby.

Piaget, J. (1960). *The psychology of intelligence.* Paterson, NJ: Littlefield, Adams.

Schwartzberg, S., Howe, M., & Barnes, M. A. (2008). *Groups: Applying the functional group model.* Philadelphia, PA: Davis.

Siegler, R. S. (1981). Developmental sequences within and between concepts. *Monographs of the Society for Research in Child Development, 46*(2), serial no. 189.

Siegler, R. S., & Eisenberg, N. (2014). *How children develop* (4th ed.). Philadelphia, PA: Lippincott, Williams and Wilkins.

Sigelman, C., & Shaffer, D. (1995). *Life-span human development* (2nd ed.). Pacific Grove, CA: Brooks/Cole.

Spencer, M., & Markstrom-Adams, C. (1990). Identity processes among racial and ethnic minority children in America. *Child Development, 61,* 290-310.

"Take a Closer Look." (1998). *Roots and Shoots Los Angeles: A curriculum packet to connect community, environment and wildlife.* (Limited publication supported by The Los Angeles Roots and Shoots Steering Committee, The Los Angeles Zoo, and The University of Southern California Department of Occupational Science and Occupational Therapy.)

YMCA. (2017). History. Retrieved from http://www.ymca.net/history/

Young, K. (1992). Work with girls and young women: Losing the purpose? *Youth Clubs, 67,* 17.

YWCA. (2017). Who we are. Retrieved from http://www.ywca.org/site/c.cuIRJ7NTKrLaG/b.7515821/k.23CE/Who_We_Are.htm

Internet Sites

4-H: http://www.4h-usa.org
4-H Afterschool: www.4hafterschool.org
YMCA: http://www.ymca.net
YWCA: http://www.ywca.org
Boys & Girls Clubs of America: http://www.bgca.org
Jane Goodall's Roots and Shoots http://www.rootsandshoots.org

20

Shelter Programming for Homeless Persons With HIV/ AIDS and Mental Illness
Exploring Skills and Knowledge Supporting Employment

LEARNING OBJECTIVES

1. To appreciate the complexity of programming necessary to meet the multiple needs of those homeless persons with HIV/AIDS who may be mentally ill

2. To examine the development of a sample program to meet the goals and multiple objectives of a selected group of homeless persons with HIV/AIDS and mental illness

3. To understand the contributions of activity analysis to the success of an occupation-centered program designed to meet multiple objectives

KEY TERMS

1. Human immunodeficiency virus (HIV)

2. Acquired immunodeficiency syndrome (AIDS)

3. Mental illness and homelessness

4. Sexually transmitted disease (STDs)

5. Shelters

6. Prevocational and vocational/pre-employment

7. Occupational balance

8. Activity analysis

Fazio, L. S. *Developing Occupation-Centered Programs With the Community, Third Edition* (pp 329-336).
© 2017 Taylor & Francis Group.

The population introduced in the title of this chapter appears to be cumbersome in description, but it is, in fact, quite common in today's shelter and mission system to find **HIV/AIDS, mental illness**, substance abuse, physical illness, and conditions associated with aging existing simultaneously in one individual who is **homeless**. This truly challenges the skills of the occupational therapy practitioner to bring to the forefront all of the academic information and experience he or she can accumulate while maintaining a focus on meaningful occupation and the self-assigned needs of the person.

Of course, successful programs can be conducted in the community for all of the aforementioned groups individually with entirely different objectives; however, in working in the community, it can be more beneficial to combine groups whenever possible and to remember that the presence of a diagnosis or disease entity has little bearing on your programming. Rather, it is your challenge to design meaningful programming for the individual and to remember that your intervention occurs within and is strongly influenced by the orientation of community.

You must also remember that, even though a population may share the condition of homelessness, this is by no means perceived in the same way by each individual. For some, it may be disabling; for others it is desirable and enabling. The condition or circumstance of homelessness represents a community of individuals who must be treated as such.

THE POPULATION/CONDITION CHARACTERISTICS OF OUR PROGRAM EXAMPLE

Although psychiatric symptoms are often linked to homelessness, the link to functional impairment may be overlooked. According to Gorde, Helfrich, and Finlayson (2004), mental illness and homelessness can create a cycle of functional impairment that results in an inability to achieve and retain the basic skills necessary for living independently (p. 693). Persons with mental illness are at particular risk for homelessness because they encounter many barriers when accessing housing services such as strict eligibility criteria, lack of transportation, inadequate resources, and cost (Gallop & Everett, 2001). Of the 3.5 million people in the United States who experience homelessness each year (Urban Institute, 2000), 61% to 91% present with psychiatric disabilities. According to the Substance Abuse and Mental Health Services Administration (SAMHSA, 2015), 20% to 25% of the homeless population in the United States suffer from some form of severe mental illness. The Mental Illness Policy Organization has reported that there are 250,000 mentally ill homeless persons (with schizophrenia or manic-depressive disorders) in the United States, based on data from a 2007 national survey (*Mental Illness/Homeless Policy*, 2008). Obtaining accurate figures for both homeless persons and those with mental illness is virtually impossible, but we do know that these individuals spend more days homeless, rate their quality of life lower than those without mental illness, and have marked problems meeting basic needs for daily living (American Psychological Association, 2016; Sullivan, Burnam, Koegel, & Hollenberg, 2000). Individuals living with schizophrenia make up a large portion of the population of the mentally ill who are homeless, and this was true for the program we describe further on. Chronicity with acute episodes is a frequent pattern, and failure to obtain and/or maintain medications is a common occurrence (albeit a result of neglect, misinformation, fear, or lack of availability). Self-medicating behaviors through street drugs or alcohol complicate and exacerbate already unpleasant symptoms, such as hallucinations and delusions. In addition, depression is a common factor and is even more likely to prompt self-medicating behaviors than perhaps the symptoms of schizophrenia. In combination with mental illness or existing alone, HIV/AIDS must also be considered. See Chapter 17 for an additional discussion of homeless populations, including those with severe and persistent mental illness.

The human immunodeficiency virus (HIV) is found in bodily fluids such as blood, semen, vaginal secretions, and breast milk. It destroys the immune system by inserting its own genetic material into white blood cells called *T cells*. Over time, T cells are destroyed and HIV replicates. The disease has four stages, the last of which is full-blown AIDS, when the body has little natural immunity left. In the past, the average time from HIV infection to AIDS was 10 years, with a person living for several months to as long as 5 years after the AIDS diagnosis. With today's interventions, persons can live much longer after developing AIDS, and a good deal longer in the HIV stage of the illness (Straub, 2007). It is thought that upwards of 30.6 million people worldwide are living with HIV/AIDS; at the end of 2006, some 1,106,400 people in the United States were estimated to have HIV/AIDS (Centers for Disease Control and Prevention, 2008; UNAIDS, 1997). Assuming that all cases are not recognized or reported, it is difficult to obtain an accurate estimate, and the official estimates are probably low. This population is also often homeless and may use street drugs and alcohol to medicate their symptoms. On a more optimistic note, according to 1997 statistics provided by the Los Angeles County Department of Health Services, the fatality rate in Los Angeles County has dropped from 95% in 1983 for advanced HIV disease to 11% in 1996, and the figures are continuing to drop (Los Angeles County Department of Health Services, 2012). Such statistics are encouraging for those with HIV and AIDS and the people who care for them.

Of course, there are numerous other **sexually transmitted diseases (STDs)** and sexual infections prevalent in the communities of the homeless of all sexually active ages. All of these conditions are spread by sexual contact. Masters, Johnson. and Kolodny (1997) describe the following sexually transmitted and sexual contact diseases: gonorrhea, syphilis, chlamydia infections, chancroid, genital herpes, viral hepatitis, genital warts, various bacterial vaginal infections, and pubic lice (also spread by other contact) (pp. 510-535). Programmers working with homeless populations should become familiar with all of these conditions to better serve their clients and to protect their own health and well-being.

THE SITE OF OUR PROGRAM EXAMPLE

The site/location of the papermaking project was within a **shelter** system consisting of seven houses, each supporting a combined mission to provide residential care and supportive housing for people in transition to independent living. There were from five to seven residents in each home, and all were considered to be homeless before coming into the residential system. To receive funded services in this particular system, residents were first required to be HIV-positive and symptomatic. Other illnesses, as described previously (i.e., alcoholism/substance abuse, mental illness), weres secondary to the HIV/AIDS diagnosis. In addition, a small number of HIV/AIDS persons came to the system on a daily basis for food, showers, medications, and activities but continued to live on the street. It should be kept in mind that for many, the desirable and preferred option was to remain homeless.

The seven houses were located within a geographic region with similar community characteristics. All were surrounded by small single-family homes with a few scattered apartment structures. Other residents of the community were largely Black, Hispanic, and Asian and would generally be considered low-income/poverty level. The seven residences could easily be linked by public transportation and on foot. This was an important characteristic that permitted programming to be established at one site while meeting the needs of all residents of the system.

ASSESSING NEED AND PLANNING THE PAPERMAKING PROJECT

Planning for the residents was not unlike other programs described in this text. The sponsoring system was engaged to provide the mission and purpose and to elicit the goals each residential advisor had for his or her residents. The goals were examined in light of the mission and purpose of the full system, and these were utilized to structure a needs assessment for the individual

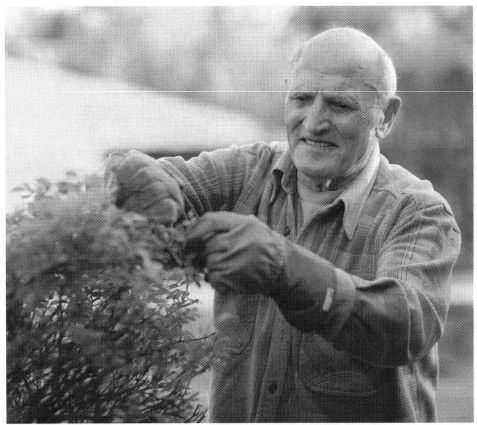

A shelter resident cleans up the yard; shared community encourages caring.

residents. Resources available from regional and county social services and private donations were examined.

Information received from these combined efforts stimulated the establishment of goals and objectives that were deemed appropriate to the needs of the shelter system and of the individuals who would be involved in the program. Shared goals were drafted around several central themes: (1) the establishment and strengthening of a community to incorporate all of the residents of the seven houses, (2) the creation of a balance of occupations demonstrated through a daily routine of independent living skills for each resident, and (3) the establishment of a venue for the testing and practice of **prevocational and vocational skills** appropriate for residents' transition to other communities of their choice and to find independent employment for some.

Objectives were then drafted with each individual who wished to participate in programming, including those who wished to remain homeless. Regardless of individual interests, each participant was required to attend one community meeting per week, conducted in each house. The meetings were intended to provide the route for self-governance and self-empowerment, which may accompany the shared responsibility of achieving positive outcomes. When the papermaking project was initiated, this meeting also became the place where group business decisions were made.

Previous to this program, the second theme of **occupational balance** and daily routine of independent living skills had had little success with residents who spent much of their time watching television, smoking, and sleeping. Some previous residents had experienced success with the third theme of pre-employment exploration, but the residential managers felt that something more was needed at a more achievable foundational level since many of the residents had never worked and/ or had never worked consistently.

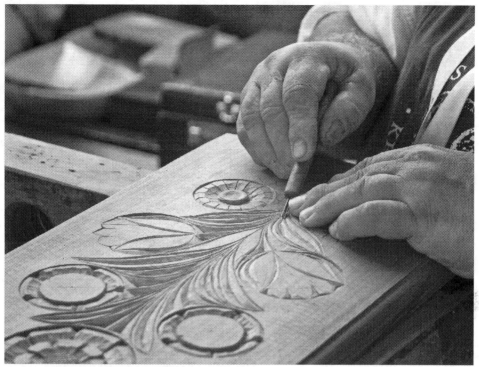

A wood carving is made for pressing handmade paper.

Following evaluation of all of the information collected in on-site interviews, through paper/pencil assessments, and after substantial library and Internet research of the population and the community systems supporting the existing programs, it was time for some substantial brainstorming between the students assigned to this opportunity and the instructor. Through this process and a review of the basic tenets of occupation and occupational therapy, it was determined that all of the themes/goals of the program could be incorporated through the use of a carefully selected activity and could also meet the therapeutic objectives of individual residents through the employment of the foundation skills of **activity analysis**. Further, the activity to be selected would have the potential to become a profit-producing endeavor.

In today's language of self-efficacy, empowerment, and personal advocacy, this conclusion may seem too simplistic to some and may provide a bit of an enlightening experience for others. Whichever it is, it is important to remind ourselves to continue to cultivate our historical roots and to recognize that some of our most significant strengths reside in that soil. The mix of a well-understood and carefully selected occupation/activity, comprehensive and skillful activity analysis, and the combination of clinical reasoning and a strong therapeutic self can be powerful in achieving occupation-centered outcomes, even within the most sophisticated paradigms.

THE SELECTION OF AN ACTIVITY TO MEET THE PROGRAM GOALS

Following lengthy discussions, it was determined that the task ahead was to select an occupational activity that would (1) produce a relatively inexpensive but marketable product (2) with good or at least tolerable profit margin, and that the production of this product would be (3) broad and flexible enough to meet the shared goals and objectives of each resident while (4) offering a realistic example of the business characteristics appropriate to umbrella the development of prevocational/vocational/employment skills.

Contiguous to the discussion was that the selected activity must be meaningful and relevant to the participants and to the potential market. Arts and crafts were considered because they can offer a certain mystique in today's mechanized and mass-produced environment. For these reasons and more, it was anticipated that they would be taken seriously by street-smart participants who likely had numerous agendas for being in the program, but perhaps none of them were the ones expressed to the planners.

Some of the students had heard of similar projects with varying populations. Suggestions were made to include the packaging of dry ingredients for a favored soup recipe, selling produce and/or flowers from a community gardening venture (perhaps also packaging the seeds from an organic garden), making candles and soap, or collecting and mixing potpourri. Constructing small wooden toys and compiling books of poems, personal journal notes, or recipes were suggested as well.

All ideas were entertained with equal enthusiasm, but when these and numerous other suggestions were measured against the desired goals and objectives, the desired characteristics of the project, potential collaborations, available space, and proposed cost, papermaking—or more accurately, paper recycling—was selected. The first step was to research papermaking and paper recycling, select an appropriate recipe, and obtain the necessary supplies and equipment. (Resources for activity analysis and papermaking/recycling are included in the Recommended Reading section at the end of this chapter.)

The next step involved the actual experimentation with recycled paper production so that all members of the student group could gain some experience with the medium before attempting an activity analysis of the steps involved. Finally, a step-by-step list of the tasks involved in the process was completed. Following some experimentation, it was determined that small packets of blank notepaper would be packaged as well as sheets of wrapping paper that would be printed with natural object impressions (such as shells, twigs, leaves, and flower petals). Following further experimentation and later consultations with the residents, it was decided to use predesigned stamps to print the name of the program on attached cards and to use raffia to tie the packages. Plastic bags were the preferred product packaging, although equipment for shrinkwrapping could be a future consideration.

The most formidable task was the completion of the full activity analysis of the process from the first step to the last, including preparing and maintaining supplies and equipment, actually making and drying the paper sheets, printing, packaging, obtaining retailers, marketing, and accounting.

The next step of this first stage was to locate space and to obtain funding for start-up. Space was provided in an empty garage at one of the residential sites and was brought to functional use through donations from a local builder's supply and several residents, students, and volunteers with suitable carpentry skills. It was determined that several corporate groups were accustomed to offering assistance to charitable groups in need through volunteer days, and these were utilized as well. A small $3,000 startup grant was received from a local philanthropic organization, which was a satisfactory sum to obtain the supplies and equipment to initiate the program. An earlier search of assets this community had to offer resulted in finding the builder's supply and resident volunteers/artists as well as existing volunteer organizations with supportive interests.

The next phase involved a fairly lengthy interview and evaluation period to determine the perceived and actual baseline skills of the residents and a matching of these to the steps of the activity. Following initiation, it was planned that the residential project would be able to support the work of a supervisory occupational therapist or occupational therapy assistant and one resident who would function as an aide. This group along with the community of participants/volunteers (including retired business entrepreneurs) would determine the future direction of the project. The occupational therapist or occupational therapy assistant would provide individual evaluation

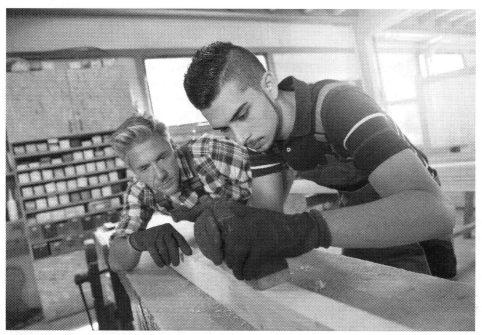

Learning furniture making from a master.

and recommendations to appropriate professionals regarding the prevocational/pre-employment and vocational/employment readiness of participants and would also monitor the evaluation of the program in general. In time, some members acquired wood carving skills to make relief plates for printing larger projects. From this, some moved on to employment in wood finishing and furniture making.

This program provides an exciting model that easily can be tailored to the needs of many populations in the community and is one that challenges us to use all of our skills as occupation-centered practitioners. Survey your community and you will find the assets as well as challenges to which this model is responsive.

SUMMARY

This chapter has continued to provide discussion of persons who are homeless—in this example, those who are homeless and living with mental illness. In addition, it has provided a description of the complex needs of homeless people with HIV/AIDS. This information connects the reader to the earlier example of youth who are homeless and the program to encourage them to practice safe sex. The problems of the homeless living with mental illness and HIV/AIDS may be further complicated by the presence of self-medicating behaviors in the form of substance abuse, and often concurrent physical illnesses. A multi-shelter program has been described that is structured around goals to establish and strengthen community, to balance individual occupations, and to create a venue for the testing and practice of prevocational/pre-employment and vocational/employment skills. This program example emphasizes the importance of one of the core skills of occupational therapy practitioners—activity analysis. When your programming involves engagement in a shared activity, a thorough analysis of that activity is the only way to ensure that it will match the individual needs of the participants while also meeting the goals of the program for all participants.

REFERENCES

American Psychological Association. (2016). *Health and homelessness*. Author. Retrieved from http://www.apa.org/pi/ses/resources/publications/homelessness-health.aspx

Centers for Disease Control and Prevention. (2008). *HIV Prevalence estimates – United States, 2006. Morbidity and Mortality Weekly Report*. October, 2008. Retrieved from http://www.cdc.gov/mmwr/; http://www.cdc.gov

Gallop, R., & Everett, B. (2001). Recognizing the signs and symptoms. In B. Everett & R. Gallop (Eds.), *The link between childhood trauma and mental illness: Effective interventions for mental health professions* (pp. 57-79). Thousand Oaks, CA: Sage.

Gorde, M., Helfrich, C. A., & Finlayson, M. L. (2004). Trauma symptoms and life skill needs of domestic violence victims. *Journal of Interpersonal Violence, 19*(6), 691-708.

Los Angeles County Department of Health Services. (2012). *Advanced HIV disease surveillance summary*. Los Angeles, CA: HIV Epidemiology Program.

Masters, W., Johnson, V., & Kolodny, R. (1997). Sexually transmitted disease and sexual infections. In W. Masters, V. Johnson, & R. Kolodny (Eds.), *Human Sexuality* (5th ed., pp. 510-537). New York, NY: Addison Wesley Longman.

Mental illness/homeless policy. (2008). Author. *Retrieved from* http://www.mentalillnesspolicy.org/

Straub, R. O. (2007). *Health Psychology: A biopsychosocial approach*. New York, NY: Worth Publishers. Reprinted in National Coalition for the Homeless. Retrieved from http://www.nationalhomeless.org/factsheets/hiv.html

Substance Abuse and Mental Health Services Administration, Center for Mental Health Services. (2015). *Homelessness*. Author. Retrieved from http://mentalhealth.samhsa.gov/cmhs/Homelessness/

Sullivan, G., Burnam, A., Koegel, P., & Hollenberg, J. (2000). Quality of life of homeless persons with mental illness: Results from the course-of-homelessness study. *Psychiatric Services, 51*(9), 1135-1141.

UNAIDS. (1997). *Report on the global HIV/AIDS epidemic*. New York, NY: Author.

Urban Institute. (2000). *A new look at homelessness in America*. Retrieved from http://www.urban.org/url.cfm?ID=900302&renderforprint=1

Recommended Reading

Lamport, N., Coffey, M., & Hersch, G. (2001). *Activity analysis and application* (4th ed.). Thorofare, NJ: SLACK Incorporated.

Thomas, H. (2012). *Occupation-based activity analysis*. Thorofare, NJ: SLACK Incorporated.

Toale, B. (1983). The *art of papermaking*. Worcester, MA: F. A. Davis.

Tubbs, C., & Drake, M. (2007). *Crafts and creative media in therapy* (3rd ed.). Thorofare, NJ: SLACK Incorporated.

Wankelman, W., & Wigg, P. (1993). *A handbook of arts and crafts* (3rd ed.). Madison, WI: Brown and Benchmark.

Watson, D. (1997). *Task analysis*. Bethesda, MD: American Occupational Therapy Association.

Watson, D. (1994). *Creative handmade paper*. Kent, UK: Search Press.

Watson, D., & Wilson, S. (2003). *Task analysis: An individual and population approach* (2nd ed.). Bethesda, MD: American Occupational Therapy Association.

21

Programming for the Homeless Adolescent in Transitional Shelter
Filmmaking for High School Credit

LEARNING OBJECTIVES

1. To appreciate the conditions that prompt running away and resulting homelessness in children and adolescents

2. To understand the particular challenges experienced by children and adolescents when living on the street

3. To identify services offered to homeless children and adolescents

4. To review the example of the development of an occupation-centered program for an adolescent shelter population

KEY TERMS

1. Homeless family

2. Family shelters

3. Homeless adolescents

4. Crisis intervention

5. Transitional living

Fazio, L. S. *Developing Occupation-Centered Programs With the Community, Third Edition* (pp 337-343).
© 2017 Taylor & Francis Group.

Homelessness is a condition that not only cuts across cultures, socioeconomic considerations, and gender, but it also does not have much relation to age or family structure. Although not nearly adequate, shelters and temporary housing are available across the country to individuals, families, and teens. The current data are limited on the numbers of homeless youths in America. Estimates have found that 1.3 to 1.7 million youths experience one night of homelessness per year, with 550,000 youths being homeless for 1 week or longer (National Alliance to End Homelessness, 2012; U.S. Department of Justice, 1999). However, there are no current national data because no government or philanthropic entity has invested in national research on homeless youths in the United States. The most accurate data available are of school-aged (largely minors) homeless youths who are still attending public schools, which does not give a complete picture of the extent of youth homelessness but constitutes important regular and national data. The National Network for Youth (n.d.) reported that, in the 2013–2014 school year and in January 2013, American communities counted 46,924 unaccompanied homeless youths living in shelters or on the street. Over 40,000 of these youths were transition-aged (48.6% unsheltered) and 6,197 were under the age of 18 years (59.3% unsheltered).

Most homeless youths have either run away, been kicked out of unstable home environments, been abandoned by their families or caregivers, been involved with public systems (foster care, juvenile justice, and mental health), or have a history of residential instability and disconnection. Many young people hide their homelessness because they do not want to become ensnared in either the child welfare or criminal justice system (National Network for Youth, n.d.). In Los Angeles County, there were approximately 82,096 homeless persons in 2004; of these, approximately 20% to 40% were single mothers and children (Just the Facts, 2004). Certainly, many families disintegrate under the pressures of homelessness.

A trends analysis of the constant flux in the job market, in the wages of the working poor, and in affordable housing in this urban area (Los Angeles) and others like it does not appear optimistic for families who currently have low incomes or whose employment skills may be inadequate. **Family shelters** are excellent communities for occupation-centered services because they provide access to a family system within the protected environment of the shelter.

Programming in such shelters can include life skills for adults and teens, employability assessment and employment skill building for adults, developmental screening and creative play opportunities for young children, and educational support services for school-aged children. Family shelters are generally nonprofit organizations with a mission to provide food, shelter, and other services to homeless families. They are often funded by city governments, foundations/corporations, and private donations. The residences may include a family bedroom, common dining room and bathrooms, a day care/play room for infants and toddlers, a tutoring/educational support room for school-aged children, and a playground. Occupation-centered services, therapeutic or formative, find a comfortable fit with this structure.

Teens may be found as part of the **homeless family**, but when they are alone and homeless, their problems and concerns are quite unique. The next program description will provide a view of the special concerns of **homeless adolescents**.

THE POPULATION CHARACTERISTICS OF OUR PROGRAM EXAMPLE

Homeless youths, who are most frequently runaways, dot the United States as they make their way to various perceived "utopias" around the country. As we have indicated, according to the U.S. Department of Health and Human Services (DHHS, 1991) and the National Network for Youth (n.d.), upwards of 1 million youths run away from home each year. Shelters of many kinds may be found in virtually every city, urban or rural, in an effort to stop or at least postpone this exodus from home. Although there are many popular destinations for runaways, Hollywood, CA, has the dubious distinction of being the "runaway capital" of this country, with estimated from 5,000 to 10,000 children and adolescents surviving on the streets and in abandoned buildings (Covenant House California [CHC], n.d.). Although runaway children and adolescents include all ethnicities, the Hollywood CHC has reported that White youths accounted for nearly half of all of their contacts in recent years (CHC, 2005).

The largest population seems to comprise those between the ages of 18 and 21 years who are too young for adult shelters and yet too old for the shelters and systems caring for minor children. Many of them "aged out" of the foster care system at age 18 years, and even though they were often ill prepared for adult life, they were released to the street. According to a 1991 study by the DHHS, 45% of homeless youths in California were in foster care in the year before they took to the streets.

It is estimated that 81% of CHC clients have been victims of some kind of abuse, which includes physical, sexual, and emotional abuse; neglect; and abandonment (CHC, 2005). Approximately 11% of these children had sex before the age of 9 years and 46% had sex before the age of 15 years. Other statistics that are significant in understanding this group include the fact that 83% have a family history of substance abuse and 74% have substance abuse problems themselves. An estimated 93% have an array of emotional disorders, which include depression, post-traumatic stress disorder, suicidal ideation, and psychosis. Most have not graduated from high school (92%) and have inadequate job skills.

Wherever there are large numbers of homeless adolescents, there are those who victimize them with promises of notoriety, money, and affection. The lure of the film industry in Los Angeles is likely one of the factors that draws so many homeless youths to California, and many of the children quickly become ensnared in pornography while waiting to "be discovered." One out of three runaway children is lured into prostitution within 48 hours of leaving home; it is estimated that nearly 30% of youths on the street have been paid for sex and that 22% have traded sex for food or shelter (CHC, 2005). Unfortunately, opportunities to become victims far exceed the available shelters and services.

When we review the developmental considerations of adolescence, it is not difficult to see how vulnerable these youths may be to the so-called temptations that are believed to accompany the perceived freedoms, attributes, and rights of adulthood. The community of homeless adolescents, wherever it exists, is a strong one, with many of the "club" characteristics noted in previous chapters. There are perhaps more covert rules among these youths than there are in the adult homeless community, and adolescents are more likely to group and support each other than are homeless adults. Considering that they are all likely to be either "running away from" or "running to" something and considering that many are being searched for by families, they tend to be less trusting, more furtive, and more secretive than homeless adults.

THE SITE OF OUR PROGRAM EXAMPLE

A fairly common model for programs targeting homeless youths is a frontline **crisis intervention** outreach program of some sort. Intervention counselors, often volunteers from the police departments or churches, go to the streets where homeless youths are likely to congregate. Crisis intervention often takes the form of assisting youths who are endangered by excessive drug use or a "bad drug trip" or those who are being pursued by pimps or pornographers. Although occupational therapy intervention is not likely to find a foothold in crisis intervention, it is an opportunity to observe and to begin to understand what this community is about, which is critical for those who wish to provide programming to this group. It is also an excellent way to become familiar with the other service providers and volunteer organizations and a way to become known to them because they are your potential allies and partners.

Beyond this front line is usually an emergency bed shelter that may also provide medical services as well as counseling. In addition, there may be a **transitional living** environment that offers support directed toward the skills necessary to live independently and to remain off the streets. Transitional living is generally reserved for those adolescents who have demonstrated the motivation, interest, and initiative to benefit from this opportunity. There are paid personnel who work in the transitional living environment who may be social workers, teachers/tutors, and sometimes occupational therapists (although you will likely have to market yourself for such a position), and there are many volunteers from the surrounding community to provide role-modeling and skill development.

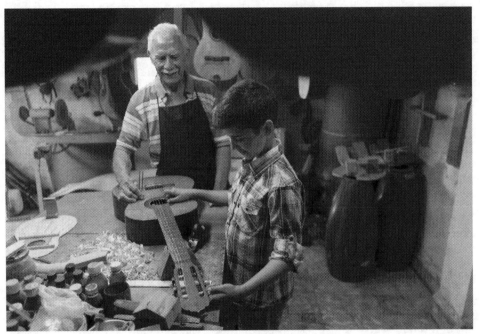

A member of the local community shares guitar-making skills with a young transitional living resident.

COVENANT HOUSE: ASSESSING NEED AND PLANNING THE PROGRAMMING

CHC is a nonprofit agency whose mission is to reach out to at-risk homeless youths living on the streets and offer them hope and opportunities to turn their lives around (CHC, n.d.). CHC is the largest privately funded agency (80% of the funding comes from private donors) in the Americas, providing shelter, food, immediate crisis care, and other services to homeless and runaway youths; it also provides care to homeless youths aged 14 to 20 years. There are two sites in California: Covenant House–Los Angeles, and Covenant House–Bay Area. Both sites are open 24 hours per day, 365 days per year, and all services are offered free. The mission of CHC was developed by the Catholic Church when the first such shelter was established in New York City in 1967.

This organization and its Los Angeles location provided an excellent partnering opportunity for student learning while also offering companion programming to support the mission of CHC. Following several evenings with the crisis-intervention teams to better understand the needs of this population and to support the research that had been done before coming into the community and preliminary discussion with CHC personnel as well as observation of existing programming, it was determined that occupation-centered providers could best match their body of knowledge and expertise with the aspect of programming that was directed toward life skills development. It was the interest of the director to offer small, individualized opportunities for learning. These opportunities were preconceived as modules with a similar format and structure to what is expected in formal education, which was a large part of the residents' day.

A needs assessment was developed and distributed to residents. It was developed according to the structure and content requested by the director and in keeping with the mission and philosophy of the facility/organization. This assessment included life skills development modules in the areas of communication, goal setting, time and task management, and sexuality. Through this assessment, which was conducted in personal interviews, specific concerns were elicited in each of the areas first noted by the director. Most of the residents were fairly disinterested in the idea of yet "another class" and were not as helpful in this stage of program development as might have been desired.

Although the occupational therapy student group conducting the needs assessment was fairly disheartened by the response, it was thought after some discussion that the respondents might be more motivated if they had a hand in selecting how the content of the modules would be disseminated or investigated, which is generally the approach of choice with all programming recipients and perhaps even more significant for teenagers. Another series of interviews gleaned an assortment of creative but often impractical (generally because of time and/or cost) ideas. It was clear, though, as mentioned in the previous chapter, that street-smart participants offered a substantial challenge for the creation of stimulating and engaging programming.

A Wealth of Assets: Community Partnering to Provide the Program

Bringing together the larger program goals and objectives that incorporated the enhancement of communication, setting realistic and manageable life goals, managing time and tasks, and exploring developmentally appropriate and safe sexuality in an informative and captivating programming package was the challenge. The response came in the form of a series of documentary videos.

Through an investigation of community assets and capacity in the form of volunteer resources of persons and companies, it was discovered that one of the local movie studios had previously offered an internship program along with high school credit to residents of the transitional living unit. With this information, the occupational therapy students prepared a proposal for the approval of the director of the shelter. Following this step, a similar proposal that outlined the program and the purpose was developed for the studio executives. Although it had different goals than the traditional internship had offered, the proposal was received positively and the studio agreed to offer the internship/high school credit format. In addition, the studio recommended the services of other college film program interns to advise and assist and to be responsible for video equipment to be loaned to the program—a collaboration that exceeded initial expectations!

The film interns supplied the technical expertise and advice, and the occupational therapy students offered the structure to make sure that the content of the scripts and the process of residents' involvement met the goals of the program established from the earlier needs assessment. A timeline was developed; tasks were determined, analyzed, and distributed; the product was developed; and the process was evaluated.

The goals of establishing realistic objectives—time and task management—were accomplished in the process of planning and scripting, filming, and editing. The goals of developing communication skills and learning about sexuality were accomplished through the group decision that the film would be a documentary of individual "life story" vignettes provided by each of the participants. Not only were individual goals met through this activity, but there were also numerous other positive outcomes related to formal education and employment exploration (e.g., discovering talents for writing, directing, and acting).

The initial format for formative program evaluation was eventually discarded in favor of a qualitative analysis of the filmed vignettes for the five participants. Since numerous practice films were made, there was substantial footage available for analysis. This was conducted both by the occupational therapy students and by the participants with shared observations of progress and identification of areas still needing improvement.

Videotaping or filmmaking is an excellent tool for occupation-centered interventions. If your community includes film students, they are most likely looking for practice opportunities and generally have access to equipment. If not, then perhaps the local television station can become involved, particularly if the programming can be developed to advance the station's public relations agendas as well as benefit participants. If no television stations are available, then consider "oral histories" and radio or audiotaping as the medium.

Even if none of these external resources/assets are available, the seemingly simple process of using a camcorder can still utilize the development of a script through the telling of personal stories or story making, and a review of the film can be a powerful evaluative tool for both respondents and students in the classroom.

This review of programming for homeless adolescents has presented some of the advantages and potential dilemmas you may find working with this community. They are perhaps the most challenging of the homeless persons for whom you may wish to develop programs. They offer all of the characteristics of the homeless alongside the particular characteristics of the developmental phase of adolescence. Frequently, these youths have been abused and neglected, and they are often the most disenfranchised of all—rejected by family systems while in many ways still children.

SUMMARY

The problems of homeless children and adolescents, whether part of a homeless family unit or alone, are complicated by their developmental characteristics and their lack of preparation for the adult roles that may be thrust upon them or that they are seeking. Communities of homeless children and adolescents resemble the structure of clubs, as discussed in previous chapters. There are often more covert rules than in adult homeless communities, and adolescents as well as younger runaway children are more likely to group together and support each other.

Children and adolescents are more difficult to engage in programs because they are often being searched for by families or are engaging in unlawful behavior, so they fear being found or identified. This chapter has described a program that shows how homeless adolescents might become engaged in an occupation-centered environment targeting the development of age-appropriate life skills. You may also wish to revisit the Denver Sanctuary Program for Homeless Teens, described in Chapter 10.

Of significance to this program is the identification and utilization of the assets and capacities of several "communities." Partnering with largely volunteer members of these multiple communities and also recognizing the stakeholders and potential partners, in large part, provided the impetus for programming success.

REFERENCES

Covenant House of California. (n.d.). Website. Retrieved from http://covenanthousecalifornia.org/

Covenant House of California. (2005). About CHC. Retrieved from www.coventhouse.org/about-chc-pg.php

Just the Facts. (2004). *Institute for the Study of Homelessness and Poverty at the Weingart Center* (August Report). Washington, DC: Author.

National Alliance to End Homelessness. (2012). *An emerging framework for ending unaccompanied youth homelessness NAEH typology.* Washington, DC: Author.

National Network for Youth. (n.d.). How many homeless youth are in America? Retrieved from http://www.nn4youth.org/learn/how-many-homeless

U.S. Department of Health and Human Services. (1991). *Runaway youth annual report.* Washington, DC: Author.

U.S. Department of Justice Office of Juvenile Justice and Delinquency Prevention. (1999). *National incidence studies of missing, abducted, runaway and thrownaway children.* Washington, DC: Author.

22

Promotion of Health, Well-Being, and Community
A Culturally Relevant Intergenerational Program for Older Adults Living in a Senior-Care Facility

---

LEARNING OBJECTIVES

1. To explore health promotion and wellness programming for older adults who are living in a senior-care institution

2. To become aware of the need for older adult programming that is culturally relevant and linked to the larger community

3. To examine ideas and theories that assist in our understanding of effective programming for older adults in institutional care

4. To examine intergenerational programming as a viable and effective mode for encouraging community in institutions for older adults

5. To become familiar with one site-linked example of an intergenerational/culturally relevant older adult program designed to support health, well-being, and a sense of community membership

---

Fazio, L. S. *Developing Occupation-Centered Programs With the Community, Third Edition* (pp 345-359).
© 2017 Taylor & Francis Group.

KEY TERMS

1. Health disparities
2. Health promotion and well-being
3. Cultural traditions
4. Aging in place/aging-friendly communities/aging in a familiar context
5. Self-determination theory (competence, autonomy, relatedness)
6. Expectancy, self-efficacy, and outcome expectations
7. Kinship and social connectedness
8. Intergenerational mentoring programs

For more than two decades, the U.S. Department of Health and Human Services (DHHS) has encouraged the use of health promotion and disease prevention objectives to improve the health of the American people (DHHS, 1990, 1998). Since the 1970s, there has been a growing social movement that encourages people of all ages to look at wellness as optimal physical, mental, and spiritual well-being. It is no surprise that the first goal of *Healthy People 2010* (DHHS, 1998) was to increase the quality as well as the years of healthy life. Today's older adult is more fully aware of this agenda and its role in preventing illness and disability, improving functioning, and living fully in the world. Granted, escalating health care costs may be a motivating factor across the economic continuum for many aging adults, but most want more than simple illness prevention. They wish to live fully, engaged in lives of choice, and all hope to live independently in their homes for all or most of their lives.

Occupational therapy practitioners endorsed the objectives of the above reports in their 2001 American Occupational Therapy Association (AOTA) official statement: *Occupational Therapy in the Promotion of Health and the Prevention of Disease and Disability* (AOTA, 2001). We know that people are living longer. Atchley (1994) predicted that by 2050, there would be about 68.5 million Americans 65 years of age and older (p. 520). In 1990, there were about 500,000 people 85 years of age and over living in long-term care facilities. At that rate of utilization and anticipating the aging of even the old-old population (aged 95 years and above), we can expect 3 million people 85 and over to need long-term care by 2050. Of course, trends in long-term care will likely evolve to shift from nursing home to more independent living spaces with less standardized menus of care and will likely encourage older adults to remain connected to their previous lives, but how will this occur and who will be involved in the orchestration of this transition? Occupational therapy practitioners seem ready to move to the forefront, as the programming example in this chapter might suggest. Engagement in occupations of choice that are linked to the larger community is key to successful living and aging.

Sultz and Young (2004) describe already evolving innovations in long-term care to meet the diverse medical needs, personal desires, and lifestyle choices of older Americans. Concepts such as aging in place, life-care communities, and high-tech home care are some of the changes that offer enriched alternatives to long-term care recipients. The future of physical aging, according to Atchley (1994), will be influenced by the impact of biomedical research, trends in morbidity and mortality, and the impact of a general movement toward wellness (p. 521). Other advancements— such as improved diagnosis, prevention, and treatment of debilitating diseases such as Alzheimer's disease and other dementias—will lead to a more viable population of aging adults.

In the United States, it is predicted that Hispanic and Asian populations will triple over the next half century and that non-Hispanic Whites will represent about one-half of the total population by 2050 (U.S. Census Bureau, 2011, 2012). Such trends will obviously call for more bilingual programming and programs to meet various cultural demands provided by a culturally diverse health promotion workforce. A culturally diverse workforce of occupational therapy practitioners adequate to meet such needs does not currently exist. As a profession, we all have some work to do to encourage academic admission and retention of ethnically diverse students or risk becoming marginalized in this evolving, culturally diverse future.

These reports and statements deal specifically with the U.S. population, but we know that aging and older adults around the world are utilizing all resources available to them to maintain a viable place on the planet. The world's population aged 65 years and older is growing by an unprecedented 800,000 people per month (He, Goodkind, & Kowal, 2016).

Global aging will likely continue well into the next century, with the numbers and proportions of older people continuing to rise in both developed and developing countries. According to the He et al. (2016), the ratio of older people to total population differs widely among countries. The United States was 32nd on a list ranking countries with a high proportion of people aged 65 years and older. Italy was the "oldest" country in 2000, with 18% of Italians having celebrated at least a 65th birthday. In many countries, the "oldest old" (aged 80 years and above) were the fastest growing component of the population.

Certainly, we know that not all of the world's older population has equal access to the social and economic factors that invite the characteristics of "aging well." Even in the United States there are wide and obvious health disparities. The Trans-National Institutes of Health (NIH) Work Group on Health Disparities has defined the term **health disparities** as "the difference in the incidence, prevalence, morbidity, mortality, and burden of diseases and other adverse health conditions that exist among specific population groups" (NIH, 1999). The NIH work group notes that "health disparities arise from a complex combination of social and economic factors, the physical environments, cultural beliefs and values, educational level, personal behaviors, and genetic susceptibilities" (1999). Previously in this text, we discussed the work of Ann Wilcock (1998). Her concepts of occupational imbalance, occupational deprivation, and occupational alienation help us to understand health disparities from an "occupation" perspective.

Occupational therapy practitioners are well positioned to offer assistance in several of these areas of disparity that will even the odds for all persons, and, for aging adults in particular. Clearly, we have ample justification from demographics alone to devote substantial funded research efforts in community programming for older adults to encourage broader education of students in matters of older adulthood, and to establish occupation-centered parameters for health promotion and wellness in our aging populations.

HEALTH PROMOTION AND WELL-BEING

The title of this chapter uses the terms *health promotion, well-being,* and *community.* From earlier discussions in this text, we know that Green and Kreuter (1991) define **health promotion** as any planned combination of educational, political, regulatory, environmental, and organizational supports for actions and conditions of living conducive to the health of persons, groups, or communities (p. 5). As long ago as 1986, the World Health Organization declared that health promotion is simply "the process of enabling people to increase control over and to improve their health" (p. iii). Complex or simplistic, by definition, *occupation* is central to health promotion, and occupation-centered practitioners are central as well.

Scaffa (2001) describes occupation-based health promotion interventions that may be conducted at an individual, group, organizational, community (societal), and governmental/policy level. Some examples of each for older adults are driving evaluation, safety checks, and perhaps compensatory instruction for the individual older adult and programs to encourage groups of older adults to remain engaged in meaningful occupation. Chapter 19 of this text provides an example of an exercise program for groups of older adults with Parkinson's disease and their significant others. Providing consultation to businesses and potential employers regarding the benefits of hiring older adults in the part-time work force; providing information on accessibility and universal design to local building suppliers, hardware stores, and contractors; and encouraging accessible public transportation in the community are examples targeting organizations. At the governmental/policy level, for example, we may promote policies that offer affordable, accessible health care for all older adults.

Well-being is defined quite simply as "the state of being healthy, happy, or prosperous (Morris, 1976, p. 1454). Anderson (1994) offers a definition perhaps more appealing to occupational therapy practitioners: "achievement of a good and satisfactory existence as *defined by the individual*" (p. 1664). Granted, these definitions are subjective, as, of course, the phenomenon of well-being should be. If we are to place "well-being" within an appropriate context according to the AOTA's *Occupational Therapy Practice Framework: Domain and Process* (2014), it would undoubtedly be in the spiritual context, but certainly informed by and interconnected with the cultural, physical, social, personal, and temporal contexts. For our purposes, it is a significant goal for intervention and a direct outcome of our health promotion efforts. The following program example links attention to all of these domains with the combined goals of health promotion and well-being.

OCCUPATION-CENTERED PROGRAMMING FOR OLDER ADULTS: LUNALILO HOME ON THE ISLAND OF O'AHU, HAWAII

This particular programming example is selected to best illustrate the encouragement of individual health and well-being by linking the institutionalized older adult to the larger cultural community. The bulk of this work was accomplished by Keali T. Lum, OTD, OTR/L, as a programming student and continued when he returned home to O'ahu (Segal, 2002). It showcases a blend of traditional program planning as described in this text with an integration of **cultural tradition** and attention to the specific characteristics of the ethnic community (Segal, 2002).

Background

Aging seniors in Hawaii are little different than many other aging populations around the world except that their population appears to be growing at a rate more than two times the national average. In 2002, there were approximately 160,601 seniors age 65 years and older, showing a 28.5% increase over 125,005 seniors living in Hawaii in 1990 (Segal, 2002). In 2015, the U.S. Census Bureau reported a total population of 1,431,603 in Hawaii, with a 16.1% increase in adults above 65 years of age. Any increases are likely due to increased health agendas targeting prevention and management of diabetes and other life-threatening illnesses linked to diet and genetic predisposition.

Not unlike other similar regions where many families live at or below the poverty line, there may be little planning for older adult years. The traditional mode of many generations living under one roof or in clustered housing is likely being undermined by the need and desire for the middle generations, particularly women/daughters, to work outside the household. If the older generation lives to require nursing care, there is little recourse. The Island of O'ahu, although sophisticated in many respects, has not created sufficient and affordable support services for this growing contingent of the population. Certainly, this is a problem, but the larger dilemma may be that, if such services were available (particularly low-income senior care housing), it is uncertain that it would meet the broader cultural needs of a population that has relied on family and tradition for sustenance and well-being since the beginning.

Lunalilo Home

Lunalilo Home provides an example of a senior-care residence and was the original site of this experiment in creative programming that focused on the cultural family traditions of the indigenous population demonstrating Hawaiian ancestry. Perhaps exotic in that this population may be confined by choice to an island, it is not unlike many we are aware of in pocketed urban areas, small towns, and rural areas throughout the United States. The characteristics of the population and the programming may be transferred to many scenarios we encounter as practitioners and programmers.

KEY ELEMENTS CONTRIBUTING TO THE PROGRAM DESIGN

Following an extensive investigation and multiple interviews with residents of Lunalilo, their family members, and members of the surrounding community, the combined needs assessment supported the initial hypothesis of the programmers, suggesting the readiness for a "renaissance" celebrating indigenous Hawaiian crafts and tradition. Central to this awareness were the curators and directors of cultural anthropology and artifacts, indigenous arts, and indigenous horticulture at the University of Hawaii, the Bishop Museum Library and Archives, and the Edith Kanaka'ole Foundation for the Preservation of Indigenous Traditions. This group provided a strong foundation of knowledge and resources to support the ideas of the programmer. In the asset identification and needs assessment process, several strong partnerships were developed who, through volunteerism and funding, would support this program's goals and continue to do so. One does not have to investigate deeply to know that many indigenous groups have lost cultural traditions, often turning them aside in favor of efficiency and current social trends. Resurrecting such tradition by accessing older adults who remember and practice them offers purposeful engagement benefiting the community at all levels.

Central ideas or organizing elements for potential programming that were gleaned during the early research and assessment process and were in danger of being lost to younger generations were deemed to be as follows:

1. Shared traditional culture, preservation of information gleaned through oral tradition/story-telling, art and craft knowledge and skills, music and dance traditions, both in archival form and to be shared with younger generations

2. The importance of kinship, family, intergenerational systems; staying connected to family and community

3. Health and wellness for aging adults (diet, activity, "meaning," efficacy, engagement, and empowerment)

Supporting Ideologies

These organizing elements have several supporting ideas and theories within their structure that provide scaffolding for the development of the day-to-day programming:

Aging in place is a phrase found in the literature of many disciplines. Siebert (2003), in her AOTA Continuing Education module *Aging in Place: Implications for Occupational Therapy*, described the values and goals of "aging in place." These values and goals are offered as autonomy, engagement, community living, and a healthy active lifestyle. Scharlach and Lehring (2016) discusses the importance of **aging-friendly communities** and how they may promote the continuity of continued engagement in life and community, and the provision of opportunities for familiar and new activities for enhanced quality of life. Generally, when we think of aging in place and aging-friendly communities, we think of older adults continuing to live in their own residences in

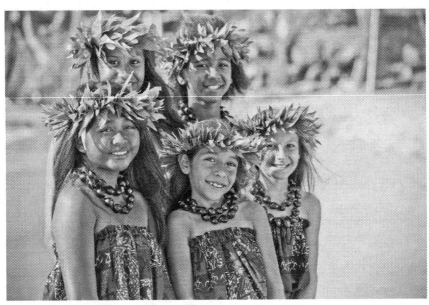

Proud children prepare to dance for family.

the community that has always supported their values and interests and in the presence of family and friends. It was the intention of the Lunalilo program to respect the notion of aging in place, but also for these residents to expand this notion to **aging in a familiar context**: that of the community and the culture.

Self-determination theory (SDT) is an approach to human motivation and personality that uses traditional empirical methods while employing an organismic metatheory that highlights the importance of humans' evolved inner resources for personality development and behavioral regulation (Ryan, Kuhl, & Deci, 1997). When people are at their fullest potential, they appear to be curious, vital, and self-motivated. They are agentic and inspired, striving to learn and extend themselves and to master new skills. However, we know that these persistent, proactive, and positive tendencies of human nature are not always apparent and perhaps not present. In thinking of older adults in institutional care, we are not likely to describe them with any of these terms. Why not? Ryan and Deci (2000) have identified three needs that, when satisfied, provide the basis for self-motivation, personality integration, optimal functioning, and, most importantly, personal well-being. These three needs are the need for competence, relatedness, and autonomy. The foundations for self-determination begin with the nature of motivation—whether one is internally motivated to function in the world with action and intention or whether one is externally pressured to act. Our interests in providing programming for older adults (or any population) is to encourage an environment, a context that fosters internal motivation observed as actions with energy and direction. We have all too often seen older institutionalized adults forced from bed to chair, to the lunch room, that then becomes the activity room, that then becomes the dinner room, followed by return to bed. Throughout this series of events, we seldom see any action from the person that appears to be intentional and certainly not one that expresses interests or values.

Our first act as therapists and programmers is to establish an environment that encourages internal motivation and opportunities for engagement in activities of interest, skill, and value that satisfy what Ryan and Deci (2000) describe as the "need for competence" (p. 69). In our programming example, this environment is rich with opportunities to engage in various components of cultural tradition that one is good at, is interested in, and values (most importantly, a "valuing" that is shared by all members of the culture). **Competence** and **autonomy** are related in that competence is fulfilled by the experience that one can effectively bring about desired effects and outcomes, and autonomy involves the perception that one's activities are endorsed by or congruent with the self. **Relatedness** then pertains to feeling that one is close and connected to significant others (Reis, Sheldon, Gable, Roscoe, & Ryan, 2000, p. 419). The ultimate outcome is a general sense of well-being.

Expectancy, **self-efficacy**, and **outcome expectations** are terms from the work of Bandura (1977a, 1977b). Related to concepts that support self-determination theory, expectancy is an important feature of self-efficacy. Expectancy is described as a value an individual places on a particular outcome. Efficacy expectations are related to competence and stem from previous and present skills and knowledge; successful accomplishment enhances one's expectation for future efforts, acting on the world with the expectation that you will be successful in your efforts. Key to "revisiting" old knowledge and skill sets is the evidence to support that the more similar the current task is to those performed successfully in the past, the greater the efficacy expectations will be (Bandura, 1977b). This is of great significance to the programming for Lunalilo in that the skills and knowledge sets of the residents were central to the selected programming. A programmer's encouragement and ability to structure (perhaps through activity analysis and adaptation) circumstances for a successful outcome are critical to the development of efficacy expectations, as well as expectations for general outcomes. Bandura (1977a) describes outcome expectations as the individual's belief that a given behavior will lead to specific outcomes. In our example, these outcomes may be praise, playful pleasures, a greater perceived sense of health, and a general sense of well-being. It is also the programmer who must orchestrate environmental expectations, what Bandura (1997a) describes as how events are related to each other and what one may expect from a given environment. It is often partnering with other individuals and groups in the community that establishes the supportive environment and solidifies expectations for program performance and success.

Kinship and the maintenance of social connectedness or relatedness (as described previously) is central to the health and well-being of people regardless of age but is perhaps most significant as adults age and may become isolated from families. Baumeister and Leary (1995) discuss relatedness as a significant component in the satisfaction of innate psychological needs. This desire for interpersonal attachments can perhaps best be satisfied in a somewhat predictable and reliable fashion through connections with family. Kendig (1986) strongly suggests that social status impacts an older person's options and abilities to form and maintain supportive bonds, whether within the boundaries of kinship or in wider circles. Over time, older adults experience reduced social opportunities as they lose power and respect and become increasingly dissimilar from those in the mainstream of adult life; this may be described as a loss of **social connectedness**. We would question, then, the impact of institutionalization and removal from mainstream family and cultural life for our population of indigenous Hawaiian individuals as we might for any older adult who is living within an institution. Our compelling question, as occupational therapy practitioners, is how we might establish programming that would encourage power, respect, and social opportunities rather than diminishing them. How can we maintain the rights and obligations associated with kinship and assist the older adult to stay connected and related toward optimal functioning and personal well-being? According to Dowd (1980), the concept of "exchange" provides a valuable way to understand the interactions that take place within informal as well as formal relationships and may, in fact, form them. Older people who are institutionalized experience a retracting social world that is marked by the withdrawal of dominant younger people who may no longer receive the returns commensurate with investments, and also of subordinate older people whose independence and self-esteem is compromised in each encounter. How can we offer programming that will encourage engagement rather than disengagement or activity and inter-relatedness rather than isolation? Clearly, if we think of establishing an exchange system, the "commodities" must be considered of importance and valued by all levels of the social network and layers of kinship. Can we think of disappearing traditions (i.e., stories, arts, crafts, music, and dance) as the valued media for exchange? Also, can we develop and encourage relationships between our Lunalilo residents (the ancestral/elder keepers of these traditions) and those institutions and persons in the community who hold power relationships that cross generations and who sanction and encourage the collection, documentation, and teaching of these traditions (i.e., the museums, the foundations, and the universities)? For every craft, art, music, dance, and oral or written tradition to continue, there must be a craftsman, an artist, a musician, a dancer, a storyteller, and a writer or teacher, perhaps not always rewarded though appreciated and generally respected. This provides a potential path to empowerment and is an important concept for a program linking art/craft knowledge and production to family and community.

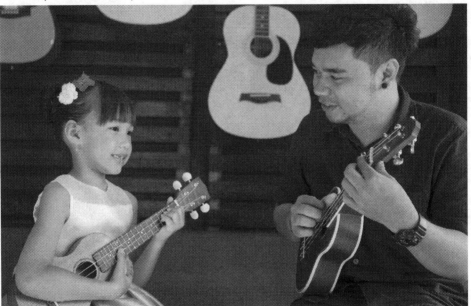

Children learn the ukulele when very young.

Intergenerational mentoring programs offer two or more generations of persons the opportunity to experience meaningful and supportive relationships that result in social and emotional fulfillment and growth. It is my preference, whenever possible, to engage at least three generations in programming of this type: the elders (in our programming example, the direct recipients of services), the middle (sons and daughters, perhaps siblings), and children through adolescence/young adulthood. These generations encompass not only family members, but friends and neighbors as well, and often strangers in the initial encounter The task then is to link generations in what becomes a shared microcosm of community, with a resulting effort toward shared goals of solidarity, integral responsibility, and better life quality for all involved.

The origins of intergenerational programming may lie in the foster grandparent programs established by the federal government in the 1960s (Newman, Ward, Smith, Wilson, & McCrea, 1997). Over time, these earlier programs have evolved into three main models: youths serving older adults, older adults serving youths, and young and old united in serving the community (Hawkins, McGuire, & Backman, 1999). Shared engagement in occupation is the common characteristic of all of these programs, and most often the benefits are mutual. It is sometimes hard to know whether the giver or the recipient of a gift enjoys the process more.

Newman et al. (1997) suggest that the original concept of intergenerational programming may have developed through recognition of the bond that develops in a family, across generations. Transfer of knowledge, values, and experience benefits both adults and children. In an exchange that is not so obvious, adults gain a sense of enhanced purpose, well-being, and life satisfaction (Newman et al., 1997, p. 4).

The term **mentoring** is used to describe a supportive relationship between a more experienced person and usually a younger, less experienced one. A mentoring relationship involves mutual caring, commitment, and trust (Taylor & Dryfoos, 1998/1999, p. 44). Such programs often involve a youth population considered to be at risk. Although still emerging, intergenerational programs have been field-tested widely and have generally been found to be effective (Kuehne, 2012). For at-risk youths in particular, such programs offered by older adults with perhaps similar life experience can present a perspective that is "rooted in survival" and provides a feeling of continuity between past, present, and future that is generally not available to children and young adults (Taylor & Dryfoos, 1998/1999, p. 44).

For most older adults, the benefits of involvement in such programs are the combined results of the opportunity to remain useful and vital and, most importantly, to make a positive difference in the life of a child/adolescent in the community (*Intergenerational Programs*, 2017). Jansen (2016) described a preschool inside a nursing home and the positive influences on both adults and children. Her observations describe a lasting effect on both adults and children to include better health and well-being for the adults and for less ageism and negativity toward older adults as children age.

For children and older adults, a common intergenerational model may involve an adult senior day care center, nursing care facility, and/or long-term care facility and an organization that provides after-school or day care programming for children from lower-income families (the YMCA is such an organization). These children may or may not be at risk; however, programming goals generally are designed to support community wellness through the promotion of healthy aging and the prevention of further illness or disability for the older adult and optimal development for the children.

In many cities across the country, adult facilities and organizations offering programming for children are coupled with ethnic, culturally circumscribed communities. Programs that utilize the mutual sharing of cultural (and perhaps religious) traditions, holidays, rituals, writings, stories, costumes, toys, etc. are particularly engaging for both groups and may be more akin to the foster grandparent programs in goals and purpose. The Lunalilo Home example is such a program, but it is more global in intergenerational scope and purpose than the typical foster grandparent programs.

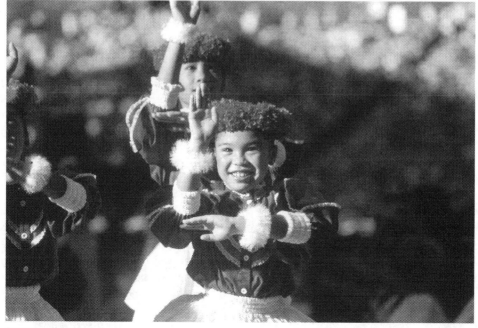

Dances tell stories.

Art, Craft, Music, Dance, and Oral Traditions—Why?

To someone of shared native Hawaiian ancestry, it may appear an obvious answer; these traditions are so linked to the expression of life that one cannot realistically separate them. It is not a unique phenomenon that all generations of an indigenous Hawaiian family engage in ceremonies and rituals involving dance and music (perhaps less likely for arts, crafts and storytelling); nevertheless, the traditions are there in the making of the flower lei (*maile*) and the music and dance instruments. One can also argue that the perhaps romantic desire for a return to a simpler life through resurrection of art, craft, and surrounding traditions can be a powerful motivator, as can the more practical notion of protecting one's heritage by protecting the objects and rituals associated with it.

The Goals to Structure Programming and Outcomes

The programming goals were generated following the comprehensive needs assessment in a focus group format, with the residents, families, and potential partners all engaging in participatory leadership. The resulting goals were powerful, subjective statements of what would be achieved. They were appropriately charismatic in an effort to attract positive attention to the program. Objectives were attached to all of the goals to provide a map to achievement of the larger goals/outcomes. Considering all of this information, organizing ideas, and literature, the following goals were established for the Lunalilo Home project:

- To empower kupuna (grandparents) living in the Lunalilo Home and residents of the adjacent communities to embrace and celebrate their cultural identities through intergenerational community-centered programming
- To foster and encourage opportunities for engagement in meaningful occupations that promote and enhance health, well-being, and the perceived quality of life for the individual and the community while preserving indigenous/native Hawaiian culture
- To perpetuate the knowledge of indigenous/native Hawaiian ancestors through the integration of activities that are imbedded with symbolic and spiritual meaning
- To build an awareness of occupational choices that facilitate, integrate, and motivate individuals to engage in respected roles appreciated and honored by the family and the community

The Programming

The programming was developed in phases that were symbolic of the spiritual context within which the native cultural arts evolved. The first phase was the community garden. It is fitting that the various arts, crafts, music, and dance traditions could be traced back to the plant materials that are so closely associated with them. Multiple generations of adults and children from families and the surrounding community worked alongside kupuna restoring and preparing the land and selecting native plants that would become musical instruments, dance skirts, fabric dyes, sculpted forms, and holiday foods. For planting and cultivating, the Native Hawaiian Community Garden was the place to begin.

Overall, the program was designed to encourage the residents of Lunalilo Home to explore occupational choices intended to promote and improve health, well-being, and the perceived quality of life while engaging with their families and those of the surrounding communities in the enjoyment and celebration of traditional Hawaiian culture. These activities ran the gamut from how to plant and tend a banana palm to the weaving of a grass skirt, construction of a ukulele, making of poi, and storytelling dance traditions. These activities formed cultural bridges to validate the knowledge and skills of residents in the cultural/social traditions of indigenous/native Hawaii by offering them the opportunities to share their knowledge and skills with their children and grandchildren and other multigenerational residents of the community. The cultural legacy of

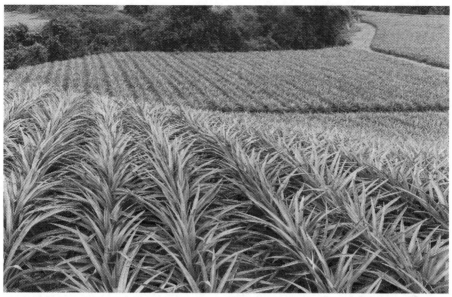

"Gardening" can take on a different meaning for different people. Pineapple fields can stretch long distances.

what it is to be "native Hawaiian" will be protected and preserved through the personal empowerment of every individual involved in the experience, both young and old.

Additional phases of programming have included the fabrication of craft implements and materials, dance implements, and musical instruments, followed by the actual production of art, crafts, dance traditions, and music. Songs and oral traditions are being collected in the development of archival material for an anticipated on-site museum. Recently, an adult day care program was added to the facility and has contributed to the ongoing programming. Further planned production and demonstrations will include flower and seed *maile lei* making, *lauhala* weaving (mats, hats, etc.), *'meke* (gourd bowls and containers), woodworking and carving, fishing tools, and feather working. Classes and demonstrations will always be cross-generational.

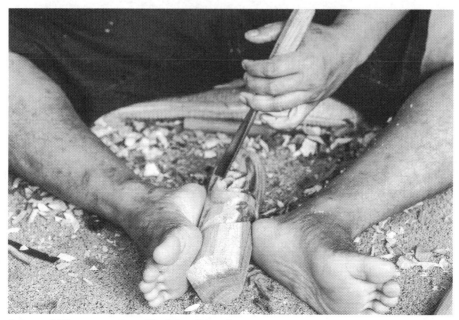

Ceremonial figures are carved in the traditional way.

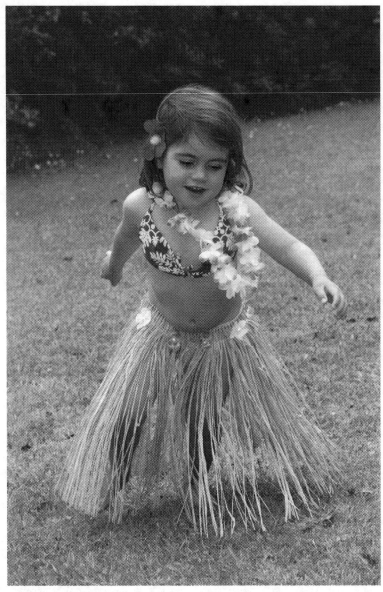

Dancing traditional hula comes early.

Program Outcomes

Present outcomes are subjectively demonstrated in connectedness to the community, resulting in the maintenance of emotional, social, and physical health and modified independent living *within* a residential facility. Regular interviews are conducted with residents, and they are encouraged to maintain journals of their daily activities with indications of perceived well-being daily and weekly. The self-determination scale of Sheldon, Ryan, and Reis (1996) may be useful in providing measures of competence and autonomy as compared with the journal entries. Should we wish, we could evaluate the level of engagement against measures of health and well-being—lowered blood pressures, reductions in pain, and reductions in the symptomatology associated with depression and perhaps dementia.

What Is Happening Now?

At this writing, exciting things are happening at the site of the original Lunalilo Home project, initiated in 2001. The work of the project has continued with the original efforts surrounding all of the agendas of the Native Hawaiian Community Garden. The garden has continued to support the arts, crafts, native foods, and cultural traditions of the Lunalilo community and has now expanded to a commercial *maile* farm (Honolulu Magazine, 2012). According to an article in the Honolulu Magazine (2012), "Big Island Farm Mahiai Ihi is bringing commercial maile back home, establishing two acres of plants in 2009, and harvesting its first crop late 2011. With the support of the community the farm is now able to produce 60 to 100 lei a month for graduations, dance events and other celebrations." According to Executive Director Keali T. Lum, OTD, OTR/L, the present mission of the enterprise is "to establish a self-sustaining community-based mahi'ai (farm) in a manner that is culturally, economically, and spiritually fulfilling for all involved. Through the cultivation of important native Hawaiian trees and plants, including the prized maile, Mahi'ai 'Ihi will support Ali'i Pauahi Hawaiian Civic Club's commitment to advancing the Hawaiian culture" (Lum, 2012).

SUMMARY

Adults are living longer and generally better than in past years. They are more knowledgeable about exercise, nutrition, stress, and wellness. Most hope to enjoy their older adult years at home and in good health. Many may be able to do so with advances in technology and information; however, there will always be those who will live out their lives in institutions designed for senior care. Occupational therapy practitioners are in an excellent position to assist older adults toward continued lives of competence, autonomy, and general well-being regardless of where they live. This chapter has offered some examples of the considerations that are necessary to provide creative and relevant programming that will assist residents of a senior care facility, and their surrounding communities, to engage in meaningful activity that will promote health, well-being, and membership in the larger community. You can easily translate some or all of these ideas to senior-care programming where you live and work.

This programming has developed and grown in large part thanks to the charismatic leadership, marketing, and persuasive agendas of the programmer, who is now the executive director of this work. His ability to identify stakeholders, to network with community partners, and to share his compelling vision with them has carried this program from its original purpose (to serve the residents of the Lunalilo Home) to its present stronghold in the community. Throughout this process, the community has flourished.

REFERENCES

American Occupational Therapy Association. (2001). *Occupational therapy in the promotion of health and the prevention of disease and disability.* Bethesda, MD: AOTA.

American Occupational Therapy Association. (2014). *Occupational therapy practice framework: Domain and process (3rd edition).* Bethesda, MD: AOTA.

Anderson, K. N. (Ed.). (1994). *Mosby's medical, nursing, and allied health dictionary* (4th ed.). St. Louis, MO: Mosby.

Atchley, R. (1994). *Social forces and aging: An introduction to social gerontology.* Belmont, CA: Wadsworth.

Bandura. A. (1977a). *Social learning theory.* Upper Saddle River, NJ: Prentice Hall.

Bandura, A. (1977b). Self-efficacy: Toward a unifying theory of behavioral change. *Psychological Review, 84,* 191-215.

Baumeister, R., & Leary, M..R. (1995). The need to belong: Desire for interpersonal attachments as a fundamental human motivation. *Psychological Bulletin, 117,* 497-529.

Dowd, J. J. (1980). *Stratification among the aged.* Monterey, CA: Brooks/Cole.

Green, L. & Kreuter, M. (1991). *Health promotion planning: An educational and environmental approach.* Mountain View, CA: Mayfield.

Hawkins, M. O., McGuire, F. A., & Backman, K. F. (Eds.). (1999). *Preparing participants for intergenerational interaction: Training for success.* New York, NY: Haworth Press.

He, W., Goodkind, D., & Kowal, P. (2016). *An aging world: 2015. International population reports.* Washington, DC: U.S. Census Bureau. Retrieved from https://census.gov/content/dam/Census/library/publications/2016/demo/p95-16-1.pdf

Honolulu Magazine. (2012). *Hawaiian grown maile lei.* Retrieved from http://www.honolulumagazine.com/Honolulu-Magazine/May-2012/Hawaiian-Grown-Maile-Lei/

Intergenerational programs: Penn State extension. (2017). State College, PA: Penn State College of Agricultural Sciences. Retrieved from http://extension.psu.edu/youth/intergenerational

Jansen, T. R. (2016). The preschool inside a nursing home. Retrieved from https://www.theatlantic.com/education/archive/2016/01/the-preschool-inside-a-nursing-home/424827/

Kendig, H. (1986). Perspectives on ageing and families. In H. Kendig (Ed.), *Ageing and families.* Sydney, Australia: Allen and Unwin.

Kuehne, V. (2012). *International programs: Understanding what we have created.* New York, NY: Routledge.

Lum, K. (2012). Mission of Mahi'ai 'Ihi. Retrieved from http://www.mahiaiihi.org

Morris, W. (Ed.). (1976). *American heritage dictionary of the English language.* Boston, MA: Houghton Mifflin.

National Institutes of Health. (1999). Trans-NIH work group on health disparities. Retrieved from http://www.nimhd.nih.gov/docs/2009-2013nih_health_disparities_strategic_plan_and_budget.pdf

Newman, S., Ward, C. R., Smith, T. B., Wilson, J. O., & McCrea, J. M. (1997). *Intergenerational programs: Past, present and future.* Washington, DC: Taylor and Francis.

Reis, H. T., Sheldon, K. M., Gable, S. L., Roscoe, J., & Ryan, R. M. (2000). Daily well-being: The role of autonomy, competence, and relatedness. *Personality and Social Psychology Bulletin, 26*(4), 419-435.

Ryan, R., & Deci, E. (2000). Self-determination theory and the facilitation of intrinsic motivation, social development, and well-being. *American Psychologist, 55*(1), 68-78.

Ryan, R. M., Kuhl, J., & Deci, E. L. (1997). Nature and autonomy: Organizational view of social and neurobiological aspects of self-regulation in behavior and development. *Development and Psychopathology, 9*, 701-728.

Scaffa, M. (2001). *Occupational therapy in community-based settings.* Philadelphia, PA: F. A. Davis.

Scharlach, A., & Lehring, A. (2016). *Creating aging-friendly communities.* New York, NY: Oxford University Press.

Segal, D. (2002). Group seeks ways to address growing needs of isle seniors. Honolulu, HI: Star Bulletin. Retrieved from http://archives.starbulletin.com/2002/02/19/news/story12.html

Sheldon, K.,M., Ryan, R.,M., & Reis, H. (1996). What makes for a good day? Competence and Autonomy in the day and in the person. *Personality and Social Psychology Bulletin, 22*, 1270-1279.

Siebert, C. (2003). Aging in place: Implications for occupational therapy. *O.T. Practice, 8*(7), 1-7.

Sultz, H., & Young, K. (2004). *Health care USA: Understanding its' organization and delivery.* Sudbury, MA: Jones and Bartlett.

Taylor, A. S., & Dryfoos, J. G. (1998/1999). Creating a safe passage: Elder mentors and vulnerable youths. *Generations, 22*(4), 43-48.

U.S. Census Bureau. (2011). America's diversity. Retrieved from https://www.census.gov/newsroom/releases/archives/2010_census/cb11-cn125.html

U.S. Census Bureau. (2012). More diversity, slower growth. Retrieved from https://www.census.gov/newsroom/releases/archives/population/cb12-243.html

U.S. Census Bureau. (2015). Fact sheet: Population/Hawaii. Retrieved from https://www.census.gov/quickfacts/table/HSG030210/15

U.S. Department of Health and Human Services. (1990). *Healthy people 2000: National health promotion and disease prevention objective.* Washington, DC: Author.

U.S. Department of Health and Human Services. (1998). *Healthy people 2010: Objectives: draft for public comment.* Washington, DC: Author.

Wilcock, A. (1998). *An occupational perspective of health.* Thorofare, NJ: SLACK Incorporated.

World Health Organization. (1986). The Ottawa charter for health promotion. *Health Promotion, I*, iii-v.

Web Resources

Big Island Farm Mahiai Ihi: http://www.mahiaiihi.org

Bishop Museum Library and Archives, Honolulu, Hawai'I (Published primary sources database: published diaries, narratives, memoirs related to 18th- and 19th-century Hawai'i): http://www.bishopmuseum.org/research/cult-stud/libarch/libbooks.html

EARTH SUN (People, culture and language of Hawai'i): http://members.aol.com/EARTHSUN/hawaii.html

Edith Kanaka'ole Foundation (Mission: to heighten indigenous Hawaiian cultural awareness and participation through its educational programs and scholarships): http://www.edithkanakaolefoundation.org/

HAWAII (History, geography, and tourism): http://www.hawaii-nation.org/

Hawaii Craftsmen (Indigenous crafts of Hawai'i): http://www.hawaiicraftsmen.org/

NAKANIOHULA (Hula supplies and Hawaiian crafts): http://www.nakaniohula.com/

VI

What Now? Responding to Trending Issues
Stories in the Making

23

Health Promotion and Wellness Programming for Older Adults Living in the Community

Sexuality, Sexual Functioning, and Intimacy

LEARNING OBJECTIVES

1. To re-evaluate the needs of older adults in maintaining health and wellness
2. To appreciate sexuality, sexual functioning, and intimacy as full components of healthy living
3. To define relevant terms associated with sexuality, sexual functioning, and intimacy
4. To become more familiar with the role of the occupational therapy practitioner in providing guidance in matters of sexuality and sexual functioning

---

KEY TERMS

1. Community mobility
2. Instrumental activities of daily living (IADLs)
3. Productive aging
4. Aging in place/aging-friendly communities
5. Longevity revolution
6. Self-management
7. Sexuality
8. Intimacy/sensuality
9. Sexual functioning/sexual dysfunction
10. PLISSIT model; (extended) PLISSIT model

Fazio, L. S. *Developing Occupation-Centered Programs With the Community, Third Edition* (pp 363-380).
© 2017 Taylor & Francis Group.

When one peruses the occupational therapy literature in recent years, it would appear that we have been fairly thorough in assessing the needs of older adults choosing to "age in place" and continue to live fully in their communities of choice. We have instruments to measure life quality and we have occupation-centered programming to help older adults access their communities safely in order to engage in those aspects of life they deem most significant to their personal interpretation of meaningful engagement (Clark et al., 1997, 2015; Stav, 2014; Stav, Hallenen, Lane, & Arbesman, 2012; Stav, Hunt, & Arbesman, 2006)

WHAT ARE THE SELF-CONCERNS OF OLDER ADULTS?

Community Mobility

Most older adults (and adults of any age) would probably list community mobility near the top of their list of important factors that help them feel independent and in control of their lives. The American Occupational Therapy Association (AOTA, 2014) has defined **community mobility** as "moving around in the community and using public or private transportation, such as driving, walking, bicycling, or accessing and riding in buses, taxicabs, or other transportation systems" (p. s28).

In the United States, for an assortment of reasons, community mobility translates to driving for most adults. The driving rehabilitation practice area has become an important and vibrant area of specialization for occupational therapists and others since the 1990s (Association of Driver Rehabilitation Specialists, 2017). We will see in Chapter 25 how important matters of driving are to returning combat veterans.

Of course, driving and community access permit one to engage in many other favored occupations, including most of the **instrumental activities of daily living (IADLs)** (AOTA, 2014, pp. s19-s20). Access to the community and the service and opportunities it offers most certainly is a predictor of perceived well-being and life quality (Stav et al., 2012). What else is important to older adults, and to their continued engagement in occupations of choice?

Safety and Fall Prevention

Most older adults will tell you that they worry about falling; they will also report that they have fewer falls than they actually do, and minimize the injuries when they do fall, but, of course, why not? Falling indicates another area where the older adult may be losing some of the markers of independence. Normal aging and the addition of medications can cause balance issues, dizziness, loss of visual acuity, and loss of muscle strength and joint mobility. All of these can certainly cause one to fall, and it is a concern for older adults and their families (Bonder & Wagner, 2001; Centers for Disease Control and Prevention [CDC], 2006).

Caldeira and Becker-Omvig (2014) offer an example of a health-promotion/fall prevention program designed and conducted by students (pp. 202-205). The major goals they established for the program represent the following concerns all such programs need to address:

- To raise awareness among seniors regarding strategies to prevent falling
- To alter dangerous behaviors in the everyday life of seniors
- To promote seniors' safety in homes and activities
- To minimize the risk of seniors falling indoors and outdoors

Fall prevention programs are always a good idea and should be included in all primary care agendas that address the needs of aging adults. Innovative programming will not only address the risks and education regarding dangerous behaviors, but will also include background in change theory to address why risks may continue to be taken by many older adults or why they become so cautious and self-protective they forget to live.

Productive Aging and Aging in Place

Clearly, safety and fall prevention are key factors in maintaining **productive aging** and in **aging in place**. National agencies concerned about "livable" communities for all ages define aging in place as "continued living in one's own home and having needed services to be safe, independent, and comfortable while growing older" (Neufeld, 2014, p. 211).

Certainly, there are changing demographics today, and they represent what Butler (2008) has described as a **longevity revolution**. This refers to a remarkable gain in life expectancy and the significant impact this will have on society overall. In the United States, people are living longer, with the number of older adults expected to increase to 72.1 million by the year 2030. This is more than twice the number than in the year 2000. Older adults aged 85 years and older are the fastest growing segment of the aging population and are expected to increase from 4.6 million in year 2000 to 9.6 million in 2030 (Hillman, 2000).

We know that when people age, they begin to experience the aftermath of the earlier years of negative health behaviors: smoking, poor nutrition, obesity, or drug and alcohol abuse, among other things. Health promotion and disease and illness prevention must begin early, and that is the intent of books such as this one. Targeting unhealthy behaviors in older adulthood is "closing the barn door when the horses have already escaped." The cost of health care for aging adults is escalating, along with their longevity. Occupational therapy practitioners are in very favorable positions to work with aging seniors to devise and coordinate **self-management** programs in which, together, they manage their long-term health conditions (e.g., the consequences of disease, negative behaviors, and genetics) by making healthy lifestyle changes in partnership with medical professionals (Lorig & Holman, 2003).

Retirement from employment, as a phenomenon, also puts older adults at risk for adverse health consequences. Occupational therapy practitioners can also intervene with this population and provide coaching to prepare potential retirees for the loss of roles and productivity and a general feeling of lack of control over their lives. Because of years of low pay and resultant financial constraints, many older adults are postponing retirement as long as possible and are often beginning to experience the effects of aging long before they leave the workforce, resulting in depression, substance abuse, and faulty relationships with spouses and families.

One additional area where occupational therapy practitioners can work alongside aging adults and their communities is as an advocate for **aging-friendly communities**. Such communities represent an initiative related to worldwide concerns of increased numbers of older adults. In a keynote address to a global online conference on creating aging-friendly communities, Scharlach (2008) pointed out the importance of communities offering continuity, compensation, and opportunity for healthy aging—opportunities for continued engagement in life and community, compensation for any supports or accommodations needed for functional limitations due to aging, and opportunities for familiar and new activities for enhanced quality of life.

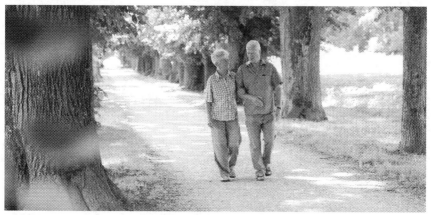

A walk together: sharing a valuable occupation.

These words—*opportunities for familiar and new activities for enhanced quality of life*—move us nicely to the focus of this chapter: sexuality, sexual functioning, and intimacy in the lives of older adults.

SEXUALITY, SEXUAL FUNCTIONING, AND INTIMACY

Sexuality is a core characteristic and formative factor for human beings (MacRae, 2010). *The Occupational Therapy Practice Framework: Domain and Process* (AOTA, 2014) lists sexual activity as an ADL. As such, it is an acceptable, billable practice area for occupational therapists. It is part of a routine evaluation of clients, and occupational therapists and occupational therapy assistants address this area in occupational therapy interventions. At last view, older adults remained very much present in occupational therapy practice, so we can assume that the issues older adults may have with sexuality, sexual functioning, and intimacy are included in an occupational therapy practitioner's repertoire. The AOTA fact sheet "Sexuality and the Role of O.T." suggests that sexuality can be addressed by occupational therapy practitioners in a great variety of settings (AOTA, 2013). Yamkovenko (2014) is Editor of the AOTA blog, "Checking the Pulse" and includes "talking about sex with clients" as a prominent topic for occupational therapy practitioners.

Intervention/remediation and modification for issues regarding sexuality can occur in such settings as homes, group homes, nursing homes, rehabilitation centers, community mental health centers, pain centers, senior centers, hospitals, retirement communities, and other venues, so we have many possibilities to choose from. A large number of the programs highlighted in this text are about health promotion, and we know there are numerous venues for programs targeting the promotion of health and wellness. Often, health and wellness programs serve up a healthy portion of advocacy alongside information, and this is probably how it should be. As occupational therapy practitioners, we can choose from a wide variety of educational programming that may include large instructional venues such as auditoriums and classrooms as well as smaller in-service training classes to assist caregivers in institutions (e.g., skilled nursing facilities appreciate and understand the sexual needs of older adults and those with diverse sexual orientations).

The National Center for Creative Aging (n.d.) tells us that productive aging is about more than volunteering, caregiving, and employment; it also refers to living life fully, socially engaged with a positive zest for life and expressing oneself creatively with the ability to achieve outcomes.

Many of the older adults we encounter as occupational therapy practitioners are representative of what we would describe as the disenfranchised in terms of education, socioeconomic status, and access to health care. Some may be spending their days caring for abandoned grandchildren or adult children who have not aged well themselves. Many in our care have experienced the effects of debilitating illnesses and conditions (strokes, diabetes, and Alzheimer's or Parkinson's disease, among other problems), but there is extensive diversity in the population of older adults, both in the United States and in other countries. Contrary to popular stereotypes, older adults as a group are more heterogeneous than both young and middle-aged adults (Hillman, 2012; Thornton, 2002). Across the populations of older adults living in their communities of choice, the needs are as diverse as the assets and capacities.

Overall, older adults today are better educated and have enough resources to make positive choices about healthy lifestyles. They have access to the world through electronic media. In general, they look and feel better than their predecessors. They may worry more about having enough money to protect the health and lifestyle they desire, but they tend to have high expectations for what it means to maintain health and well-being, even though they are not necessarily free of the management of chronic illness such as diabetes and hypertension. For these older adults, maintaining safety with railings and grab bars and ensuring accessibility to home and bathrooms is often self-motivated and initiated and accomplished with the aid of their handyman, contractor, or the local hardware store. They have many strengths and assets.

Health service practitioners, with occupational therapy practitioners among them, often focus on the loss of physical and cognitive functioning that older adults may experience, but not on the loss of opportunity/access for emotional health and well-being, which is equally devastating. Our emphasis here is on emotional health in the form of opportunities for intimacy, and sexual expression/sexual functioning. As mentioned previously, the *Occupational Therapy Practice Framework* (AOTA, 2014, p. s19) includes sexual activity as an "ADL" and defines it as "engaging in activities that result in sexual satisfaction and/or meet relational or reproductive needs." However, I would suggest that it is a good deal more than that; rather, we think of it as an "IADL" defined as "activities to support daily life within the home and community that often require more complex interactions than those used in ADLs" (p. s19). We might even be able to make a case for it under the category of "play." According to Parham and Fazio (1997), "play is any spontaneous or organized activity that provides enjoyment, entertainment, amusement, or diversion" (p. 252). Many adults, including older adults, would like this definition!

Terminology Used to Frame Our Discussions of Older Adult Sexuality

Among the key words for this chapter are three broad terms that serve to frame our current discussion: intimacy, sexuality, and sexual functioning. To those, we will now add sexual expression/sensuality and sexual dysfunction. **Intimacy** can be defined as "the quality of the interpersonal relationships among two people in a romantic relationship, who may or may not be actively engaged in sexual relations; it represents interpersonal satisfaction and subjective feelings of closeness" (Hillman, 2000, p. 11). Masters, Johnson, and Kolodny (1995) offer this definition of intimacy: "a process in which two caring people share as freely as possible in the exchange of feelings, thoughts, and actions...it is marked by a mutual sense of acceptance, commitment, tenderness, and trust" (p. 329). Szuchman and Muscarella (2000) connect intimacy with love. According to these authors, intimacy, passion, and decision/commitment form a triangle that is conceptualized as love (p. 234). They see the intimacy component as primarily emotional or affective, involving feelings of warmth, closeness, connection, and bondedness within a love relationship.

Sexuality is defined as a broad term that indicates any combination of sexual behavior, sensual activity, emotional intimacy, or sense of sexual identity (Hillman, 2012, p. 11). Bonder and Wagner (2001) suggest that sexuality also includes the way we think about ourselves as sexual beings, and the corresponding gender roles and behaviors, need for intimacy, ideas about reproduction, and feelings of excitement and pleasure that are associated with sex. For these authors, sexuality also includes the entire range of sexual behaviors as well as the decision to be celibate (p. 219).

Sensuality can be defined as the experience of pleasure from one's senses, leading to an increased awareness of and appreciation for one's own body (Hillman, 2012, p. 12). Sensual pleasure can be experienced with or without another person and can include such sensory activities as a massage, a hot bath or shower, listening to music, and engaging in or appreciating art. While sensual activities may induce sexual excitement, that is not the goal.

Sexual functioning refers to the ability to have and maintain an erection for males and to reach orgasm and the ability to reach orgasm in females with or without penetration by the male. As practitioners, we may be more familiar with the term **sexual dysfunction**, which includes a myriad of disorders and symptoms; however, most population-based surveys do include some assessment of erectile dysfunction for men and difficulty with lubrication (e.g., vaginal dryness) for women (Hillman, 2012). An American Association of Retired Persons (AARP) 2010 national survey reported that, of the respondents who were sexually active, about 56% of males aged 70 and above self-reported erectile dysfunction; only 3% of females in the same age group reported having difficulty with vaginal dryness. Of these individuals, 26% of the men and 27% of the women reported sexual satisfaction. Since this was a self-report survey, it is unclear exactly what led these respondents to seek or not seek treatment, although many reported not seeking treatment either

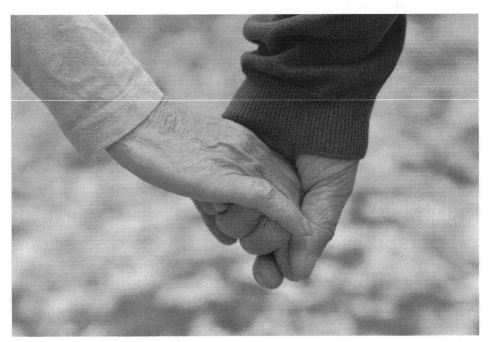

Intimacy is often reflected in touch.

because they felt uncomfortable discussing sexual issues or because the cost of seeking treatment was too high.

Practicing Occupational Therapy Within the Realm of Sexuality

Thus, with the inclusion in the *Occupational Therapy Practice Framework* (AOTA, 2014), we know that we can practice in this area, but few occupational therapy practitioners choose to do so, either because of unclear roles, the lack of practice standards, or a general discomfort with the topic. In addition, most occupational therapy educational programs offer only very limited information regarding sexuality content; this is most often included only as it relates to physical dysfunction. In fact, many conditions and illnesses that are common among those in late adulthood and that can affect sexual functioning are likely to present themselves as physical problems. See Table 23-1 for some of the more common illnesses that affect sexual arousal or desire that may be common to older adults.

Occupational therapy practitioners are likely to be asked questions about problems with sexual functioning because we may be seeing older adults who are experiencing both chronic and acute illnesses accompanying the aging process. In addition, many medications frequently prescribed for older patients such as antihypertensives, tranquilizers, and antidepressants may have sexual side effects to include decreased libido and ejaculatory difficulties. See Table 23-2 for some common prescription medications with possible sexual side effects.

The use of alcohol and other drugs, even heavy smoking, may adversely affect sexual arousal and performance at any age. However, there may be a cumulative effect on long-time heavy drinkers. Excessive and chronic use of alcohol and drugs to aid sleeping can further complicate the older adult's life.

TABLE 23-1
COMMON ILLNESSES ASSOCIATED WITH AGING THAT AFFECT SEXUAL AROUSAL OR DESIRE
• Cardiac disease, including coronary artery disease, post-coronary recovery, high blood pressure
• Cardiovascular accident (stroke)
• Liver problems, including hepatitis and cirrhosis
• Kidney problems, including nephritis, renal failure, dialysis (radical prostatectomy)
• Peripheral neuropathies (diabetes mellitus, alcoholic neuropathy, and multiple sclerosis)
• Pulmonary diseases; degenerative diseases
• Arthritis and other connective tissue diseases
• Diabetes and amputation
• Thyroid diseases
• Head injuries
• Parkinson's disease
• Malignancies
Sources: Bonder & Wagner, 2001; Hillman, 2012; Kellett, 2000; Sipski & Alexander, 1997.

TABLE 23-2
PRESCRIPTION MEDICATIONS WITH POSSIBLE SEXUAL SIDE EFFECTS
• Antihypertensives (sympatholytic, or adrenergic-inhibiting, drugs [e.g., reserpine] and diuretics [e.g., thiazides or spironolactone]): Resulting in erectile dysfunction and some loss of desire
• Tranquilizer, anxiolytic (e.g., Valium [diazepam], Xanax [alprazolam], Ativan [lorazepam]): Resulting in changes in libido; erectile dysfunction
• Antidepressant (e.g., Prozac [fluoxetine], Zoloft [sertraline], Paxil [paroxetine], Effexor [venlafaxine]): Resulting in changes in libido; delayed orgasm/ejaculation
Sources: Hillman, 2012; Weiner & Rosen, 1997.

The PLISSIT Model to Guide Our Responses to Sexual Concerns

The **PLISSIT model** (Annon, 1976) provides some direction about our roles. It was developed by Annon to address the sexual well-being needs of individuals with acquired disability or chronic illness. The PLISSIT model sets out four levels of involvement that can be used to help health care practitioners identify their role in the assessment and evaluation of an individual's sexual well-being needs.

The four levels of intervention are as follows (Annon, 1976, p. 4):

1. Permission (P)

2. Limited information (LI)

3. Specific suggestions (SS)

4. Intensive therapy (IT)

Annon (1976) believed that most people experiencing sexual problems can resolve them if they are given permission to be sexual, to desire sexual activity, and to discuss sexuality; if they receive limited information about sexual matters; and if they are given specific suggestions about ways to address sexual problems. Taylor and Davis (2007) have reported that most practitioners bypass the permission level and go directly to limited information in the form of a booklet or pamphlet. Occupational therapists and nurse practitioners often do this, particularly if they have been working with a particular diagnosis and begin to think that one solution fits everyone. Giving permission means that you are open for a discussion.

Taylor and Davis (2007) later developed the **extended PLISSIT model**. This revision emphasizes the role that permission giving plays at all stages. Permission giving involves normalizing sexuality; for example, "Many people with this condition have concerns about sexuality. Is there anything you would like to talk about or ask?" This revision not only recommends explicit permission giving as a core feature of each of the other stages, but also the incorporation of reflection as a means of increasing self-awareness by challenging assumptions clients may have. As noted previously, the original PLISSIT model identified the four levels of intervention. The first two levels are appropriate for entry-level occupational therapy practitioners to use; the third level is also appropriate assuming the practitioner has obtained accurate knowledge to offer specific suggestions. The fourth level is beyond our general entry-level education and knowledge and is generally reserved for those trained in counseling/sex therapy (Leiblum & Segraves, 2000). If you would like to know more about the problems sex therapists address, please review the Additional References at the close of the chapter.

In the 1960s and 1970s, when I was first practicing, occupational therapists had few models for practice in sexuality and sexual functioning; therefore, I chose to obtain an advanced degree in counseling/sex therapy in order to obtain the specialized knowledge to practice in this area in order to extend my options and will return to thoughts about the validity/benefits of this decision as it relates to present occupational therapy practices.

WHAT DO WE KNOW ABOUT SEXUALITY AND HOW DO WE KNOW IT?

The first empirical studies to provide information about the sexual practices of older adults were conducted in the 1940s and 1950s by Kinsey and his colleagues (1948, 1953). This was the first organized group of studies that involved extensive interviews to find out what people were doing and thinking about sex. Results of the studies included information to suggest that men over the age of 60 years engaged in intercourse slightly more than once per week on average, with no sudden decline related to aging. Women over age 60 years did so less frequently but with patterns similar to those they reported in their late teenage years.

In 1966, Masters and Johnson reported that men and women were biologically capable of engaging in sexual intercourse at any age. Depending on the sex of the individual, there are specific physiologic changes that occur during the act of intercourse. A significant outcome of their research was laboratory documentation of these changes, resulting in a model of sexual response— the "normal sexual response cycle"—as shown in Table 23-3.

Aging can alter the normal sexual response cycle. For men, normal physiologic changes occurring with the aging process in the response cycle may include a decline in testosterone, decline in sperm production, and changes in the amount and consistency of seminal ejaculate. Also present are diminished force of ejaculation, likely increase in the size of the prostate gland, longer periods

TABLE 23-3
THE NORMAL SEXUAL RESPONSE CYCLE
• Excitement
• Plateau
• Orgasm
• Resolution
Source: Masters & Johnson, 1966.

of time to stimulate sexual excitement and erections, as well as less frequent ejaculations and longer refractory periods. For women, although there are likely changes in natural vaginal secretions and longer periods of time to achieve sexual excitement, the response cycle is largely unchanged with aging.

A more recent study conducted by the 2010 AARP Survey of Midlife and Older Adults (Fisher, 2010) included large samples of men and women between the ages of 45 and 90 years. This study oversampled Black and Hispanic men and women, who had been under-represented in the earlier studies. The findings suggested that both older women and older men participated in vaginal sex and masturbation well into their 80s and 90s; however, they were less likely to participate than middle-aged men and women. Rates of participation in foreplay remain consistent across age, and it is interesting to note that foreplay as well as remaining in embrace following sexual engagement are often considered measures of intimacy. Significantly, more Hispanic men report participation in weekly vaginal sex than non-Hispanic men.

Further findings indicate that approximately 10% of aging men and women report a sexual orientation other than heterosexual. About 6% of men and 1% of women indicate that they have multiple sex partners, while less than 5% report usually or always using condoms. Variability in condom use and misinterpretation of the risk of STDs has been a significant factor in needs assessments previous to designing sexuality programming for older adults.

It is important to remember that, in all of these findings, we should distinguish average from normal in interpreting the reports of frequencies and behaviors. Most of these results neglect information regarding whether the older adults surveyed were satisfied with their sexual relationships. We do not know whether they desired more or less sexual contact, had consistent access to a consenting sexual partner, and were healthy enough to engage in certain sexual activities.

What Is Sexual Health for Older Adults?

We are all getting older. The changes in sexual interest and function that accompany aging, as well as the sexual concerns of aging adults, are a topic that is both personally and professionally relevant. Most survey studies of older adults find that they remain interested in an active and varied sex life, although sexual frequency and activity do tend to decline with aging (Chao, et al., 2011; Hinchliff & Gott, 2008; Leiblum & Segraves, 2000; Schwartz, 2015). There are wide differences, however, and it is important not to stereotype older adults as disengaged and sexually disinterested.

The most salient marker of aging in women is menopause, occurring at around age 50 years (Hillman, 2000). Most women notice changes in their physical appearance as well as in their sexual response. Lack of lubrication and diminished sexual desire are common complaints among both heterosexual and homosexual women. Hormone replacement of both estrogen and androgen can prove helpful in reducing vaginal atrophy and in increasing sexual interest and sensitivity (Leiblum & Segraves, 2000). In recent years, there has been controversy over hormone replacement and connections made to both breast cancer and heart disease; thus, many women resort to over-the-counter vaginal lubricants and various herbal remedies for accompanying menopausal "hot flashes" and sleeplessness.

Changes in men with aging are not dissimilar to the changes occurring in women, but they occur more gradually. Most notably, erectile performance declines and, for some men, there is less penile sensitivity. The force and frequency of desire for sexual release decrease in older men (Kontula & Haavio-Mannila, 2009). Vasoactive agents are a viable treatment for many men, but it is important to determine the interest and desire of the female partner prior to initiating pharmacological intervention. Leiblum and Rosen (2000) devoted an introductory chapter to "Sex Therapy in the Age of Viagra" in the third edition of their text, *Principles and Practice of Sex Therapy*. There are now commonplace advertisements in print and on television strongly linking erectile function to health and quality of life. Although there is no present female equivalent of Viagra, women partners of older men are clearly present in the advertisements and look aptly pleased with their partner's choice. On March 29, 1998, sildenafil citrate (Viagra) was approved as the first orally active agent for the treatment of erectile dysfunction (Leiblum & Rosen, 2000). Today, "the little blue pill" is widely available from primary care physicians, sexual medicine specialists, and urologists as well as the Internet. There is no doubt that erectile dysfunction can attain monumental status in relationships, but it is well known that medical and pharmacological treatments do not address or resolve relationship problems and these psychological and relationship factors are frequently the major source of sexual inhibition or distress in the first place (Leiblum, 1999).

Leiblum and Seagraves (2000) report that older couples experience much of the same sexual complaints as younger couples. Problems with sexual desire discrepancy, arousal difficulties, erectile failure, anorgasmia, early or delayed ejaculation, pain with intercourse, script incompatibility ("why don't you do what I want you to do?"), and problematic sexual communication and technique are common. Many older couples would like to try new and interesting things, and it appears that if sex was a source of pleasure and gratification during early and middle adulthood, it will probably continue to be an important source of life satisfaction as one grows older. For others in long partnered relationships, predictability often replaces spontaneity, and sexual encounters may become routine and perfunctory. Sometimes, simply providing specific information about reviving the couple relationship and rewriting the sexual script can make a difference.

On the other hand, it is important to acknowledge that there are many older adults and couples who grew up in a post-Victorian society and in fundamental and traditional households in which sexually proscriptive values and beliefs persist. For these older adults, there were so many restricted sex acts in their youth that they, particularly women, are often glad to have the opportunity to "retire" from sex.

Sometimes, the biggest problem for older men and women is the lack or loss of a partner. Grief about both physical and psychological losses may have to comprise part of the therapy with this population. In fact, it is often the loss of a life partner that prompts the need for community program intervention with a sexuality component or module. Many chronic diseases and the use of varied medications inhibit or interfere with the sexual response of older adults, but psychological factors are often implicated as well. It is a mistake to prematurely conclude that organic factors are the primary culprits in the sexual complaints of either older men or older women without taking a thorough sexual history of both partners in a couple. When health care providers, including occupational therapy practitioners, are attempting to use the PLISSIT permission and limited information model to address questions regarding sexuality and sexual practices, it is easy to be pulled into relationship problems and sometimes co-occurring psychological and psychiatric problems. You can avoid this, but you need to practice your communication/active listening skills. I cannot emphasize this enough: the issue that is presented to you is often not the actual issue, and you will need to use skillful communication in order to stay within your practice guidelines. It is more likely that this can happen when you are working one-on-one with a patient than when you are conducting a community program for a larger group.

OUR ATTITUDES AND BELIEFS ABOUT AGING AND SEXUAL EXPRESSION

As we have indicated, we are an aging population. Nevertheless, despite their increasing presence (and perceived power) and the ever-growing number of articles and interest in successful aging, older adults are often victims of negative stereotypes that associate aging with images of fragility, incompetence, and disengagement. Young adults, in particular, continue to believe that older adults are sad, sick, and asexual, with little energy or enthusiasm for social or intellectual pursuits. Most young adults and even some middle-aged adults find it difficult to imagine their parents and grandparents as sexually interested and active.

Historically, sexual relations among older people were viewed as evil, immoral, perverse, inappropriate, impossible, and comical (Covey, 1989; Hillman, 2012). During the Middle Ages in Europe, the Roman Catholic Church played a central role in shaping beliefs about elderly sexuality. At the core was the prohibition that sexual intercourse was reserved for procreation only, and this applied to people of all ages. Aristotle, learned thinker and teacher of a much earlier time, wrote that sexual activity ceased for women at menopause and for men after their fifth decade of life (Stone, 1977). The standards for men and women were different. Older men who still managed to have an active sex life were believed to gain social status and even an increase in their length of life. In contrast, if an older woman was thought to have sex in her later years, it was only through trickery aided by witchcraft (Stone, 1977). The confusion many Puritans felt around sexuality, particularly the sexual activity of older women, undoubtedly fueled the flames of many witch burnings.

Today, often blamed on the media and advertising, sexual expression is clearly acceptable among those who present the physical attributes prized by popular culture. Not only are older adults restricted (unless they are attractive and/or wealthy, and the two are likely linked), but also those who are younger but not thought to be attractive by the culture or not in good health are restricted as well. According to Hillman (2012), our "youth-oriented culture" views the process of aging as something of a tragic, narcissistic injury instead of as an opportunity for personal growth and change (p. 37). Unfortunately many older adults internalize and generalize these negative attitudes toward their own sexuality. The clinicians' attitudes regarding sexuality among the elderly are often negative as well, reinforcing their patients' attitudes. However, Hillman (2012) is optimistic about a growing field of clinical interest in elderly sexuality, although it is a slow progression (p. 179).

Sexuality practice with older adults is complicated at best. There is much variation in how we feel about sexuality, sexual functioning, and intimacy. Most people have strong opinions about who they believe is entitled to participation and who is not. The average person would probably prefer that sexual engagement be limited to only a few, and these few are identified early on by the culture and society. Needless to say, most practitioners (including physicians) and those who are interested in health maintenance may prefer to steer clear of this area (Gott, Hinchliff, & Galena, 2004).

We know that opinion and comfort levels vary widely among practitioners when it comes to discussions regarding sexuality and sexual expression with our younger patients and clients (i.e., spine-injured clients wanting to resume sexual practices with their partners, midlife patients with coronary artery disease or cancer, adolescents on the autistic spectrum who are curious about masturbation, etc.), and we can only imagine how complicated discussions of sexual practices may be with older adults. Most occupational therapy practitioners would likely prefer to limit their practices with older adults to those concerns we highlighted at the opening of this chapter. Some of your comfort in discussing sexual concerns with any client comes with practice and life experience. The more you increase your own knowledge of sexual practices and sexual information, the more confidence you will have in response to client/patient questions. It is important that practitioners recognize their own strengths and limitations and acknowledge the limits of their own comfort zone and competence. When necessary, refer patients to others who are more able to address their individual need; unfortunately, there is often no one else available.

Based on the work of White (1982), the Aging Sexual Knowledge and Attitudes Scale (ASKAS) continues to be used extensively among older adults, adult children of older adults, college students, doctoral-level psychology students, medical students, and care providers. The knowledge subtest of the ASKAS includes 35 items and is recommended to anyone who anticipates talking with older adults about sexuality or simply as necessary information any clinician working with older adults should have. See the appendix of this chapter for sample knowledge items from the ASKAS. The full scale is also published in Hillman (2012, pp. 49-52).

PROFESSIONAL DEVELOPMENT AND EDUCATION IN SEXUALITY

If you wish to expand your knowledge of sexuality, you may choose to explore some of the professional societies and journals that support and publish research and clinical applications, such as sex education and therapy. The Society for the Scientific Study of Sexuality, established in 1957, is the oldest organization in the United States that is devoted to the professional study of human sexuality (www.sexscience.org). The society's official publication, *The Journal of Sex Research*, is devoted to the selection and distribution of empirical research and other scientific writings in contemporary sexual science. The society also publishes the *Annual Review of Sex Research*.

Sex education and related topics are the focus of the Sexuality Information and Education Council of the United States (SIECUS) (siecus.org). SIECUS is a national nonprofit organization founded in 1964 to develop, collect, and disseminate information about human sexuality; to promote comprehensive sexuality education; and to advocate the right of individuals to make responsible sexual choices. SIECUS maintains a comprehensive sexuality library and publishes numerous pamphlets, booklets, and bibliographies for professionals and the general public. They publish a bimonthly journal, the *SIECUS Report*. The sister organization in Canada is called the Sex Information and Education Council of Canada (SIECCAN). SIECCAN publishes the quarterly journal the *Canadian Journal of Human Sexuality*.

The American Association of Sex Educators, Counselors, and Therapists (AASECT) was founded in 1967. AASECT is devoted to promoting understanding of human sexuality and healthy sexual behavior. This organization certifies qualified health and mental health practitioners in dealing expertly and ethically with the sexuality concerns of individuals and couples and offers a broad range of education and training activities. AASECT publishes the *Journal of Sex Education and Therapy* (http://www.aasect.org/). In addition to the previously mentioned journals, there are others that address different aspects of sexuality: *the Journal of the History of Sexuality; Sexualities: Studies in Culture and Society, Sexuality and Culture; the Journal of Psychology and Human Sexuality; Journal of Lesbian and Gay Studies; Journal of Homosexuality; Journal of Social Work and Human Sexuality;* and *Sexuality and Disability*, to name a few. You may also wish to review the Additional References at the close of the chapter for recommended reading.

I indicated previously that I took an advanced degree in counseling with an emphasis in sexuality that included 1 year's internship with both individual clients and couples, as well as a postdoctoral internship in group practice with spinal injury clients of all ages, genders, and sexual preferences, and their partners. At the time, this credential permitted me to practice as an occupational therapist, a sex therapist, and a counselor. My confidence grew enormously from all of the practice exposure, but the curriculum really offered me only resources and direction. I am offering you, here, similar resources, those from which I learned the most; and now, for you as occupational therapy practitioners, the door is open and the advanced degree is not needed unless you wish to do sex therapy and attempt to treat sexual dysfunction.

OCCUPATION-CENTERED PROGRAMMING WITH ISSUES OF SEXUALITY AND SEXUAL FUNCTIONING IN OLDER ADULTS

As with any potential community programming, we approach issues of sexuality in much the same way as we have approached other issues in this text. First, is there a "need" for intervention services? Can we as occupational therapy practitioners meet that need? If we believe we can meet the need, how will we do it? We also find the capacities and assets in our community, our clients, and in our stakeholders.

Briefly discussed here will be a programming example that will help demonstrate the previously described process: An evolving curriculum on sexuality and aging for an adult community education center (has also been incorporated as a module within a program for adults/older adults who have lost a significant other).

Skills- and Knowledge-Building Workshop on Sexuality—Then

The Early Programming

In the early 1980s, one of my clients asked if I would provide a program for older adults that would help them better understand their own sexuality and also help them appreciate changes that may be expected with aging and be prepared to distinguish those changes that may indicate problems that can be remedied. So, I did. To summarize the programming for an edition of *Community Programs for the Health Impaired Elderly*, I wrote the following:

> Community programs serving the elderly are becoming actively involved in the support of comprehensive wellness to meet the changing needs of the aging adult. An occupational therapy perspective enjoys compatibility with community wellness programs by recognizing the community as an arena for practice and by encouraging a broad view of wellness to include many occupational roles for the aging adult. [This paper] addresses the expression of sexuality as a component of occupational behavior through a description of a program designed to assist the aging adult to (1) become more aware of the processes of normal sexual development, (2) become more aware of changes that are likely to occur in sexual needs and functions with aging, (3) understand the impact of illness, disability and medications on sexual functioning, and (4) view sexuality within one's occupational profile. (Fazio, 1988, p. 59).

The first series of programs were relatively well received, attended by more women than men, and likely of most interest to the participants who wished "to fix" their partners. As I continued to develop educational programming, I found that an adult education lecture/discussion model worked well, accompanied by smaller discussion groups that brought anonymous questions and concerns back to the larger class. The goals of the first program were: (1) educational: to gain accurate information on sexuality and aging; (2) attitude adjustment—to gain acceptance and understanding of one's own sexuality and that of others; and (3) awareness—to be more fully cognizant of one's life roles and the ability to alter them if needed. The general purpose was to provide accurate information on sexuality and aging for males and females and to offer a supportive and facilitative climate for sharing concerns and questions regarding sexuality and occupational roles (Fazio, 1988).

In the same time frame, occupational therapist Maureen Neistadt (1986) published a module on sexuality counseling for adults with disabilities in the *American Journal of Occupational Therapy*. Thereafter, I began to include modules on sexuality for my students at Texas Woman's University, and I knew of other occupational therapy faculty who were doing the same. Then, the bottom seemed to fall out of sex, at least for occupational therapists— they lost interest! Of course, we know that was not likely the case, but students did seem to become a bit more conservative over the years, a bit more squeamish, and, for the first time in my experience, were asking to be excused from classes discussing sexuality. As the world became bombarded with sex, students seemed to retreat from the topic, and maybe that is the reason.

Skills- and Knowledge-Building Workshop on Sexuality—Now

As I have continued to do workshops on sexuality, sexual functioning, and intimacy, many of the same questions are still being asked. Today, my participants are often health care providers who want more accurate information (Bauer, McAuliffe, and Chenco, 2013). Nursing homes are seeking education for their staff because residents are having sex all around them (Scott, 2015). In these times of abundant information about everything, all one has to do is go to the Internet. However, you might want to take a look at what is out there in regard to sexuality—it would instill confusion in the most sophisticated viewer. Often, workshop participants (particularly older adults) will say that it is far easier not to get out there and not to participate at all. In my earlier programming, no one wanted to know how to put on a condom, particularly older adults who were past childbearing age. In fact, much of the earlier programming was about finding ways to educate adolescents about the need to wear condoms to avoid teen pregnancies. STDs were certainly out there, but most people thought that they themselves were somehow not at risk (LaVail, 2010). Many people still think that. Today, it is not uncommon for older adults to ask about STDs and condom use, particularly if they have just lost a long-time spouse, but they may choose not to engage in intercourse rather than wear a condom.

Today, the oldest old, defined as those 85 to 89 years of age in the United States, comprise more than 2.5 women for every man (Hillman, 2012, pp. 4-5). Therefore, one of the commonly asked questions of this group is how to deal with the perceived stigma of dating younger men. Society has already defined the "cougar" as the pursuer, not the pursued, which leaves the older woman in the relationship in a vulnerable position. In many ways, the questions today lend themselves very well to the PLISSIT model supporting "permission" and "limited information."

Programming for a Specific Diagnostic Group

A good way to begin programming in the area of sexuality is to include the topic as a module along with other needs of a particular population. A program for post-coronary clients, for example, can occur in an outpatient facility and has been successful offered in a health and wellness club/facility and/or a YMCA. Modules, in addition to sexuality, may include graduated exercise, nutrition, weight loss, and yoga/relaxation. Other population-specific multitopic programs might include those for post-prostatectomy (bowel and bladder function and sexuality); post-mastectomy (body image, sexuality, wardrobe, exercise); and others you may think of.

SUMMARY

This chapter proposes that sexual functioning and intimacy are important considerations for the health and well-being of older adults living in their communities of choice. Occupational therapy practitioners work closely, often intimately, with older adults. They are in a position to listen to the sexual concerns of older adult clients and patients and to offer them both permission and limited information as they seek out answers to their concerns and questions regarding sexuality and intimacy. There is substantial need for occupational therapy to embrace this practice area, first in the curriculum of professional educational programs, and then in advocacy for a practice niche. This chapter also provides information and resources to occupational therapy practitioners who wish to improve their foundational knowledge of sexual issues and concerns of older adults and provides some ideas for community-centered programming. Approaches to programming are no different than what you find in previous chapters. You retain the same formula with the same considerations—your population and their needs and assets are different.

This chapter also contains some cautions with regard to the sometimes fuzzy lines between what the occupational therapy practitioner, the sex therapist, and the counselor can do when clients bring concerns of a sexual nature to the clinician. Most of our community programs are intended to provide education (limited information) and offer a safe place for people to ask questions and to be listened to. Sexuality and intimacy is most often offered as a module or portion of programming that focuses on loss of a life partner or is specific to a group of clients with similar sexual concerns (post-prostatectomy, amputations, cardiovascular incidents/surgeries, breast cancer, and Parkinson's disease, among others).

REFERENCES

American Association of Retired Persons. (2010). *Social media and technology use among adults 50+.* Washington, DC: Author. Retrieved from http://assets.aarp.org/rgcenter/general/socmedia.pdf

American Occupational Therapy Association. (2013). Sexuality and the role of occupational therapy. Retrieved from http://www.aota.org/about-occupational-therapy/professionals/RDP/sexuality.aspx

American Occupational Therapy Association. (2014). Occupational therapy practice framework: Domain and process (3rd ed.). *American Journal of Occupational Therapy, 68*(Suppl 1), s1-s48.

Association for Driver Rehabilitation Specialists. (2017). Who we are. Retrieved from http://www.aded.net/

Annon, J. (1976). The PLISSIT model: a proposed conceptual scheme for the behavioural treatment of sexual problems. *Journal of Sex Education and Therapy, 2*(1), 1-15.

Bauer, M., McAuliffe, L., & Chenco, R. N. (2013). Sexuality in older adults: Effect of an education intervention on attitudes and beliefs of residential aged care staff. *Educational Gerontology, 39*(2), 82- 91.

Bonder, B., & Wagner, M. (2001). *Functional performance in older adults* (2nd ed.). Philadelphia, PA: Davis.

Butler, R. N. (2008). *The longevity revolution: The benefits and challenges of living a long life.* New York, NY: Public Affairs.

Caldeira, R. M., & Becker-Omvig, M. (2014). *Fall prevention.* In M. Scaffa & S. M. Reitz (Eds.), *Occupational therapy in community-based practice settings* (2nd ed., pp. 201-209). Philadelphia, PA: F. A. Davis.

Centers for Disease Control and Prevention. (2006). Fatalities and injuries from falls among older adults—United States, 1993-2003 and 2001-2005. *Morbidity and Mortality Weekly Report, 55*(45), 1221-1224.

Chao, J. Lin, Y., Ma, M., Lai, C., Ku, Y., Kuo, W., & Chao, L. (2011). Relationship among sexual desire, sexual satisfaction, and quality of life in middle-aged and older adults. *Journal of Sex and Marital Therapy, 37*(5), 386-403.

Clark, F., Azen, S. P., Zemke, R., Jackson, J., Carlson, M., Mandel, D., & Lipson, L. (1997). Occupational therapy for independent-living older adults: A randomized controlled trial. *Journal of the American Medical Association, 278,* 1321-1326.

Clark, F., Blanchard, J, Sleight, A, Cogan, A, Florindez, L, Gleason, S, Heymann, R., . . .Vigen, C (2015). *Lifestyle redesign: Guidelines for implementation of the intervention assessed for effectiveness in the USC Well Elderly Studies* (2nd ed.). Bethesda, MD: AOTA Press.

Covey, H. C. (1989). Perceptions and attitudes toward sexuality of the elderly during the middle ages. *The Gerontologist, 29,* 93-100.

Fazio, L. S. (1988). Sexuality and aging: A community wellness program. In E. Taira (Ed.), *Community programs for the health impaired elderly* (pp. 59-68). New York, NY: Haworth Press.

Fisher, L. L. (2010). *Sex, romance, and relationships: AARP survey of midlife and older adults.* Washington. DC: AARP.

Gott, M., Hinchliff, S., & Galena, E. (2004). General practitioner attitudes to discussing sexual health issues with older people. *Social science and medicine, 58*(11), 2093-3103.

Hillman, J. (2000). *Clinical perspectives on elderly sexuality.* New York, NY: Kluwer Academic/Plenum Publishers.

Hillman, J. (2012). *Sexuality and aging: Clinical perspectives.* New York, NY: Springer Publishers.

Hinchliff, S., & Gott, M. (2008). Challenging social myths and stereotypes of women and aging: Heterosexual women talk about sex. *Journal of Women and Aging, 20*(102), 65- 81

Kellett, J. (2000). Older adult sexuality. In L. Szuchman & F. Muscarella, *Psychological perspectives on human sexuality.* Hoboken, NJ: John Wiley and Sons.

Kinsey, A. C., Pomeroy, W. B., & Martin, E. E. (1948). *Sexual behavior in the human male.* Philadelphia, PA: Saunders.

Kinsey, A. C., Pomeroy, W. B., Martin, E. E., & Gebhard, P. H. (1953). *Sexual behavior in the human female.* Philadelphia, PA: Saunders.

Kontula, O., & Haavio-Mannila, E. (2009). The impact of aging on human sexual activity and sexual desire. *Journal of Sex Research, 46*(1), 46-56.

LaVail, K. H. (2010). Coverage of older adults and HIV/AIDS: Risk information for an invisible population. *Communication Quarterly, 58*(2), 170-187.

Leiblum, S. (1999). After Viagra: Bridging the gap between pharmacologic treatment and an active sexual life. *Journal of Clinical Psychiatry, 60*(7), 32-36.

Leiblum, S., & Rosen, R. (Eds.). (2000). *Principles and practice of sex therapy* (3rd ed.). New York, NY: Guilford Press.

Leiblum, S., & Segraves, R. (2000). Sex therapy with aging adults. In S. Leiblum & R. Rosen (Eds.), *Principles and practice of sex therapy* (3rd ed., pp. 423-444). New York, NY: Guilford Press.

Lorig, K. R., & Holman, H. R. (2003). *Self-management education: History, definition, outcomes, and mechanisms.* Annals of Behavior Medicine, 26, 1-7.

MacRae, N. (2010). Sexuality and aging. In R. H. Robnett & W. C. Chop (Eds.), *Gerontology for the health care professional* (pp. 235- 258). Sudbury, MA: Jones and Bartlett.

Masters, W. H., & Johnson., V. E. (1966). *Human sexual response.* Boston, MA: Little, Brown.

Masters, W. H., Johnson, V. E., & Kolodny, R. C. (1995). *Human Sexuality* (5th ed.). New York, NY: Longman.

National Center for Creative Aging. (n.d.) *Productive aging.* Retrieved from http://artsandaging.org/index.php?id=7

Neistadt, M. E. (1986). "Sexuality counseling for adults with disabilities: A module for an occupational therapy curriculum." *American Journal of Occupational Therapy, 40*, 8.

Neufeld, P. (2014). Aging in place and naturally occurring retirement communities. In M. Scaffa & S. M. Reitz (Eds.), *Occupational therapy in community-based practice settings* (2nd ed., pp. 210-221), Philadelphia, PA: F. A. Davis.

Parham, L. D., & Fazio, L. S. (Eds.). (1997). *Play in occupational therapy for children.* St. Louis, MO: Mosby.

Scharlach, A. (2008). *Why our communities must become more aging-friendly.* Keynote address presented at creating aging-friendly communities online conference; February 20, 2008. Retrieved from http://icohere.com/aging-friendly/program.htm

Schwartz, P. (2015). How to have sex after 50. In e-book: *Better sex: AARP's guide to sex after 50.* Retrieved from http://www.aarp.org/home-family/sex-intimacy/info-2015/sex-questions-libido-stds-schwartz.html

Scott, P. (2015, June). Sex in the nursing home. *AARP Bulletin/Real Possibilities.* Washington, DC: AARP.

Sipski, M., & Alexander, C. J. (1997). Basic sexual function over time. In M. Sipski & C. J. Alexander (Eds.), *Sexual function in people with disability and chronic illness* (pp. 75-83). Gaithersburg, MD: Aspen.

Stav, W. B. (2014). *Driving and community mobility for older adults.* In M. Scaffa & S. M. Reitz (Eds.), *Occupational therapy in community-based practice settings* (2nd ed., pp. 167-179). Philadelphia, PA: F. A. Davis.

Stav, W. B., Hallenen, T., Lane, J., & Arbesman, M. (2012). Systematic review of occupational engagement and health outcomes among community-dwelling older adults. *American Journal of Occupational Therapy, 66*(3), 301-310.

Stav, W. B., Hunt, L., & Arbesman, M. (2006). *Driving and community mobility for older adults: Occupational therapy practice guidelines.* Bethesda, MD: American Occupational Therapy Association Press.

Stone, L. (1977). *The family, sex, and marriage in England, 1500-1800.* New York, NY: Harper and Row.

Szuchman, L., & Muscarella, F. (2000). *Psychological perspectives on human sexuality.* Hoboken, NJ: John Wiley and Sons.

Taylor, B., & Davis, S. (2007). The extended PLISSIT model for addressing the sexual well-being of individuals with an acquired disability or chronic illness. *Sex and Disability, 25*, 135-139.

Thornton, J. (2002). Myths of aging or ageist stereotypes. *Educational Gerontology, 28*(4), 301- 312.

Weiner, D., & Rosen, R. (1997). Medications and their impact. In M. Sipski & C. J. Alexander (Eds.), *Sexual function in people with disability and chronic illness* (pp. 85-118). Gaithersburg, MD: Aspen.

White, C. B. (1982). A scale for the assessment of attitudes and knowledge regarding sexuality in the aged. *Archives of Sexual Behavior, 11*, 491-502.

Yamkovenko, S. (Ed.). (2014). Talking about sex: Man who was paralyzed says sex just as important as walking again. *AOTA Blogs: Checking the Pulse.* Retrieved from https://otconnections.aota.org/aota_blogs/b/pulsecheck/archive/2014/08/06/talking-about-sex-man-who-was-paralyzed-says-sex-just-as-important-as-walking-again.aspx

Additional References

Sexuality and Sexual Functioning/Disability

Comfort, A. (1978). *Sexual consequences of disability.* Philadelphia, PA: George Stickley Co.

Ellis, K., & Dennison, C. (2014). *Sex and intimacy for wounded veterans.* The Sager Group.

Fegan, L., Rauch, A., & McCarthy, W. (1993). *Sexuality and people with intellectual disability.* Baltimore, MD: Brooks.

Hebert, L. (1994). *Sex and Back Pain.* Greenville, ME: IMPACC US. http://www.impaccusa.com

Hein, K., & Digeronimo, T. (1989). *AIDS: A guide for teens.* Mount Vernon, NY: Consumer's Union.

Mooney, T., Cole, T., & Chilgren, R. (1975). *Sexual options for paraplegics and quadriplegics.* Boston, MA: Little, Brown and Co.

Selkirk, E. (1994). *Sex for beginners.* New York, NY: Writer's and Reader's Publishing.

Wainrib, B., & Haber, S. (2000). *Men, women, and prostate cancer.* Oakland, CA: New Harbinger Publications.

Sex Therapy

Kaplan, H. S. (1974). *The new sex therapy.* New York, NY: Brunner/Mazel.

Kaplan, H. S. (1995). *The sexual desire disorders: Dysfunctional regulation of sexual motivation.* New York, NY: Brunner/Mazel.

Leiblum, S., & Pervin, L. (1980). *Principles and practice of sex therapy.* New York, NY: Guilford Press.

Leiblum, S., & Rosen, R. (Eds.). (2000). *Principles and practice of sex therapy* (3rd ed.). New York, NY: Guilford Press.

LoPiccolo, J., & LoPiccolo, L. (1978). *Handbook of sex therapy.* New York, NY: Plenum Press.

Appendices

(Appendix A)

The Aging Sexual Knowledge and Attitudes Scale (ASKAS): A Self-Test for Knowledge

The items here were selected from the ASKAS, the original work of C. B. White (1982), as reprinted in Hillman (2012, pp. 49-52). For your reference, the item numbers below correspond to the full scale.

Answer the following True (or) False

2. Males over the age of 65 typically take longer to attain an erection of their penis than do younger males.
4. The firmness of erection in aged males is often less than that of younger persons.
7. The older female may experience painful vaginal intercourse due to reduced elasticity of the vagina and reduced vaginal lubrication.
8. Sexuality is typically a lifelong need.
9. Sexual behavior in older people increases the risk of heart attack.
11. The relatively more sexually active younger people tend to become, the relatively more sexually active they remain as older adults.
13. Sexual activity may be psychologically beneficial to older person participants.
16. Prescription drugs may alter a person's sex drive.
22. Barbiturates, tranquilizers, and alcohol may lower the sexual arousal levels of aged persons and interfere with sexual responsiveness.
29. The ending of sexual activity in old age is most likely and primarily due to social and psychological causes rather than biological and physical causes.
35. Masturbation in older males and females has beneficial effects on the maintenance of sexual responsiveness.

Key: The Aging Sexual Knowledge and Attitudes Scale (ASKAS): Selected Sample Items (as above)

2. (True) It takes more time for an older man to have an erection, related in large part to the increased time it takes to provide increased blood flow to the penis.
4. (True) Conservative estimates suggest that up to one-half of U.S. men over the age of 65 have some degree of erectile dysfunction (ED) due in large part to changes in the blood flow to the penis.
7. (True) Vaginal dryness can often be alleviated with over-the-counter lubricants (KY Jelly); or prescription lubricants and hormone therapies.
8. (True) The biological urge to engage in sexual (and sensual) activity does not appear to diminish significantly with age.
9. (False) Unless an older adult is under a physician's orders to limit his or her physical activity, sexual activity can be actively persued without fear of life-threatening exertion. Among healthy older adults, sexual activity can provide some of the benefits of cardiovascular exercise.
11. (True) One predictor of an older adult's sexual activity is his or her prior level of sexual activity.
13. (True) Participation in foreplay, including kissing, hugging, and caressing appears to remain consistent throughout later life. Many older adults cite that they enjoy their sexual relationships even more than they did when they were younger.

16. (True) A variety of prescription medications for depression, blood pressure, and diabetes can negatively impact on an older person's level of sexual interest and sexual functioning.

22. (True) Many over-the-counter medications and substances can alter sexual function. Because older adults metabolize alcohol more slowly than younger adults due to changes in body composition (increased fat-to-muscle ratios) and a general decline in liver function, even one or two alcoholic drinks can negatively affect sexual performance. Nicotine also has been related to erectile dysfunction among older men.

29. (True) Many of the physical problems associated with aging can be addressed; however, many older adults are affected by societal myths that perceive them as asexual.

35. (True) For men, masturbation can improve blood flow to the penis and help prevent future incidents of erectile dysfunction. For women, masturbation has been shown to increase blood flow to the vaginal area and promote premenopausal levels of lubrication.

(Appendix B)

Suggested Interview Questions Regarding Sexuality and Sexual Practices in Older Adults (Adapted from Hillman, 2012, pp. 53-55.)

The following selected interview questions can be useful to guide programming content for occupational therapy practitioners, and others who wish to program in this area. It is important that you do not ask questions you are not prepared to address, or know someone who can and will for a referral.

1. What would you consider a satisfactory sex life? Some people are satisfied while other people are dissatisfied with their sex lives. How do you feel about your sex life?

2. How long has it been since you have engaged in any sexual activity?

3. Do you have any current sexual partners?

4. Does your religion influence how you feel about sex or influence your current sexual activities in any way? Can you tell me about your religious views?

5. Having sex means different things to different people. For some people it means having sexual intercourse and to others it means holding hands. What different types of intimate sexual activity do you engage in?

6. How often do you masturbate or touch yourself to feel good? How do you feel about it? (This is often a good opportunity to tell an older adult about the potential emotional and physical benefits of masturbation.)

7. As people age, they sometimes experience pain or discomfort during sexual intercourse. Do you ever experience such pain or discomfort? Have you discussed this with anyone (your partner or a health care provider), or have you tried to do anything about it?

8. The average person experiences some kind of sexual difficulty at some point in their life. Could you tell me about any trouble or problems that you, or a partner of yours, may have had in the past?

9. Some people experience changes in their body as they age, either slowly over time or more suddenly through illness or surgery. How do you feel about your body? How does your partner feel about your body?

10. Do you use any lubricating gels or liquids when you engage in sex? What kind do you use? (Does the client use something inappropriate like an oil-based lubricant such as Vaseline with a condom, or does he/she use something water soluble like KY jelly?)

11. Have you ever used condoms when you have sex? Do you use condoms now? Why or why not? How does your partner(s) feel about condoms?

12. Do you feel you know enough about sexually transmitted diseases? If not, what would you like to know?

13. Do you have enough privacy for the sexual activities that you want to engage in?

14. Is there anything about your sex life that you wish were different?

15. Do you ever feel hurt or threatened by your (a) partner?

16. How easy or difficult is it for you to talk about your sexual behavior with your partner? Your physician? With me right now? (You can inform patients that they are doing a wonderful job talking about such a personal topic, if in fact they are. This is also an opportunity to talk about how many people feel uneasy talking about sexual matters and to empathize with their fears and concerns.)

17. Many people have fantasies about sex. What kind of sexual fantasies can you tell me about?

18. People often have questions they would like to ask about sex. Do you have some questions about sexual activity that you would like to ask me?

24

Human Trafficking and Exploitation
Considerations for Community Programming

LEARNING OBJECTIVES

1. To define human trafficking and exploitation

2. To identify the forms of human trafficking

3. To gain a foundational understanding of the factors that contribute to human trafficking, including cultural, social, political, and economic

4. To identify some of the psychological, health, and social consequences of human trafficking

5. To describe some of the existing services (educational, preventative, mental health, legal, and social) targeting victims of human trafficking

6. To begin to frame occupation-centered community interventions for victims of human trafficking and sexual exploitation

---

KEY TERMS

1. Trafficking of persons/human trafficking

2. Human smuggling

3. Sex trafficking/commercial sex acts

4. Domestic minor sex trafficking

5. Bonded labor/forced labor

6. Child labor/child conscription

(continued)

Fazio, L. S. *Developing Occupation-Centered Programs With the Community, Third Edition* (pp 381-392).
© 2017 Taylor & Francis Group.

7. Prostitution/pornography/child sex tourism

8. MutiMurder/organ trafficking

9. Post-traumatic stress disorder (PTSD)

10. The QUALIFIED program

11. Dwelle Collaborative

12. "Putting the Pieces Back Together" (program)

This chapter begins to explore the world of human trafficking and the aftermath—what happens to the victims of trafficking. In Chapter 25, we will talk about the needs of military combat soldiers and veterans. These may appear to be widely disparate populations; however, they share a common factor: the prevalence of post-traumatic stress disorder (PTSD) and the changes in functional abilities that PTSD brings about.

Of course, these populations are different, and the individuals within them differ. They also present differently within communities, but they often have in common a reluctance to be identified and to acknowledge their needs. Why do you need to know about the forms of trafficking? That is because you live on the planet and we, as care providers and programmers, have an obligation to keep our eyes open and know what is happening around us. We can no longer, if we ever could, refuse to recognize the concerns and problems that surround us. You may sleep in a warm, safe bed at night; however, when you consider our global population, you are among the few who enjoy this luxury.

Human trafficking is a severe human rights violation. Occupational therapy practitioners subscribe to the idea of social justice, but what can we do? One way for us to begin is to educate ourselves and our respective disciplines about the global nature of human trafficking. Trafficking humans for labor and sex is not a new social problem; it has always existed, on every continent. Most countries were settled and developed by individuals who were forcibly taken from their families and homes to work for minimal or no wages (Bales, Trodd, & Kent, 2009; Batstone, 2007). In the United States at least, every schoolchild learns about our history of slavery and it is often romanticized, although less so today. Bales and Soodalter (2009) tell us that, in 1850, slaves were highly valued, and the cost of a slave was equivalent to about $40,000 today. (Today, the cost of a slave has fallen to an average of about $100 (Bales & Soodalter, 2009, preface). In this context, the value of a life has sadly declined. Individuals have always been exploited either because they were excluded from the common language and culture (with its accompanying advantages) and/or were victims of poverty. In the 1970s, the number of foreign-born sex workers in Europe increased, with a large percentage originating from Southeast Asia. By the 1980s, more women from Africa and South America were entering into the sex trade in Europe (Hepburn & Simon, 2013). However, it was probably not until the 1990s that human trafficking gained global media attention, particularly as it related to women from eastern Europe and the former Soviet Union.

Likely, about this time, the issue of sex trafficking was being perceived differently as one that victimized women who were white and innocent, and it also included children. Although human trafficking has always existed, it has begun to gain increased attention as a result of awareness and outreach efforts (Bales, 2007; Congressional Research Service, 2015). It is now seen not only as a human rights issue, but it has also garnered the attention of feminists, religious conservatives, labor activists, immigration specialists, and the mental health professions, including, quite recently, occupational therapy practitioners (Suh & Bae, 2015).

Background

As of 2005, human trafficking had reached the status of a global phenomenon and had reaped an annual worldwide profit of $44.3 billion. It affected more than 12.3 million persons (Hepburn & Simon, 2013). The International Labor Organization (ILO, 2006) estimated that 43% of victims were trafficked for commercial sexual exploitation, 32% for forced labor, and the remaining 25% for a mixture of both or for undetermined reasons. More recently, ILO global estimates have risen to 20.9 million victims. About 68% are victims of forced labor exploitation and 22% are victims of forced sexual exploitation. The remaining 10% are in state-imposed forms of forced labor such as that imposed by rebel armed forces, state militaries, and prisons with conditions that conflict with ILO standards (ILO, 2012, p. 13). The estimates in the United States are fairly unclear, as they are globally, but some approximate that 14,500 to 17,000 individuals are illegally transported to the United States every year for the purpose of exploitation (Hepburn & Simon, 2013).

There are many definitions of human trafficking. The United Nations Protocol to Prevent, Suppress, and Punish Trafficking in Persons, Especially Women and Children, is the worldwide standard for anti-trafficking law. The protocol, which supplements the 2000 United Nations Convention against Transnational Organized Crime, contains three elements that define the **trafficking of persons (human trafficking)**:

1. The first element is the act of trafficking, which is the recruitment, transportation, transfer, harboring, or receipt of persons.

2. The second, the means of trafficking, is the threat or use of force or other forms of coercion, abduction, fraud, deception, abuse of power, or vulnerability, or giving payments or benefits to a person in control of the victim.

3. The third, the purpose of trafficking, is exploitation. This includes, at a minimum, sexual exploitation, including the exploitation of the prostitution of others, forced labor or services, slavery or practices similar to slavery, servitude, or the removal or organs (United Nations Office on Drugs and Crime [UNODC], 2004, p. 42).

In considering this definition, it is important to distinguish human trafficking from **human smuggling**. Human smuggling involves an individual being brought into the country through illegal means, but is voluntary. The individual has also provided some remuneration to another individual to accomplish this goal. While the outcomes of this relationship are often negative, it was initiated by the individual (Hepburn & Simon, 2013, pp. 157-158).

In many cases, women and children are considered the typical victims of human trafficking. Bales and Soodalter (2009) suggest that women are more vulnerable to trafficking due to the lack of social safety nets in many developing countries. Coupled with women's subordinate social statuses in many cultures and accompanying vulnerability, this leads to the feminization of poverty; although many men are also victims of human trafficking.

FORMS OF TRAFFICKING

Sex Trafficking

The Victims of Trafficking and Violence Protection Act (VTVPA) of 2000 (PL 106-386) is a U.S. federal statute passed by Congress to address the issue of human trafficking; it offers protection for the victims of human trafficking. This statute defines **sex trafficking** as "the recruitment, harboring, transportation, provision, or obtaining of a person for the purpose of a commercial sex act" (Hepburn & Simon, 2013, p. 4; Kora, 2009, p. 2). A **commercial sex act** is "any sex act on account of which anything of value is given to or received by any person" (Hepburn & Simon, 2013, p. 16).

In other words, it involves the illegal transport of humans into another country to be exploited in a sexual manner for financial gain. Victims of sex trafficking can be forced into prostitution, stripping, pornography, escort services, and other sexual services. Victims may be adult women, men, or children, although there is a higher prevalence of women and girls. The term **domestic minor sex trafficking** has become a popular term used to connote the buying, selling, and/or trading of children for sexual services within the country, not internationally (Bales, 2004).

In the United States, the children most vulnerable to domestic minor sex trafficking are those who are homeless, abused, runaways, and/or in child protective services. One study estimates about 30% of shelter youth and 70% of street youth are victims of commercial sexual exploitation. They may be coerced into prostitution for "survival sex" to meet daily needs for food, shelter, or drugs (Belles, 2015). It is often through our existing community programming for these children and teenagers that we encounter victims of sexual exploitation and trafficking; this, however, is frequently not identified as such. Nationally, 450,000 children run away from home each year, and 1 in 3 teens will be lured into sex trafficking within 48 hours of leaving home. The average age is 12 to 14 years for girls; and 11 to 13 years for boys. The hidden nature of the crime makes exact numbers difficult to come by.

Bonded Labor/Forced Labor

Perhaps of less immediate interest to occupation-centered programmers, victims of **bonded and forced labor** are nevertheless victims of human trafficking. The United Nations has defined debt bondage as "the status or condition arising from a pledge by a debtor of his personal services or of those of a person under his control as security for the debt" (UNODC, 2012). Essentially, because the individual does not have money as collateral for a debt owed, the individual pledges his or her labor or that of a child for an unspecified amount of time (Flanagan, 2015; ILO, 2006, 2012). These individuals may be transported or trafficked into another country for forced labor. Although this is often first seen as a welcome relief from debt, victims do not realize that they will never be able to pay the loans. Sometimes, these "debts" are passed down from one generation to the next (Hepburn & Simon, 2013, p. 429). Bonded laborers are found across the world, working in brick kilns, mines, stone quarries, factories, and on farms. In January 2009, the U.S. government broadened its anti-trafficking law to include a specific definition of forced labor, further increasing the protections granted under the statute (U.S. Department of State, 2010). In the United States, individuals may be trafficked to work long hours in garment factories, restaurants, and other manufacturing sectors. Migrant workers are at a high risk of being forced into labor.

Many nations have only recently introduced forced labor as a form of human trafficking to their criminal codes; unfortunately, many law enforcement officers are unfamiliar with how to recognize and protect potential victims. The result is that victims are not recognized and face arrest and punishment for offenses they committed as a result of their trafficking experience, such as immigration violation (Hepburn & Simon, 2013, p. 430).

In the United States, forced labor is predominantly found in five sectors (U.S. Department of State, 2010):

1. Prostitution and the sex industry (46%)

2. Domestic servitude (27%)

3. Agriculture (10%)

4. Sweatshops and factories (5%)

5. Restaurant and hotel work (4%)

It is speculated that most of the forced labor occurs in California, Florida, New York, and Texas, all major routes for international travel. Domestic servitude refers to a category of domestic workers (usually women, especially young women) who work as servants, housekeepers, maids, and/or caregivers in private homes. Often, they are lured by the promise of a good education and work;

however, when they arrive in the United States, their passports or identification papers are taken away (sometimes, they are told "for safekeeping") and they are forced to pay off their travel debt plus other bogus expenses before being able to retrieve their papers. Seldom do they speak or read English; therefore, their exploitation is easy.

Child Labor

Child trafficking is not as common in the United States as it is in many third world countries, where children and infants are bonded and sold (Hepburn & Simon, 2013). Child labor can be viewed as a specific form of bonded labor or forced labor; however, not all child laborers have been trafficked. **Child labor** is defined by the ILO as economic labor performed by a child younger than 15 years of age (ILO, 2006). Child labor goes hand in hand with poverty. The ILO (2006) estimates that there are 168 million child laborers in the world. The largest numbers of child laborers are found in Asia and the Pacific region.

Although adult-supervised "child work" may be beneficial for the socialization, education, and development of children, it is distinguished from child labor, which is exploitative; involves long hours; is poorly compensated; and produces physical, social, and psychological stress that will hamper the child's development (Hepburn & Simon, 2013, pp. 213- 214).

Child Conscription

In some cases of trafficking, children are kidnapped and trafficked as soldiers. It is estimated that at any one time, 250,000 to 300,000 children younger than 18 years of age are serving as child soldiers (Hepburn & Simon, 2013, pp. 115-116; United Nations High Commissioner for Refugees, 2000). Child soldiers are cheap, easily molded to obey without question, and are more likely to kill fearlessly and recklessly than adults. **Child conscription** exists in many third world countries but may be more common and involve larger numbers in Colombia and Iraq (Coalition to Stop the Use of Child Soldiers, 2008; Hepburn & Simon, 2013, pp. 118-119, 135).

Child Pornography and Prostitution

The trafficking of children (persons under the age of 18 years) is a concern in relation to both prostitution and pornography. **Prostitution** may be defined as the activity of "one who solicits and accepts payment for sex." In the case of child prostitution, the solicitation and acceptance of payment is done by another, the seller (Estes & Weiner, 2002). **Pornography** refers to written, graphic, or other forms of communication intended to sexually excite and stimulate another. In most cases of child engagement in pornography, it is for the purpose of making film or photographic images (CBS News, 2004; Estes & Weiner, 2002). Under the law for punishing acts related to child prostitution and child pornography and for protecting children, production and distribution of child pornography is illegal, but possession is not (Johnston, 2009). According to the National Police Agency (NPA; U.S. Department of State, 2012), 11,361 persons were arrested in violation of the law in 2007. Of those, 984 were arrested for child prostitution offenses, which included online dating services and telephone clubs, and 377 were arrested for child pornography offenses, including cases that involved the Internet (U.S. Department of State, 2012).

The Central Intelligence Agency (CIA, 2012) estimates that 50,000 women and children are trafficked each year throughout the United States for commercial sexual exploitation. Estes and Weiner (2002), in the report *The Commercial Sexual Exploitation of Children in the U.S.; Canada and Mexico*, estimate that, as of 2001, there were between 244,000 and 325,000 U.S. youths at risk (p. 150). These numbers have undoubtedly increased over time. Lack of regulation within the U.S. sex industry exacerbates the problem. Although prostitution is illegal except in the state of Nevada, the operation of strip clubs and the sale of adult pornography is legal but largely unregulated.

Legal pornography (not child pornography) is constitutionally protected under the first amendment; it is pervasive in the United States and is linked to some of the biggest U.S. corporations, including Time Warner, Hilton, Westin, AT&T, and Marriott (CBS News, 2004; University of Nevada, 2012). The general lack of regulation results in the illegal use of underage and trafficked persons (men, women, and children). There is often a misconception among Americans that human trafficking for any purpose within the United States is an underground industry whose victims and abusers are exclusively immigrants. In fact, trafficking occurs in every state (victims and perpetrators), "hidden in plain sight" (Bales & Soodalter, 2009; Hepburn & Simon, 2013). It should be remembered that not all underage prostitutes are trafficked, and they may or may not seek assistance. Many of these underage prostitutes, boys and girls, who are living on the street see prostitution as an easy way to provide food and sometimes drugs (Hinman, 2011).

Child Sex Tourism

Child sex tourism is a form of exploitation that often takes place outside of the United States, but at the hands of U.S. citizens and legal residents. This form of exploitation involves Western men traveling to Southeast Asia, particularly Thailand, to pay for sex with children (Hepburn & Simon, 2013). The humanitarian organization World Vision, which collaborates with the U.S. State Department and U.S. Immigration and Customs Enforcement (ICE), estimates that there are 2 million children enslaved worldwide in the commercial sex trade. It also estimates that U.S. citizens make up 25% of child sex tourists globally and up to 80% of child sex tourists in Latin America (World Vision, 2009).

In response to the exploitation of children via sex tourism by U.S. citizens and residents, the U.S. government enacted the Prosecutorial Remedies and Other Tools to End the Exploitation of Children Today (PRO-TECT) Act of 2003 to prosecute citizens who go abroad and pay to have sex with a minor. Another program, Operation Twisted Traveler, was launched in February 2009. This program is a collaborative effort with Cambodia to identify, arrest, and prosecute U.S. citizens and legal residents who travel to Cambodia for child sex tourism (U.S. Department of Justice, 2009).

Organ Trafficking and MutiMurders

Perhaps one of the most frightening forms of human trafficking occurs in the name of traditional medicine, primarily in South Africa. **MutiMurder** (*Muti* is the word commonly used for traditional medicine in South Africa) involves abducting people, killing them, and harvesting their body parts for use in ritual or cult practices. Experts estimate that somewhere between 12 to 300 MutiMurders occur per year in South Africa (Hepburn & Simon, 2013). This practice seems very remote to us; more likely you may have heard of a somewhat related practice, that of organ trafficking.

Organ trafficking refers to the practice of harvesting and selling human organs, generally without the death of the donor. Syria is a source nation for organ trafficking to other nations. It is difficult to determine exact numbers for this form of human trafficking; however, in 2010, 11 traffickers were arrested for trafficking organs from Syria to Egypt. Part of a larger syndicate, the traffickers bought and sold kidneys harvested from more than 150 persons living in slums in 2009 (Hepburn & Simon, 2013).

Most often, traffickers do not kill their victims; rather, they offer them money to remove a kidney (the organ of choice in most cases) and then sell the kidney to someone in need of a transplant. Frequently, however, the donor receives a smaller sum than was promised or no pay at all. In 2010, an organ-trafficking ring was discovered in Israel with recipients of kidneys in Europe, Ecuador, and the Phillipines. Most often, trafficking of organs is accomplished only with the collusion of official personnel (including medical personnel and hospitals). In the United States, organ trafficking likely exists but is not well documented. However, it is not uncommon for U.S. citizens who can afford to do so to leave the country for organ transplants in other countries where trafficked organs are available.

What Is the Impact on Victims of Trafficking, and What Can Occupation-Centered Programmers Offer?

The realities of victims of human trafficking are difficult to comprehend, and it is often wondered why they appear to remain silent and compliant with their traffickers. The "silence compliance model" was established to explore the factors that promote victims' seeming willingness to comply to their trafficker's demands (Flanagan, 2015).

This model has three categories: coercion, collusion, and contrition. Victims are first coerced, then brutalized and threatened, and basic necessities of life are withheld from them. This results in silence and creates a sense of helplessness. They are isolated and encouraged to have a false sense of "belonging" and dependence on the trafficker. Ultimately, victims feel ashamed and stigmatized.

Psychological and Mental Health Consequences

Victims of trafficking experience a host of psychological and emotional problems. **PTSD** is common given the trauma most victims experience (physical and/or sexual violence and abuse often on a daily basis). See Chapter 25 for a discussion of PTSD. Trafficked victims experience extreme fear from their capture, through transit, and after they arrive at their destination. They are often deprived of food and water. Often, they are not only afraid for themselves, but for the safety of their families as well. Depression, anxiety, and PTSD are often the result.

Substance abuse is often common among victims. Trafficked women have reported that traffickers forced them to use drugs and/or alcohol so they could work longer hours, take on more clients, and/or perform sexual acts that were not normal for them. Other victims used substances simply to cope.

Children who are trafficked for labor are frequently beaten and abused. Those who are trafficked for sex fluctuate through a range of emotions from despair, shame, guilt, hopelessness, anxiety, and fear (Estes & Weiner, 2002). Some engage in self-destructive/self-mutilating behaviors and have attempted suicide. HIV infection and other STDs are common among all sexually exploited victims (men, women, and children). Sexual violence may increase a woman's chances to acquire the virus as a result of open abrasions and injuries to the vagina. Cases of unwanted pregnancies, forced abortion, pelvic inflammatory disease, and subsequent infertility are not uncommon.

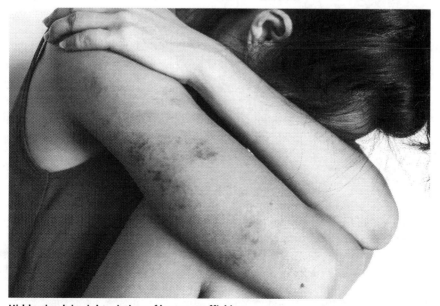

Hidden in plain sight: victims of human trafficking.

Education and Advocacy

Education is believed to be a key factor in the prevention of human trafficking. Raising awareness through advertisements, campaigns, and other creative vehicles regarding recruitment threats, the various deception techniques employed, the different forms and agendas of human trafficking, and the consequences of human trafficking can decrease the incidence.

Because the general public often believes that human trafficking is a problem that occurs only in developing countries, there is a clear need for public education, particularly to ensure the safety of young children and women both in and outside of the United States. The U.S. Administration for Children and Families has published brochures and posters about human trafficking (see website at the end of this chapter). Posting these brochures or posters increases the possibility that a trafficked victim will self-report. Identifying human trafficking victims is not easy. Anyone wishing to help must navigate and collaborate with a complex set of government, social service, mental health, and nongovernmental/nonprofit entities. It is never recommended that you attempt to intervene if you suspect someone is being trafficked; instead, go to the police or similar authority. The websites recommended in this chapter can be helpful in offering suggestions for what you should do. Remember, traffickers are dangerous.

Advocacy for the protection of victims of human trafficking and to create greater awareness of the problem is best done in cooperation with like-minded organizations. Please see the Additional Resources section at the end of this chapter to enhance your efforts.

Programming Examples

A Consulting Model: Career Bridging

Human trafficking is no stranger to the City of Los Angeles, and all categories exist (Los Angeles Police Department, 2015). When trafficking victims are rescued in Los Angeles and elsewhere, a great deal of practical day-to-day assistance is required: housing, transportation, food, clothing, medical care, dental care, financial assistance, legal aid, educational training, and—for those who wish to return to their homeland—reunification. It is unrealistic to think that any one person or organization should try to do everything; practitioners should connect, coordinate, and case manage these services as much as possible. The care provider first analyzes the assets and opportunities available to match the needs of the former victims, and this is what two entrepreneurial occupational therapists, graduates of the University of Southern California, Esther Suh, MA, OTR/L and Esther Bae, MA, OTR/L are doing.

QUALIFIED is a job-training, support, and placement program being developed in partnership with four nonprofit agencies that serve the greater Los Angeles region: Freedom and Fashion, Bedrock Creek, Two Wings, and Dwelle Collaborative (Suh & Bae, 2015a).

> The mission of QUALIFIED is to "train, mentor and match survivors of human trafficking with meaningful and lasting employment"; and the aim of the program is to utilize a multifaceted and holistic approach to bring sustainable employment to survivors of human trafficking in Los Angeles County, California (Suh & Bae, 2015a, p. 1).

> Each partner in this collaboration focuses on one aspect of the solution: Two Wings runs and manages all aspects of the 12-week job training academy in order to equip participants with the tools and skills needed for successful employment; **Dwelle Collaborative** provides and manages a group of occupational therapy volunteers who help foster a successful transition from training to workplace by providing occupational therapy consultation for 6 to 9 months during the initial stages of employment; while Bedrock Creek targets governmental and corporate partnerships to systematically provide clients with better job accessibility and retention. The Dwelle Collaborative houses the QUALIFIED program that encourages successful community integration focusing primarily on beauty centered business opportunities that provide job/career training.

According to Suh and Bae (2015b) what sets QUALIFIED apart from other staffing agencies is the occupational therapy component of the program. Each participant is matched, one on one, with a licensed occupational therapist who provides up to 9 months of direct consultation to promote a successful transition into the participant's place of employment. According to the originators, as continued planning and implementation progresses, various models are considered to guide programming, including a supported employment model and life design theory. According to Iannelli and Wilding (2007), work provides a sense of responsibility, self-worth, and identity. Leufstadius, Erlandsson, and Eklund (2006) add to this the building of a positive sense of the future, offering a stabilizing effect, and promoting improved health and well-being—all of which are important to those who have experienced trafficking. "Designing lives" and various coaching models are utilized to determine the most effective intervention map.

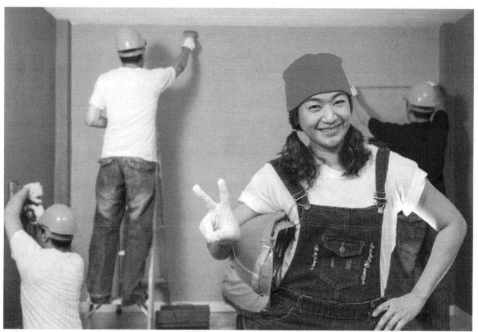

Skills, confidence, and opportunity open a door to a new life.

Qualifications for program participants/mentees include having demonstrated consistent participation and attendance in a preceding program, currently seeing or having access to a psychotherapist, living in stable housing, having submitted an application and completed an interview (Suh & Bae, 2015b). Thus far, occupational therapy mentors have assisted with troubleshooting multiple issues that occur in the participant's workplace, helping to overcome any barriers that are affecting the participant's ability to find a rhythm in new daily routines, and identifying consistent themes in the participants' lives that might affect (or enhance and strengthen) their success in transition.

Currently, program phases include the following:

- Phase 1: Job Training (12 weeks of academy and 6 weeks of internship)
- Phase 2: Job Placement (interviews with businesses in various industries)
- Phase 3: Job Support (9 months of direct occupational therapy consultation)

Occupational therapy consultation sessions are organized in small groups to include not only individual consultation time, but also small-group activities such as daily routine/living activity knowledge and skills (i.e., cooking, shopping, exercise, grooming and dressing for work, etc.). At this writing, the first group of participants has participated in a formal graduation ceremony indicating successful completion of their program (personal communication, Esther Suh and Esther Bae, May 2016).

A Group Model for Programming

Another program mentioned in recent literature was designed for adolescent girls who were sexually exploited. This program was conducted by researchers Kristine Hickle and Dominique Roe-Sepowitz. They designed an adapted group intervention originally for female prisoners who had been abused, and they wanted to know if it could help adolescent girls who had experienced or were at risk for sexual exploitation. Their design was a group intervention called **"Putting the Pieces Back Together"** (Hickle & Roe-Sepowitz, 2014).

They conducted a pilot study with 10 young women, each of whom had been trafficked, had engaged in survival sex (i.e., trading sex for resources like shelter or food), or had a history of abuse. The researchers identified four parts of "Putting the Pieces Back Together" that were instrumental to helping sexually exploited girls move through their recovery. These included educating participants about domestic minor sex trafficking, providing opportunities for youth to help and support each other, using dialogue as a tool for reducing feelings of stigma and shame, and developing skills to deal with powerful feelings. Participants reported that the group process helped them heal, feel less alone in their journey, and talk about their sexual exploitation in a safe space.

Some of the recommendations for those who would like to offer the "Putting the Pieces Back Together" group model are as follows:

- Front-line people such as caseworkers, social workers, and therapists need to know how to identify young women who have been trafficked, have traded sex for resources, or are at risk of either form of sexual exploitation. Correctly identifying victims, in turn, can help staff members make appropriate referrals to intervention.
- Group members need a safe place to discuss the traumatic experiences associated with their exploitation even if they are receiving treatment for issues like substance abuse or self-harm.
- The presence of a co-facilitator who is a sex trafficking survivor helps group members feel more comfortable in opening up about their own experiences.

The previously mentioned research offers an encouraging model that can be used by occupational therapy practitioners as well. Occupational therapy practitioners are more likely to encourage a group response through engagement in an activity or activities to prepare group members for participation in processing their experiences, but the outcome can be similar.

SUMMARY

This chapter has discussed human trafficking and has presented it as a trending issue that is of interest to occupational therapy practitioners as well as other care providers. The discussion is presented first of all to raise awareness and to increase knowledge of the multiple forms of trafficking and to encourage you to become an advocate for the education of others who may not be informed. It is also presented for the sake of the victims themselves. Be reminded that it is never recommended that you make any attempt to intervene if you suspect someone is being trafficked; instead, go to the police or other similar authority and review the recommended websites for suggestions about how to proceed safely.

It would appear that intervention programming for victims of sexual exploitation/human trafficking is only beginning, and this is not surprising considering how seldom these victims identify themselves and ask for assistance. However, they can be found in shelters, substance abuse programming sites, and detention centers, and it is often at these locations where we, occupational therapy practitioners, encounter them.

The reader is encouraged to review the references and websites to become better informed regarding these populations and the partners and stakeholders who are offering services to them and to consider program design for one or more of these groups.

REFERENCES

Bales, K. (2004). *Disposable people.* Berkeley, CA: University of California Press.

Bales, K. (2007). *Ending slavery: How we free today's slaves.* Berkeley, CA: University of California Press.

Bales, K., & Soodalter, R. (2009). *The slave next door: Human trafficking and slavery in America today.* Berkeley, CA: University of California Press.

Bales, K., Trodd, Z., & Kent, A. (2009). *Modern slavery: The secret world of 27 million people.* Oxford, UK: OneWorld Publications.

Batstone, D. B. (2007). *Not for sale: The return of global slave trade—How we can fight it.* San Francisco, CA: Harper Colllins.

Belles, N. (2015). *In our backyard: Human trafficking in America and what we can do to stop it.* Grand Rapids, MI: Baker Books.

CBS News. (2004). *Porn in the U.S.A. 60 minutes.* Retrieved from http://www.cbsnews.com/news/porn-in-the-usa-21-11-2003/

Central Intelligence Agency. (2012). *The trafficking of women and children.* Washington, DC: Author.

Coalition to Stop the Use of Child Soldiers. (2008). *Guide to the optional protocol on the involvement of children in armed conflict.* Retrieved from https://www.unicef.org/protection/option_protocol_conflict.pdf

Congressional Research Service (2015). *Sex trafficking of children in the U.S.: Overview and issues for Congress.* Washington, DC: Author.

Estes, R. J., & Weiner, N. A. (2002). *The commercial sexual exploitation of children in the U.S., Canada and Mexico.* Philadelphia, PA: University of Pennsylvania School of Social Work, Center for the Study of Youth Policy.

Flanagan, A. (2015). Human trafficking and exploitation continuing education module. *Continuing Education for Texas Counselors and Therapists.* Retrieved from www.NetCE.com/CTH15

Hepburn, S., & Simon, R. (2013). *Human trafficking around the world.* New York, NY: Columbia University Press.

Hickle, K., & Roe-Sepowitz, D. (2014). Putting the pieces back together: A group intervention for sexually exploited adolescent girls. *Social Work with Groups, 37*(2), 9-12.

Hinman, K. (2011). Lost boys. *LA Weekly, 17*(10), 10-19.

Iannelli, S., & Wilding, C. (2007). Health enhancing effects of engaging in productive occupation. *Australia's Occupational Therapy Journal, 54*, 285-293.

International Labor Organization. (2006). *Forced labor statistics.* Retrieved from http://digitalcommons.ilr.cornell.edu/cgi/viewcontent.cgi?article=1019&context=forcedlabor

International Labor Organization. (2012). *ILO global estimate of forced labor: Results and methodology.* Geneva: Author.

Kora, S. (2009). *Sex trafficking: Inside the business of modern slavery.* New York, NY: Columbia University Press.

Leufstaduis, C., Erlandsson, L. K., & Eklund, M. (2006). Time use and daily activities in people with persistent mental illness. *Occupational Therapy International, 13*, 123-141.

Los Angeles Police Department (2015). Human trafficking section. Retrieved from http://www.lapdonline.org/detective_bureau/content_basic_view/51926

Suh, E., & Bae, E. (2015a). A role for occupational therapy in human trafficking interventions. Presented at OTAC 2015 Conference Presentation, Fall 2015, Sacramento, CA.

Suh, E., & Bae, E. (2015b). *Qualified L.A. Occupational Therapy Mentor Manual.* Los Angeles, CA: Dwelle Collaborative Publishing.

United Nations High Commissioner for Refugees. (2000). *Convention on the Rights of the Child.* Retrieved from http://www.unhcr.org/en-us/prostitution/children/50f941fe9/united-nations-convention-right-child-cnc.html

United Nations Office on Drugs and Crime. (2004). *United Nations Convention against transnational organized crime and the protocols thereto.* New York, NY: Author.

United Nations Office on Drugs and Crime. (2012). *Signatories to the CTOC Trafficking Protocol.* New York, NY: Author.

University of Nevada. (2012). *Sex industry and sex workers in Nevada.* Retrieved from http://digitalscholarship.unlv.edu/social_health_nevada_reports/48/

U.S. Department of Justice. (2009). Three American men accused of traveling to Cambodia to have sex with children now en route to United States to face prosecution on federal "sex tourism: Charges. Press release. Federal Bureau of Investigation (FBI). Retrieved from http://www.cbsnews.com/news/operation-twisted-traveler/

U.S. Department of State. (2010). *Trafficking in persons report.* Retrieved from www.state.gov/documents/organization/123357.pdf

U.S. Department of State. (2012). 2012 *report to the Congress: Federal child pornography offenses.* Retrieved from http://www.ussc.gov/research/congressional-reports/2012-report-congress-federal-child-pornography-offenses

World Vision. (2009). *Child sex exploitation in South East Asia.* Retrieved from https://www.academia.edu/6229117/Article_Illicit_Supply_and_Demand_Child_Sex_Exploitation_in_South_East_Asia

Additional Resources

http://humantrafficking.change.org
http://www.freetheslaves.net
http://www.polarisproject.org/take-action
http://www.stopthetraffic.org

National Human Trafficking Hotline: 1-888-373-7888 (or) text "HELP" to BeFree (233733)

25

Exploring Programming for Returning Combat Veterans and Families of Veterans

LEARNING OBJECTIVES

1. To distinguish contemporary military terminology that is used to describe this population

2. To begin to understand the specific conditions of Operation Enduring Freedom (OEF) and Operation Iraqi Freedom (OIF)

3. To appreciate the concerns of the families of returning soldiers and veterans

4. To understand the characteristics of post-traumatic stress disorder (PTSD) as it is experienced by many returning soldiers and veterans

5. To become familiar with several directions that may be taken to design and develop programming for soldiers and veterans

KEY TERMS

1. Post-traumatic stress disorder (PTSD)

2. Operation Iraqi Freedom (OIF)

3. Operation Enduring Freedom (OEF)

4. Warrior transition units (WTUs)

5. Traumatic brain injury (TBI)

6. Military culture

7. Wounded Warrior Project (WWP)

8. Soldier 2020

9. Polytrauma

10. Garrison

11. Deployed/deployment

Fazio, L. S. *Developing Occupation-Centered Programs With the Community, Third Edition* (pp 393-409).
© 2017 Taylor & Francis Group.

This chapter is intended to give you a brief overview of the needs of both deployed and returning military men and women. We could describe this group as a trending area of practice for community-centered occupational therapy practitioners, but, in fact, our profession has been helping combat soldiers and veterans since its early years. Beginning in World War I, 55 occupational therapy reconstruction aides worked in France and Germany to enable soldiers to return to either active service or paid employment following discharge from service. The most common injuries in those days included orthopedic trauma and neuropsychiatric disorders (McDaniel, 1968; Quiroga, 1995).

In addition to the services provided behind the lines at base hospitals, occupational therapy was conducted experimentally at a neuropsychiatric hospital in the forward area. The experiment lasted only 2 weeks, but the medical officer in charge considered this "workshop treatment" to be successful, returning men to duty who had previously been slated to go to a base hospital for further treatment (McDaniel, 1968, p. 90). According to Nochajski and Reitz (2014), a somewhat similar trial program was implemented in Afghanistan in 2010 to provide occupational therapy evaluation and intervention services to military personnel immediately following mild head injuries.

Historically, occupational therapy practitioners have played a significant role in the rehabilitation and reintegration of service members. Early on, a condition called "shell shock" was common, (which would now probably be classified as **post-traumatic stress disorder**, or **PTSD**) this was not a formal diagnosis until 1980, with effective treatments to follow much later (Mochenhaupt, 2015). Crafts were used partly as a diversion and, in some cases, to help the soldier develop skills that could help him earn a living after recovery (Quiroga, 1995). Again, during WWII, occupational therapists helped soldiers with psychological trauma return to work and civilian life. During this time, the therapists increased the scope of practice to include activities of daily living (ADLs), training in the use of prostheses, fabricating orthotics, and leading groups (Gritzer & Arluke, 1985).

In this chapter, several recent research studies and program/intervention descriptions have been selected to provide an overview of both the needs of today's deployed and returning veterans and, in some cases, their spouses and families. Arguably, the experience of needs surrounding each of our wars and conflicts have been and are different. As these wars have become more creative in the use of technology and innovation, our programming has required more knowledge and creative innovation as well.

Today, we have more information and more tools, and our scope of practice is broader. As a result, we have an obligation to advocate for the utilization of our services to soldiers, returning soldiers, and their families. These are communities in need.

BACKGROUND

What Are the Statistics?

Military service in Iraq and Afghanistan has resulted not only in extended deployments, but higher rates of survival from wounds (Seal et al., 2009; Tanielian & Jaycox, 2008). Some 1.64 million U.S. troops have been deployed for **Operation Iraqi Freedom (OIF)** and **Operation Enduring Freedom (OEF)** since 2001 (Tanielian & Jaycox, 2008). Approximately one-third will struggle with at least one of the following injuries: PTSD; traumatic brain injury (TBI), and major depression (Tanielian & Jaycox, 2008). This generation of military service members is unique compared with those who have served in other conflicts in terms of the large number who survive serious injuries. This is because of advancements in armor as well as in medical treatment. Of course, improvised explosive devices on roadsides have caused a large number of deaths and injuries (63% of the total). These devices have contributed to the rising issue of blast injuries, which are the primary cause of TBI among active duty service members (Defense and Veterans Brain Injury Center, 2012; Defense Manpower Data Center, 2011).

In part, because of the complicated injuries, and in order to facilitate the transition of military service personnel back to active service or to civilian life, 35 **warrior transition units (WTUs)** were developed by the army to better meet the rehabilitation and vocational training needs of injured soldiers. These WTUs were designed for soldiers who required more than 6 months of medical care and were located close to medical treatment facilities across the United States as well as in a few international locations. The intent was to train them to return to active military duty or to gain civilian employment (Erickson, Secrest, & Gray, 2008).

Injury rates for **TBI** and PTSD are increasing among soldiers, as are suicide rates, according to U.S. Army data (Rivero, 2010). There were 115 suicides in 2007 and at least 128 in 2008. In 2009, there were 249 suicides and 1713 attempted suicides (NIH, 2014; Starr, 2010). In 2012, more active duty service members died of suicide (349) than in combat (295) (Chappell, 2013). **Military culture** indoctrinates service members to identify themselves as part of a team or unit and to strive to perform their duties well for the betterment of the entire unit. Unit cohesion is necessary for effective mission accomplishment, and no soldier wants to be the weak link in the chain. Service members with untreated mental health issues may erroneously feel like liabilities to their units. In addition to not seeking treatment to avoid judgment by their peers and senior leaders, they may feel that suicide is an easier choice (Bryan, Jennings, Jobes, & Bradley, 2012). Today, through efforts to educate leaders, the current message of the military is that seeking care is a courageous step in improving the safety and effectiveness of the individual service member and the unit.

All of these statistics point to an increasing need for transitional services before and during deployment as well as prior to and following return stateside. Nochajski and Reitz (2014) point out that, even though the army has increased its efforts in this area in recent years, civilian occupational therapy practitioners need to be aware of the possibility of groups of wounded warriors in their communities who may no longer be receiving services from the military (p. 250). They advise community-based occupational therapy practitioners to seek funding and support for program development to aid wounded warriors, but also, before they do so, to make efforts to understand the military lifestyle and culture as well as the work of military occupational therapists (Nochajski & Reitz, 2014, p. 250).

An unprecedented number of service personnel are returning home seriously wounded or disabled. The most common conditions are TBI, amputations, and PTSD. From 2001 to 2011, approximately 42,000 service members returned home injured (Wounded Warrior Project, 2011). The **Wounded Warrior Project (WWP)** was founded in 2003 to raise awareness of the needs of injured service members, providing programs and services to meet those needs, and facilitating the transition and reintegration of injured and disabled service members into their communities and civilian life (Wounded Warrior Project, 2011). Provided services include rehabilitation, peer support, counseling, adapted sports and recreation, technology training, employment assistance, and advocacy and education of service personnel and their families. All services are free to persons with service-related illnesses, wounds, injuries, and disabilities incurred after the terrorist attacks on U.S. soil on September 11, 2001.

Recent studies have indicated that one-fifth of Operation Enduring Freedom (OEF) and Operation Iraqi Freedom (OIF) veterans are diagnosed with PTSD (Seal, Bertenthal, Miner, Sen, & Marmar, 2007), although these findings likely underestimate the true prevalence of the disorder (Tanielian & Jaycox, 2008). What is PTSD? According to the *Diagnostic and Statistical Manual of Mental Disorders*, "PTSD is a severe, potentially chronic and disabling disorder that develops in some persons following exposure to a traumatic event involving actual or threatened death, serious injury, or sexual assault" (American Psychiatric Association, 2013). Some of the more common symptoms include intrusive thoughts, nightmares and flashbacks of traumatic events, avoidance of trauma reminders, hypervigilance, and sleep disturbance. Persistence of symptoms beyond 1 month post-trauma suggests PTSD (American Psychiatric Association, 2013). Exposure to multiple traumatic events and serious physical injury as well as to real or threatened death is not uncommon during deployment and can lead to PTSD.

PTSD and depression frequently occur together, and both diagnoses are associated with functional and social disruption, including weakened interpersonal relationships and diminished psychological resilience and self-efficacy (Gros, Price, Magruder, & Fruek, 2012). Three key symptoms that must be present for a diagnosis of PTSD are re-experiencing trauma, avoidance and numbing, and hypervigilance (National Center for PTSD, 2006). Other problems may also exist, such as difficulty sleeping, headaches, nightmares, anger, hopelessness, and irritability (National Center for PTSD, 2006). Some returning veterans engage in high-risk behaviors such as speeding, substance abuse, or aggressive acts to satisfy feelings of invincibility or to seek an "adrenaline rush." High-intensity sports such as surfing appear to provide a socially acceptable alternative to risk-taking behaviors (Diehm & Armatas, 2004; Rogers, Mallinson, & Peppers, 2014).

WOMEN IN THE UNITED STATES ARMY

Women in Australia, Canada, Denmark, Israel, Germany, New Zealand, Norway, and France have served in direct combat roles for years (Mulrine, 2013). In the United States, women have been active contributors since the Civil War. In 1948, Congress passed the Women's Armed Services Integration Act, which permitted women to directly enlist or be commissioned into the U.S. Armed Services, albeit with restrictions on job assignments. Since then, the number of women in the military has continued to grow. In 1983, women comprised 9.8% of the army, whereas in 2013, women made up 16% of the total army (active duty, reserves, and National Guard) (U.S. Army, n.d.). Of the women in the army, a large number belong to health care–related units (37%), with a small percentage playing support roles in tactical operations units (11%) (Escobar, 2013).

Recent History of Women in Combat

In 1994, the United States opened additional combat support positions to female soldiers; however, a ground combat exclusion policy was signed into law, prohibiting direct combat service (McNulty, 2012). There were undoubtedly many reasons for women's exclusion from direct combat service, from cultural traditions and beliefs to anatomical and physiological differences between males and females that could affect a female soldier's ability to meet the rigorous training and operational demands of military service (Bell, Mangione, Hemenway, Amoroso, & Jones, 1996; Springer & Ross, 2011).

The service of women in combat support roles became an especially integral asset with the beginning of the Global War on Terror in 2003. Special "Lioness" teams of female soldiers would accompany all-male combat units to conduct missions of "search and engagement" of Iraqi women and children (McNulty, 2012). Owing to strict religious laws in these geographical areas forbidding males from engaging with females, these teams of women were needed to execute sociopolitically correct interactions with the local people.

These women were vulnerable to injury; however, they did not receive the same combat training as their male counterparts. As the need for the Lioness teams grew, a training program was initiated and, with training, women's roles expanded. By 2009, the Lioness teams had an advanced training program and were attached to an infantry unit for 20 to 60 days, engaging in 3 to 4 missions per week (McNulty, 2012). The name *Lioness teams* was changed to *Female Engagement Teams*, and the army continues to use them.

Women also serve in a variety of indirect roles—as medics, photographers, military police, security forces, and drivers—that place them close to combat action.

Soldier 2020

Occupational therapy is helping the U.S. Army take a task-analysis approach to evaluating the training and physical standards for combat military occupational specialists (MOSs) (Luken, Dy, & Yancosek, 2015). This comprehensive evaluation, called **Soldier 2020**, was developed in response to the 2013 lifting of the ban on women in direct combat roles. This program is the army's analytical approach to evaluate and update the training required for all MOSs, starting with those that involve direct combat. Based on this work, as of January 2016, senior military officers were prepared to determine whether the ban will remain in effect or whether exceptions are necessary as well as how to integrate women into combat MOSs if the ban is permanently lifted (Sheftick, 2014).

Occupational therapy practitioners' perspective on Soldier 2020 is framed around the fundamental occupational therapy skill of task/activity analysis. Soldier 2020 is currently under way, and a team of investigators from various backgrounds, including occupational therapy, are using task analysis to identify the client factors and performance skills needed to develop gender- and age-neutral physical performance standards for each specific MOS (Sullivan, 2013).

For occupational therapy practitioners and community programming planners examining the history of women in the military, there are a number of unanswered questions. Will their return home bring the same concerns that we have seen with male "wounded warriors," or will women return with different injuries? Women have different life roles than men in their 20s and 30s. For many, these are childbearing years and years spent in the direct care of a family. Many women may try to balance all of these roles (as they often do in civilian life), but at what cost? The progress of women in military life is well worth watching, and we will need to raise our awareness and that of others as we best prepare to meet their needs in our design and planning of community interventions.

TRANSITIONING TO CIVILIAN LIFE WITH ILLNESS AND INJURIES

Occupational Therapy Programming

Active Duty Occupational Therapy Programming: Polytrauma

Walter Reed National Military Medical Center is one of many military facilities serving active duty service members, retirees, and their family members. Walter Reed is a comprehensive medical facility providing services to those injured in OIF and OEF. Service members injured in a war zone typically sustain **polytrauma**, defined by the Department of Veterans Affairs as "injuries to multiple body parts and organs occurring as a result of blast-related wounds" (Barnett, 2014, p. 14). Common polytrauma injuries include TBI, amputations, spinal cord injury, fractures, PTSD, and visual and auditory impairments.

Intervention programs are offered by both military and nonmilitary occupational therapists and occupational therapy assistants (generalists and specialists). Treatment programs include ADLs, sexual health/self-image/relationships, cognitive rehabilitation, hand therapy, assistive technology, meaningful leisure activities, safe driving, and mental health. Often, wounded warriors stay for extended periods; therefore, occupational therapy practitioners have the opportunity to build positive therapeutic relationships from inpatient to outpatient and while their patients are staying in transitional base housing. An article by Barnett (2014) tells the story of one service member from the onset of his injuries on the battlefield through his rehabilitation process. You are encouraged to read it for a full appreciation of what occupational therapy practitioners can do.

Sexuality and Intimacy

Another of the self-care areas where transition to civilian life has been particularly challenging for wounded returning soldiers and veterans with polytrauma is that of sexuality and intimacy. Occupational therapists Kathryn Ellis, MOT, OTR/L, and Caitlin Dennison, MOT, OTR/L, are working in the Washington, DC area with a specialty practice serving military service members. Their practice addresses the concerns of sex and intimacy for wounded veterans, and they have written a handbook/guide to accompany their practice, titled *Sex and Intimacy for Wounded Veterans: A Guide to Embracing Change* (Ellis & Dennison, 2014). The handbook offers an optimistic problem-solving approach for re-engagement in sexual activity and intimacy, with or without adaptations and modifications. The intention of the guide is to educate service members, veterans, families, significant others, and clinicians regarding sexual health following significant physical injury. The authors provide this compelling message: "regardless of injury, sexual pleasure with yourself or with a partner is a realistic goal, as is the ability to form intimate relationships with others" (Ellis & Dennison, 2014, introduction).

An important reminder to occupational therapists who wish to develop this kind of specialty practice is that you would begin, as you would with re-engagement in any occupation, with a detailed activity analysis followed by the adaptations or modifications needed to accomplish the task (Ellis & Dennison, 214, p. 29).

Transitioning With Posttraumatic Stress Disorder and Traumatic Brain Injury: The Experience of "Driving"

Hwang and colleagues (2014) describe programming to meet the needs of returning service members who are experiencing problems following deployment that affect their reintegration into their former civilian roles. One of the significant occupational challenges faced by these veterans is driving. According to the U.S. Department of Veterans Affairs (2012), the leading cause of death of veterans in the first years after returning home from combat is motor vehicle crashes. The reasons for this are complicated, as we have noted in discussing risk-taking tendencies and unsafe behaviors earlier in this chapter. Hwang et al. (2014) have examined the literature and propose 4 explanations for unsafe driving behavior in veterans of OIF/OED: (1) driving stress, (2) substance and alcohol abuse, (3) posttraumatic stress disorder (PTSD), and (4) TBI. Plach and Sells (2013) reported that the occupation of driving or riding in vehicles was identified as among the top 5 challenges by 33% of the participants in their Canadian Occupational Performance Measure (COPM) study.

A previous qualitative inquiry into the experiences of uninjured and undiagnosed OEF/OIF veterans returning home led to some interesting information in regard to driving (Kim, Nakama, Noble, & Peyton, 2011). These researchers determined that returning combat veterans did indeed experience high levels of anxiety and stress when driving again in the United States, and this was not necessarily found to be related to risk-taking, head injury, or PTSD. Rather, it was in response to driving transition from combat driving restrictions, such as convoy rules, and the constant threat of roadside violence. Also mentioned was difficulty when driving in traffic, in close proximity to other vehicles. Others have attributed post-deployment driving stress to the evasive or battlefield driving tactics taught to military personnel before deployment, including driving at high speeds, driving off-road, ignoring traffic signals and signs, and not wearing a seat belt (Lew, Amick, Kraft, Stein, & Cifu, 2010; Stern, Prudencio, & Sadler, 2011). These driving behaviors, taught as lifesaving techniques, are so strongly reinforced during deployment that they may become automatic driving habits.

Hwang et al. (2014) took their earlier qualitative work further and quantified driving stress and the related driving and occupational limitations among OIF/OEF veterans. It is their finding that this may constitute a "new disability" emerging for rehabilitation professionals, including occupational therapy practitioners, to address. In addition to TBI and PTSD, post-deployment driving issues merit further research as an obstacle to veterans' transition and reintegration into civilian society. The ability to drive safely is critical to participation in work; education; and social, recreational, and community activities. Some veterans recognize that they have driving issues and choose to live their lives avoiding driving, while others resume driving despite their awareness of being at risk for impaired driving safety as well as endangering passengers. Neither solution is a good one. A carefully planned and articulated driving assessment and driving program that takes into consideration psychosocial issues and uses a cognitive-behavioral approach is recommended by Hwang et al. (2014).

Targeting the Symptoms of Combat Stress

Certainly, we know that PTSD is a significant problem for returning veterans. We have numerous reported figures for how many returning veterans suffer from PTSD and/or depression (RAND Center for Military Health Policy Research, 2008). Many do not seek treatment, and the consequences are substance abuse, domestic violence, divorce, job loss, financial problems, homelessness, and suicide (National Center for PTSD, 2006).

The Psychosocial Rehabilitation and Recovery Center at the San Francisco VA Hospital supports veterans who have mental illnesses and is an example of a VA support service to aid those in transition to civilian life. Occupational therapy programming offers a class-style format that promotes community integration through symptom management, communication, coping, and life skills. Also offered are anger management, stress management, and health and wellness education and support (San Francisco VA Medical Center, 2010).

Some would suggest that traditional mental health care may be insufficient to address most PTSD problems, much of it being talk therapy alone (Ogden, Minton, & Pain, 2006) that may even increase dysregulation. Some clinicians and researchers now believe that people with PTSD need physical experiences to counter the chronic sense of emotional and physical helplessness that frequently results from trauma (Levine, 1997; Ogden et al., 2006).

Yoga, which incorporates both breath work and movement, is becoming increasingly recognized as an effective treatment modality for reducing the symptoms of PTSD (Miller, 2016; Pollack, 2010). A pilot study at Walter Reed Medical Center found that yoga nidra (a form of deep relaxation) resulted in a reduction in symptom severity on the Post-traumatic Stress Disorder Checklist; among the symptoms reduced were insomnia, depression, anxiety, and fear (Miller, 2016; Weathers, Litz, Herman, Huska, & Keane, 1993). Stoller, Grevel, Cimini, Fowler, and Koomar (2012) conducted an investigation to examine the effects of sensory-enhanced hatha yoga on symptoms of combat stress in deployed military personnel. They found that this modality was effective in reducing state and trait anxiety and suggest that the method may be useful in deployed environments as well for individuals with sleep difficulties, which is a significant problem for many. Yoga has been accepted by the occupational therapy profession as an evidence-based treatment that, with proper training, can be incorporated into the therapeutic process as a preparatory or purposeful activity (American Occupational Therapy Association, 2005). Yoga used alongside sensory-based theories and practices can be a useful tool for reducing hyperarousal and improving self-regulation in adult populations as well as offering an effective intervention to address symptoms of combat stress before they develop into PTSD.

Issues of Transition and Occupational Performance

Two recent publications by occupational therapists describe studies examining the occupational performance issues facing young U.S. veterans (aged 20 to 29 years) who have served in Iraq and Afghanistan (Plach & Sells, 2013; Speicher, Walter, & Chard, 2014). Speicher et al. (2014) describe an interdisciplinary residential treatment program for PTSD and TBI. There were 26 veterans in their program, which lasted for 6 to 8 weeks. These researchers support collaboration among disciplines and suggest that, because of symptom overlap, the interaction between PTSD, major depressive disorder, and TBI is complicated and not fully understood, making overall functional improvement perhaps a greater priority than the specialty treatment of individual symptoms. They also administered the Beck Depression Inventory and a PTSD checklist before and after treatment. Plach and Sells (2013) included screening for PTSD, TBI, major depression, and alcohol abuse or dependency in their study. Both studies used the COPM to obtain measures of occupational performance areas (Law et al., 2005).

Speicher et al. (2014) were interested in these measures as they influenced an interdisciplinary residential treatment model, and Plach and Sells (2013) recruited participants from a university campus and through the state Department of Veterans Affairs. The purpose of their study was to uncover young veterans' perspectives on their perceived problem areas, the presence or absence of mental health disorders and brain injuries, and their motivation for participation in the occupations of daily life. The study identified occupational performance challenges faced by today's young veterans when reintegrating into the community, including relationships, school, physical health, sleeping, and driving (Plach & Sells, 2013). In the challenges identified on the COPM, driving was reported to be most challenging of the self-care category at 70%, followed closely by sleeping at 67%. School was identified as being of greatest challenge, under "productivity," at 93%; and under "leisure," relationships were at 80% (particularly during the first year back from service). Both studies reported similar challenges/problem areas (i.e., self-care, productivity, and leisure-social participation). Plach and Sells (2013) suggest that occupational therapy practitioners who specialize in mental health can play a significant role in directly addressing veterans' needs. Group experiences in stress reduction and anger management, relaxation, balance in daily occupations, and sleep have also been reported to be beneficial (Reger & Moore, 2006). These are programs that lend themselves well to community models (college campuses and workplaces). Plach and Sells (2013) also remind us of the importance of the therapeutic relationship, and the creation of a trusting climate for self-disclosure. For those experiencing PTSD, most practitioners would suggest that avoidance of questions that force memories are key. It is advised not to ask someone to reveal details of his or her trauma, which may potentially cause further trauma and distress. These researchers introduced the term *occupational freedom*, which they define as "the opportunity and ability to choose and participate in activities that are meaningful to an individual" (Plach & Sells, 2013, p. 79); they suggest that during the transition from active duty, from military roles to civilian roles, service members may experience a diminished sense of occupational freedom. Occupational therapy practitioners working in communities can be prepared to focus their programming assessments in these areas of need where the context of their communities is both a challenge and an opportunity for veterans.

SOLDIERS TRANSITIONING BOTH WITHIN AND OUT OF MILITARY SERVICE PROGRAMMING ON AND OFF THE MILITARY BASE

Many occupational therapy programs are being developed to meet the needs of transitioning veterans/wounded warriors, both in and out of the military, as well as in between. Some of these programs provide multiple avenues directed toward transition and may be designed to intervene with community reintegration, warrior transition units, specialized driving services, and community mobility services.

Sheffield (2009) discusses a joint venture between Scripps Memorial Hospital and Camp Pendleton near San Diego, CA. This program provides specialized driving services and community mobility services as well as a day treatment program for wounded warriors.

Carly Rogers, OTD, OTR/L, and the Jimmy Miller Memorial Foundation are also extending services to the Camp Pendleton Wounded Warriors through a high-intensity surfing sports program both at Camp Pendleton and Manhattan Beach, CA. The Jimmy Miller Foundation (http:// JimmyMillerFoundation.org) currently serves marines of the Wounded Warrior Battalions at Camp Pendleton and 29 Palms with ocean therapy sessions coupled with occupational therapy–led processing sessions. The aim of the program is to raise perceived self-efficacy, encourage self-advocacy, and aid the process of recovery. When necessary, adaptations permit everyone to be successful. This program combines surfing performance, focused group processing, and social participation to create opportunities for veterans to examine ways in which their individual values, abilities, and experiences can support successful transition to civilian life (Rogers et al., 2014).

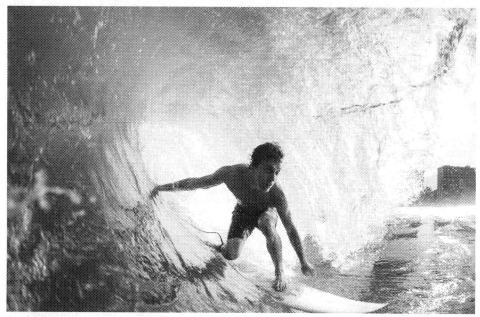

Catching a wave.

Programs Initiated by Veterans

Sometimes, the most compelling and successful programs are started by those who have been touched by need themselves. One such program, *Companions for Heroes*, was initiated by David Sharpe. Sharpe served in the U.S.A.F. Security Force, where he endured several traumatic incidents. He thought he was fine, but after returning home, he began to notice changes, as did his family. Eight years later, he was diagnosed by the Department of Veterans Affairs with PTSD. During this difficult time, he was introduced to a rescue puppy. In his words, "this puppy changed my life," and he went on to establish a nonprofit to bring together those suffering from PTSD and shelter/rescue animals. *Companions for Heroes* is an animal-assisted activity. The vision of this nonprofit is to "help every American hero and save every shelter or rescue animal from euthanasia" (Sharpe, 2015).

Archi's Acres, Inc., is a farming enterprise that uses hydroponic technology to grow organic produce. It is headquartered in Escondido, CA, and is owned and operated by Collin and Karen Archipley. Colin is a retired combat-decorated marine sergeant. The Archipleys founded Archi's Acres in 2006 with 2 core objectives: to develop a business that would provide business ownership opportunities for veterans and to create a viable, sustainable organic produce farming business. The business is certified by the U.S. Department of Agriculture as an organic greenhouse

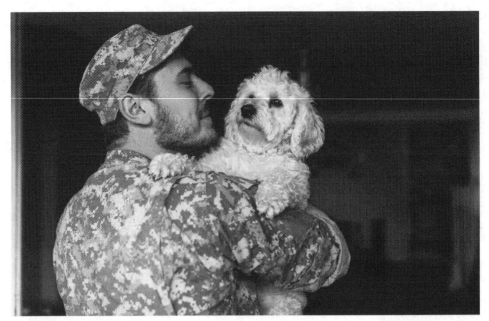

Bringing a rescue puppy home.

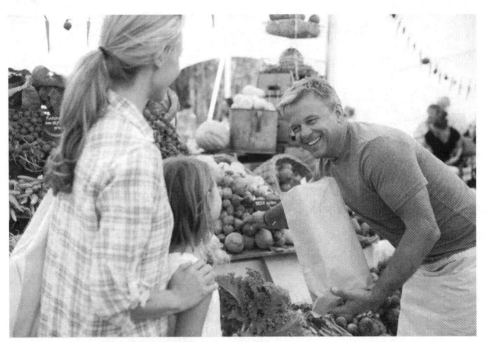

A veteran sells what he grows with pride and accomplishment.

operation; it grows basil, cut kale, chard, and other produce. The methods of crop production are efficient and maximize the locally available natural resources and local sales distribution channels.

The Archipleys have partnered with California's Poly Pomona College of the Extended University to create a one-of-a-kind, fully accredited agricultural certificate program. It is a 6-week program modeled after Archi's Acres Veteran's Sustainable Agriculture Training, an agricultural entrepreneurial incubator. The certificate program includes 6 Cal Poly Pomona courses, which earn students 17 units of academic credit. Some of the course offerings include sustainable farming production methods, agricultural irrigation planning and techniques, hydro-organics, greenhouse design, farm ownership and management, business plan development, and an introduction to the agricultural marketplace and network. Courses are offered nights and weekends; a daytime option is also available.

Some of the participants are transitioning service men and women, some are active duty personnel, as well as members of the general public. Since 2009, more than 300 people have graduated to become farm owners and workers, soil testers, restaurateurs, and owners of food companies (Archipley, 2015).

In 2004, Iraq veteran Drew Cameron took a papermaking workshop at the Community College of Vermont in Burlington. Recently returning from active duty, he was desperately searching for something; "I boozed a lot; I was super-aggravated and anxious," he recalled. "I felt like I had to get the hell out of somewhere, but I didn't know where that was" (Moses, 2015, p. 23). Papermaking turned out to be his salvation. Since that time, it has become the salvation of thousands of other veterans seeking to understand and reconcile their military experiences. In 2007, Cameron founded the Combat Paper Project with Drew Matott, the teacher in the Vermont papermaking class. In Combat Paper workshops, veterans, others connected to the military, and members of the community cut up military uniforms and make paper out of them, which often becomes the basis of artwork and journals of poetry and essays. Over several days, while they make paper, workshop participants may tell their stories and begin to process their time in uniform.

Today, Combat Paper has 4 affiliates in San Francisco, Nevada, New Jersey, and New York State. There is almost always a Combat Paper workshop somewhere; they have happened in 29 states and 6 countries. Veterans from virtually every conflict since World War II have taken part. Combat Paper artwork is in 32 public collections. According to Cameron, "the act of taking a uniform that has all of these encoded experiences in the material—what actually happened, how do we relate to it, physical geography, and so on—and transforming it into paper is profound" (Moses, 2015, p. 9).

Advocacy for Supporting Military Personnel and their Families

Cogan (2014) provides an area for needed advocacy in her discussion of the needs of military families. She brings up an interesting point in recognizing that service and the draft are no longer mandatory; thus, today's military force serves voluntarily and differs demographically from all previous military conflicts. According to the U.S. Department of Defense (2013), 36% of active-duty service members are married with children, and more than 6% are single parents. In this conflict, unlike past ones, the immediate impact of the deployment cycle extends beyond the service member and into family life. Moreover, long-term effects of multiple deployments on families, especially those with young children, are as of yet unknown.

Family-centered programs do exist (Lester et al., 2012); however, Cogan (2014) suggests that these do not target the drastic changes in daily living skills and habits needed to successfully navigate the civilian world after deployment, nor do they fully address changes in family roles, routines, and expectations that develop during the course of a deployment cycle. Cogan goes on to recommend that the profession take action on behalf of military families to include the following (2014, pp. 481-482):

- Develop and test the efficacy of occupational therapy programs for military-connected families
- Ensure that the identification of military status is standard in all occupational therapy evaluations
- Advocate for a larger role for occupational therapy in mental health
- Build understanding of the profession's diverse scope of practice

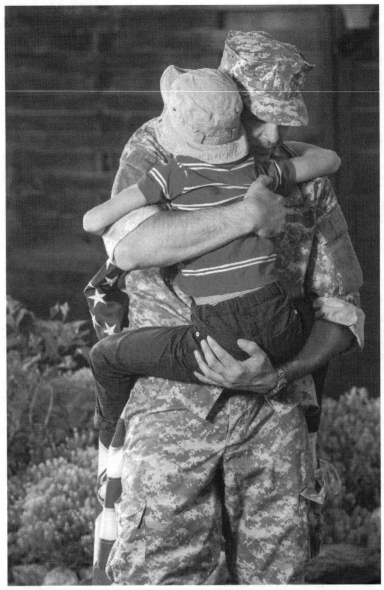

Coming home.

Programs to Raise Awareness

Occupational therapy practitioners stationed at San Antonio, TX, Military Medical Center, part of the Brooke Army Medical Center Command, have emphasized the role of occupational therapy in behavioral health through a public awareness campaign (Mummert, Wilson, & Yancosek, 2014). Operation "Your Life Counts" was sponsored by the nonprofit Yellow Ribbon Fund, focused on reducing suicidal behaviors among military personnel and their families.

Orange construction cones were decorated by clients in the behavioral health clinics who received occupational therapy services related to coping skills, altruism, available resources, and the importance of resiliency (Mummet et al., 2014, p. 13). Each cone offered a positive message that contributed to the Your Life Counts campaign. In military behavioral health treatment settings, occupational therapy practitioners provide combat stress prevention interventions in **deployed** (military/combat locations) and **garrisoned** (nondeployed) environments in in- and outpatient settings.

A special edition of *Inside Sargent* (the magazine of Boston University's Sargent College) highlights the work of two occupational therapy graduates, Brady and Jackson (2012-2013). Brady is concerned that wounded warriors might not always get the help they need to transition back to civilian life or to serve their country again. In response to this need, she is developing an online course to train occupational therapists to work with the wounded warrior population. One of her concerns is that civilian occupational therapists may not understand military culture and, therefore, may not be prepared to help as efficiently and effectively as they might. Her course is designed to bridge the gap by providing the additional education the occupational therapist will need to best work with soldiers. Alongside offering education about military culture and expectations, her course addresses military-specific issues, including how to treat combat-related injuries, typical mild TBI symptoms to look for, and how to understand military language for more effective communication.

Jackson is also a Boston University graduate and an advocate for understanding army-specific occupational therapy. She has spent a year interviewing army occupational therapists in order to create brochures to distribute at 5 major military bases. Her aim is to minimize the debilitating effects of conditions such as TBI that are treatable with occupational therapy and to educate army health care professionals to recognize opportunities for prompt referrals to occupational therapy services.

Both of these efforts represent strong advocacy programs to support best practice for occupational therapy practitioners and to provide the care that wounded warriors require and deserve. Occupation-centered community programs can take many forms, but all have similar agendas: to support our clients and our profession, saying thank you to both.

Another program designed to advocate for veterans and to raise general awareness of the service they had provided to the country was a Veterans Day Appreciation Reception: Honoring Those Who Served. The reception was held for the University of Southern California academic community as a partnership between the Marshall Military Veteran's Association, an organization within the Marshall Graduate School of Business comprising students who have served in the armed forces, and the Chan Division of Occupational Science and Occupational Therapy. The initial idea and the development efforts were conducted by L. Hoang, C. Hsu, C. Ugalde, and T. Woo as a community-programming project when they were occupational therapy students (Hoang & Hsu, 2008). For this first reception, there were approximately 60 veterans from various generations and military branches. Of those attending, there were 5 Vietnam War veterans, one of whom said that in the 20 years of working for the university, he had never been recognized or thanked for his service. The event brought together the broader university community, including faculty, staff, and students, as well as friends and families of veterans.

Many of the student veterans said they had pretty much isolated themselves and had no idea there were so many veterans on campus. In the needs assessment process previous to the decision to offer an "appreciation reception," it was learned that the student veterans on campus felt isolated from other students and wanted to establish a connection with other veterans as well. The Marshall Military Veteran's Association proved to be a valuable and strong partner alongside the occupational therapy student group. Together, these organizations developed a network that brought together veterans from all majors and courses of study at the university. A social network was established for the USC veterans community to support themselves, those who had graduated, and those who would attend the university in the future. At the time of this writing, the Veteran's Day Appreciation Reception continues to honor those who served. It is now sponsored by the Chan Division of Occupational Science and Occupational Therapy, University of Southern California.

The Glass Book Project: Advocacy of a Different Kind

The Glass Book Project is a conceptual creation of artist Nick Kline in collaboration with project partner Witness Justice and other artists, writers, survivors, students, and community organizations (Glass Book Project, 2010). It could be described as a community (students in this case) awareness program to bring understanding to the thrill-seeking behaviors of returning veterans (for both the students and the veterans). The communities can vary, but awareness and understanding is the goal.

In the Glass Book Project, survivors (in this case veterans) meet with students to share their trauma experience and explain how certain behaviors helped them cope. This discussion occurred following organized trauma education. The coping behaviors (sometimes labeled as *symptoms of mental or other illness*) are often a means of survival and resilience. The project helps students shift perspective from "What's wrong with you?" to "What happened to you?" and away from victim blaming, making books that reflect (glass books) the survivor's point of view.

The books made of glass (generally polymer resin) have been exhibited all over the United States. The Glass Book Project has been hailed as one of the top mental health innovations in the country, facilitating meaningful social change for survivors and building community understanding of the nature and impact of trauma. This particular example of the "glass books" project offered a collection of glass books titled: *120 MPH-Thrill Seeking After Combat.* This collection focuses on the impact that combat stress and trauma can have on American veterans by looking at thrill seeking and risky behavior (i.e., speeding, promiscuity, extreme sports, etc.) as a response to trauma.

This new book collection was made by students in the Department of Art, Culture, and Media at Rutgers University-Newark. The students initiated the "books" by selecting an object that they thought appropriately represented their informed take-away from veterans and the sometimes risky things they would do after reintegration. Following the project, one student commented that she "didn't realize that all soldiers have to figure out how to transition from war to home; I thought only a few experienced PTSD. I didn't know much, just from movies and TV, and it's not like that."

SUMMARY

Radomski and Brininger (2014), guest editors for the *American Journal of Occupational Therapy* special issue on occupational therapy for service members and veterans, call for the profession to continue to transform lives by using traditional and novel therapeutic occupations to address occupational dysfunction in all recipients of occupational therapy services and to mobilize around the need for rigorous study of our impact on recovery, resilience, and reintegration (p. 380).

These authors, writing in 2014, indicate that the critical needs of service members and veterans can be expected to peak in the next several decades. They call on occupational therapy to develop and enhance intervention and research. They propose that most clinicians have or will provide services to veterans or their family members at some point in their careers. They call on our professional association to advocate for services and funding that support the needs of service members and veterans. Perhaps most importantly, every occupational therapy practitioner can commit to staying informed about the ongoing needs of service members, veterans, and their families.

In support of the previous sentence, to help occupational therapy practitioners stay informed about the needs of the military, returning military veterans, and their families, this chapter has gathered recent work by occupational therapists and others who have made a commitment to provide care to one or more of these groups. It is also hoped that the reader will see how the needs of these populations can be well served in their communities and that you will be encouraged to try out one of these ideas in your community practice or to design new interventions. When you do, write about it and/or talk about it, or provide a poster or a presentation for your local conference. Occupational therapy practitioners can make a significant difference in the lives of this population. We have done so for a very long time; we have a legacy and an obligation to help.

REFERENCES

American Occupational Therapy Association. (2005). Complementary and alternative medicine (CAM) position paper. *American Journal of Occupational Therapy, 59*, 653-655.

American Psychiatric Association. (2013). *Diagnostic and Statistical Manual of Mental Disorders* (5th ed.). Washington, DC: Author.

Archipley, C. (2015). Cal poly's sustainable agriculture training at Archi's Acres. *Archi's Acres, Inc.* Retrieved from http://archisacres.com/page/sat-program

Barnett, F. (2014). Running the gamut: Polytrauma occupational therapy services at Walter Reed National Military Medical Center. *OT Practice, 19*(8), 14-19.

Bell, N., Mangione, T., Hemenway, D., Amoroso, P., & Jones, B. (1996). *High injury rates among female army trainees: A function of gender?* Natick, MA: U.S. Army Research Institution of Environmental Medicine.

Brady, J., & Jackson, K. (2012-2013). Military mission. *Inside Sargent. Magazine of Boston University, Sargent College,* 9.

Bryan, C. J., Jennings, K. W., Jobes, D. A., & Bradley, J. C. (2012). Understanding and preventing military suicide. *Archives of Suicide Research, 16*, 95-110.

Chappell, B. (2013). *U.S. Military's suicide rate surpassed combat deaths in 2012.* Retrieved from http://www.npr.org/blogs/the two-way/2013/01/14/169364733/u-s-militarys-suicide-rate-surpassed-combat-deaths-in-2012

Cogan, A. (2014). The issue is—supporting our military families: A case for a larger role for occupational therapy in prevention and mental health care. *American Journal of Occupational Therapy, 68*, 478-483.

Defense and Veterans Brain Injury Center. (2011). *TBI and the military.* Retrieved from http://dvbic.dcoe.mil/tbi-military

Defense Manpower Data Center. (2012). *Casualty summary by reason, October 7, 2001 through February 28, 2011.* Retrieved from https://fas.org/sgp/crs/natsec/RL32492.pdf

Diehm, R., & Armatas, C. (2004). Surfing: An avenue for socially acceptable risk-taking, satisfying needs for sensation seeking and experience seeking. *Personality and Individual Differences, 36*, 663-677.

Ellis, K., & Dennison, C. (2014). *Sex and intimacy for wounded veterans: A guide to embracing change.* Washington, DC: The Sager Group LLC.

Erickson, M. W., Secrest, D. S., & Gray, A. L. (2008). Army occupational therapists in the warrior transition unit. *OT Practice, 13*(13), 10-14.

Escobar, J. (2013). Breaking the Keular ceiling. *Military Review, 93*(2), 70-78.

Glass Book Project. (2010). *National GlassBook Project begins by breaking barriers in New Jersey.* Retrieved from http://www.ncdsv.org/images/NatlGlassBookProjectBeginsBreakingBarriers_1-27-10.pdf

Gros, D. F., Price, M., Magruder, K. M., & Fruek, B. C. (2012). Symptom overlap in posttraumatic stress disorder and major depression. *Psychiatry Research, 196*, 267-270.

Gritzer, G., & Arluke, A. (1985). *The making of rehabilitation: A political economy of medical specialization, 1890-1980.* Berkeley, CA: University of California Press.

Hoang, L., & Hsu, C. (2008). OTs in the community: Veterans Day appreciation reception honoring those who served. *Occupational Therapy Association of California, 33*(9), 14.

Hwang, E. J., Peyton, C., Kim, D., Nakama-Sato, K. & Noble, A. (2014). Postdeployment driving stress and related occupational limitations among veterans of operation Iraqi freedom and operation enduring freedom. *American Journal of Occupational Therapy, 68*(4), 386-394.

Kim, D. K, Nakama, K. K., Noble, A. E., & Peyton, C. G. (2011). *Experiences of combat veterans upon reentrance into the civilian society* [unpublished manuscript]. Dominguez Hills, CA: Department of Occupational Therapy, California State University.

Law, M., Baptiste, S., Carswell, A., McColl, M. A., Polatajko, H., & Pollack, M. (2005). *Canadian occupational performance measure* (4th ed.). Ottawa, Ontario, Canada: CAOT Publications ACE.

Lester, P., Saltzman, W. R., Woodward, K., Glover, D., Leskin, G.A., Bursch, B., & Beardslee, W. (2012). Evaluation of a family-centered prevention intervention for military children and families facing wartime deployments. *American Journal of Public Health, 102*(Suppl 1), S48-S54.

Levine, P. A. (1997). *Waking the tiger; healing trauma.* Berkeley, CA: North Atlantic.

Lew, H. L., Amick, M. M., Kraft, M., Stein, M. B., & Cifu, D. X. (2010). Potential driving issues in combat returnees. *NeuroRehabilitation, 26*, 271-278.

Luken, M., Dy, L., & Yancosek, K. (2015). Soldier 2020: Evaluating female fighters' training and operational demands. *OT Practice, 20*(6), 21-23.

McDaniel, M. L. (1968). Occupational therapists before World War II (1917-1940). In H. S. Lee & M. L McDaniel (Eds.), *Army Medical Specialist Corps* (pp. 69-97). Washington, DC: Office of the Surgeon General, Department of the Army. Retrieved from http://history.amedd.army.mil/corps/medical_spec/chapteriv.html

McNulty, S. S. (2012). Myth busted: Women are serving in ground combat positions. *Air Force Law Review, 68,* 119-165.

Miller, R. (2016). *Yoga Nidra Integrative Restoration Institute.* Retrieved from https://www.irest.us/

Mochenhaupt, B. (2015). The long shadow of PTSD. *AARP Bulletin/Real Possibilities.* Retrieved from http://www.aarp.org/health/conditions-treatments/info-2015/veterans-with-ptsd.html

Moses, M. (2015). *The power of paper* (p. 9). New York, NY: American Craft.

Mulrine, A. (2013). 8 other nations that send women to combat. *National Geographic News.* Retrieved from http://news.nationalgeographic.com/news/2013/13/130125-women-combat-world-australia-israel-canada-norway/

Mummert, C., Wilson, A., & Yancosek, K. (2014). Helping prevent military suicides—Operation your life counts. *OT Practice, 19*(22), 13-15.

National Center for PTSD. (2006). *Returning from the war zone: A guide for families of military members.* Retrieved from http://www.ptsd.va.gov/public/PTSD-overview/reintegration/returning_from_the_war_zone_guides.asp

National Institute of Health. (2014). Suicide in the military. Retrieved from https://www.nimh.nih.gov/news/science-news/2014/suicide-in-the-military-army-nih-funded-study-points-to-risk-and-protective-factors.shtml

Nochajski, S.M., & Reitz, S.M. (2014). Work and career transitions. In M .E. Scaffa & S. M. Reitz (Eds.), *Occupational therapy in community-based practice settings* (pp. 243-256). Philadelphia, PA: F. A. Davis.

Ogden, P., Minton, K., & Pain, C. (2006). *Trauma and the body: A sensorimotor approach to psychotherapy.* New York, NY: Norton.

Plach, H. L., & Sells, C. H. (2013). Occupational performance needs of young veterans. *American Journal of Occupational Therapy, 67,* 73-81.

Pollack, N. (2010). Warriors at peace. *Yoga Journal, 230,* 74-77.

Quiroga, V. (1995). *Occupational therapy: The first 30 years.* Bethesda, MD: American Occupational Therapy Association.

Radomski, M. V., & Brininger, T. L. (2014). From the desk of the guest editor—Occupational therapy for servicemember and veteran recovery, resilience, and reintegration: Opportunities for societal contribution and professional transformation. *American Journal of Occupational Therapy, 68,* 379-380.

RAND Center for Military Health Policy Research. (2008). *Invisible wounds: Mental health and cognitive care needs of America's returning veterans.* Retrieved from www.rand.org/pubs/monographs/MG720/

Reger, G. M., & Moore, B.A. (2006). Combat operational stress control in Iraq: Lessons learned during operation Iraqi freedom. *Military Psychology, 18,* 297-307.

Rivero, C. (2010, July 18). Invisible wounds. In G. Jaffee (Ed.), Diagnosis: Battlewound. *Washington Post,* pp. A1, A6-A7; Washington, DC.

Rogers, C., Mallinson, T., & Peppers, D. (2014). High-intensity sports for posttraumatic stress disorder and depression: Feasibility study of ocean therapy with veterans of operation enduring freedom and operation Iraqi freedom. *American Journal of Occupational Therapy, 68*(4), 395-404.

San Francisco VA Medical Center. (2010). *Psychosocial rehabilitation and recovery center.* Retrieved from http://www.SANFRANCISCO.va.gov/SANFRANCISCO/services/prrc.asp

Seal, K. H., Bertenthal, D. Miner, C. R., Sen, S., & Marmar, C. (2007). Bringing the war back home: Mental health disorders among 103,788 US veterans returning from Iraq and Afghanistan seen at Department of Veterans Affairs facilities. *Archives of Internal Medicine, 167,* 476-482.

Seal, K. H., Metzler, T. J., Gima, K. S., Bertenthal, D., Maguen, S., & Marmar, C. R. (2009). Trends and risk factors for mental health diagnoses among Iraq and Afghanistan veterans using Department of Veterans Affairs health care, 2002-2008. *American Journal of Public Health, 99,* 1651-1658.

Sharpe, D. (2015). *Companions for Heroes.* Retrieved from http://companionsforheroes.org/

Sheffield, F. (2009). Driving rehabilitation for wounded warriors. *OT Practice, 14*(19), 14-18).

Sheftick, G. (2014). *Women volunteers needed for ranger course assessment.* Retrieved from http://army.mil/article/133641

Speicher, S. M., Walter, K. H., & Chard, K. M. (2014). Interdisciplinary residential treatment of posttraumatic stress disorder and traumatic brain injury. Effects on symptom severity and occupational performance and satisfaction. *American Journal of Occupational Therapy, 68,* 412-421.

Springer, B. A., & Ross, A. E. (2011). *Musculoskeletal injuries in military women.* Retrieved from http://www.cs.amedd.army.mil/FileDownloadpublic.aspx?docid=b42d1acd-0b32-4d26-8e22-4a518be998f7

Starr, B. (2010). *Report: High-risk behavior contributes to rising army suicide rate.* CNN. Retrieved from http://cnn.com/2010/US/07/29/army.suicides.index.html?section = cnn_latest

Stern, E., Prudencio, T., & Sadler, E. (2011). Shifting gears: Helping service members return to the road. *OT Practice, 16*(2), 6-7.

Stoller, C., Grevel, J., Cimini, L., Fowler, M. & Koomar, J. (2012). Effects of sensory-enhanced yoga on symptoms of combat stress in deployed military personnel. *American Journal of Occupational Therapy, 66,* 59-68.

Sullivan, K. (2013). *Army chief of staff visits USARIEM.* Retrieved from http://www.usariem.army.mil/index.cfm/media/news/article/2013/11222013

Tanielian, T., & Jaycox, L. H. (Eds.). (2008). *Invisible wounds of war: Psychological and cognitive injuries, their consequences, and services to assist recovery.* Santa Monica, CA: RAND Corporation.

U.S. Army. (n.d.). *Women in the Army.* Retrieved from www.army.mil/women/index.html

U.S. Department of Defense. (2013). *2013 demographics: Profile of the military community.* Retrieved from http://download.militaryonesource.mil/12038/MOS/Reports/2013-Demographics-Report.pdf

U.S. Department of Veterans Affairs. (2012). VA, DOT, DOD steer vets toward safe driving. Retrieved from https://www.va.gov/opa/pressrel/pressrelease.cfm?id=1643

Weathers, F., Litz, B., Herman, D., Huska, J. & Keane, T. (1993). "The PTSD checklist (PCL): Reliability, validity, and diagnostic utility." Paper presented at the 9th Annual Convention of the International Society for Traumatic Stress Studies, July 1993, San Antonio, Texas.

Wounded Warriors Project. (2011). *To honor and empower wounded warriors.* Retrieved from http://woundedwarriorproject.org/mission.aspx

Community-Based Arts
Opportunities for
Occupation-Centered Practitioners

LEARNING OBJECTIVES

1. To become more fully aware of the many options for practice in the community utilizing the arts

2. To become familiar with the terms that are being used by artists and craftsmen who are working within their communities of interest.

3. To understand how the arts can be used to bring about social change

4. To appreciate the arts and accompanying programming as a tool for advocacy

5. To develop an appreciation for the nature of collaboration and participation in art making

6. To appreciate how a therapist's background and interests can influence and shape his or her work in the community

7. To investigate "arts and craft" as a metaphor for the utilization of "self" in practice

---

KEY TERMS

1. Makers; do it yourself (DIY); makerspaces; craftsmen

2. Clowning/circus arts and creative drama

3. Restorative justice programs

4. Art therapy/art as therapy

5. Social-change artist

6. Community-based arts

7. Collaborative art making

8. Participatory arts practices

9. Theater of the Oppressed Workshops

10. Art and craft as metaphor

Fazio, L. S. *Developing Occupation-Centered Programs With the Community, Third Edition* (pp 411-431).
© 2017 Taylor & Francis Group.

Occupational therapy was founded on the belief in the healing power of engagement in occupation, and early occupation included "craft" and, in the beginning, often the "crafting" of work in general workshops, as in France during World War I (Quiroga, 1995, p. 272). Sometimes, craft was seen as engagement in order to create a diversion from one's pain and/or a rehabilitative process and later as a bridge to effect intervention in the encouragement of muscle and joint strength and motion in order to help an injured person return to those things in life he or she wanted and needed to do. Occupational therapy students were recruited from craft/vocational education, the arts, and psychology and sociology. We continue to see many students come to occupational therapy with rich backgrounds in crafted works: dance, music of all kinds, drama, art and craft, and clowning and circus arts, to name a few. Occupational therapy can provide a platform for the practice of these crafts in designing and conducting therapeutic programs for all ages and all disabilities; however, it is often the case that they are not encouraged to do this, but rather are guided away from these creative interests. In the process, the profession has lost significant talent. This chapter highlights a courageous few who have used their creative skills and interests to craft innovative programming intended to help individuals, groups, and the larger community. It is hoped that these examples will encourage more occupational therapists to devise new practices with their own carefully developed and nourished talents and skills.

For a number of years, art and craft were the favored media for encouraging psychiatric clients to "bring the unconscious" to the surface so that psychiatrists could help them deal with their conflicts. Psychoanalytic interpretations of color choices and media, symbol, line, and form occupied the attention of psychiatrists and occupational therapists. Occupational therapy curricula included fine arts and crafts of all kinds. Many occupational therapy academic programs also included drama, dance, and music. The choices were purposely varied and inviting—who would/ could refuse such pleasures?—and, coincidentally, meet therapeutic goals. Of course, we know what happened next: art and craft are not "scientific," so the outcomes of this type of therapy were questioned since they could not be readily documented or measured. The medical community was changing and we, as a profession, changed with it.

Art therapists replaced occupational therapists as the handmaidens of psychiatry and psychoanalysis; music therapists became popular in geriatric facilities and other institutional venues. Dance and drama (the expressive arts) as therapy hung on in some isolated settings. Of course, there were still artists and craftsmen, but arts and crafts as a therapeutic intervention were rapidly disappearing.

Well, hello to the early 2000s—the dawning era of the "**maker**" and the "**do it yourself**" (**DIY**) entrepreneur! Actually, it may be impossible to suggest a year when this began to happen; as with all waves and movements, it was subtle, and so was the early "arts and crafts" movement accompanying our origins as a therapeutic practice. The second arts and crafts wave came in the 1960s, as reflected in the music and writings of that time, in the antiwar protests, and the families who took to the mountains of New England to establish communes or to a Volkswagen bus to find a better, more responsible way to live in the world. Political unrest and distrust of the government drifted into a lack of trust for most things associated with a generalized lack of attention to quality and detail. Craft was elevated in both quality and attention. *The American Craftsman's Council*, alongside many guilds and universities, developed a rhetoric that proposed "craft" as an art. Of particular interest was the work of potters and clay artists who began to develop decorative work, some of which would appear to be functional but was not (i.e., teapots with closed spouts and lids). To shorten the story, crafts took a position a bit more equal to the arts, and craftsmen gained strength in many ways. When you think about professional or even DIY craftsmen, they often differ from the canvas artists in that they generally occupy a strong presence in their communities and interface with the community on many levels. Clay artists, fabric artists and weavers, glass artists, and leather and multimedia workers are more likely to buy local goods to support their work, and they are the ones most seen at craft fairs and events. Many supplement their craft by being teachers. The community craftsman is someone to be reckoned with, and we will continue to see how their voices are being heard today. Survey research conducted by the Craft and Hobby Association (CHA) found that people engage in "crafts" because it provides a creative outlet, offers a sense of accomplishment, promotes relaxation, provides a challenge, and serves as a way to learn something new (CHA, 2015). They also discovered that more than half of all households in the United States have at least one member who crafts. People who do crafts are often part of a "craft" community; these communities frequently do charitable work and often preserve traditional art forms (Ponder, 2013). Ryan Jones (2015), editor of *Handmade Business*, suggests that when the economy began to drift and people lost their jobs, many turned to their hobbies as a way to supplement their incomes, so DIY may have had an economic push as well. Some of these crafters have entered the market by setting up booths at holiday events and local markets. Some have ventured online with their own web sites, and some are on e-commerce websites such as Etsy.com, which specializes in handmade and vintage items. According to the CHA, this has led to a $30 billion industry in the United States for the businesses that make and sell craft supplies.

WHY CRAFT?

The "Makers"

In 1979, Carla Needleman wrote, "why are so many people taking up crafts? What are they seeking? And, how can they find it?" (Needleman, 1979, bookjacket). Needleman examined the curious nature of craftsmanship and how each piece of work is somehow an extension of one's self. We could ask the same questions today, although today we have some pretty good ideas about the why, what, and wherefore of craft. I suppose we could say that we seem to have the ability to construct worlds and create lives that we either cannot tolerate or manage, or we come to a point where we simply choose not to. We seek an escape; but more than that, we seek to make "meaning."

Various authors have suggestions for why crafts. The arts have become very important to us; if you doubt it, take a look at the world of the makers. Those who craft create all manner of things—the organic farms with accompanying cattle, pigs, goats, and chickens—and their bounty: grass-fed beef, and pork; cheeses, milk, and eggs; and for the senses: flowers, herbs, and seeds and the by-products of bees and honey. The new indigo farmers in the southern United States and the tea plantations in Oregon suggest more than farmers, explorers, and risk-takers as well—the "new craftsman"—not only farmers, but chefs, restaurant and food truck owners, as well as potters, weavers, woodworkers, blacksmiths, and countless others who "make." These new makers are most often college graduates, technology savvy, business-oriented, and true to their craft and their lifestyles. They are of all ages and ethnicities. Where do you find them? Everywhere. They live in the country, in the cities, and in the suburbs. Theirs is a "way of life" not bound by locale. They represent sustainability at its origins. Important in their language is the use of the word *community*; community that is inclusionary. They are not really trending; it appears they will stay as long as the planet does. Another term you may see when people are talking and writing about makers is **maker spaces.** This is the name for collaborative workshops/workspaces that are showing up around the United States. As an example, Kelley Roy founded ADX in 2011, a collaborative work space in Portland, OR, for woodworkers, metallurgists, boat builders, and other hands-on creatives (*Sunset Magazine*, 2015). These maker spaces differ from one-purpose shops. Artists and craftsmen are purposely brought together so that they can learn and benefit from one another. This particular maker space takes on commercial projects and all come together to make them happen, bringing their own perspectives and expertise to the work.

This community of makers extends its lifestyle to others who may not wish to immerse themselves, but rather prefer to dip a toe into the therapy of "making." We, as occupational therapy practitioners, may wish to include this world of makers into our own lives and into the lives of our clients, patients, and program participants. There is no embarrassment here, the proud phrase is,

"I do crafts! I'm a crafter." There are several sources to follow to learn more about the makers: for example, Sunset Publishing Corporation (sunset.com), the American Craft Council (americancraftmag.org), and Martha Stewart Living (marthastewart.com).

FINDING SOLACE AND HEALING THROUGH ARTS AND CRAFTS

Not unlike the arts and crafts movement of the late 19th century in Britain (and later adopted in America) that had as one agenda the improvement of both commercial design and the restoration of craftsmanship (Cummings & Kaplan, 1993), we are currently experiencing something similar today. We are in an age of mass manufacture, when so many goods are designed by computers and made by machines. As a result, there is a terrific nostalgia and appetite for the handmade, the imperfect, the thing that bears the marks of its human creator. Moreover, knowing the origins of a thing and seeing it develop prompts trust in the product, whether it is perfect or imperfect (deBotton & Armstrong, 2015). These authors go on to say that we may love crafts today precisely because there is such a shortage of them. They promise to rebalance us. Crafts are a symptom of our overly technological culture (deBottom & Armstrong, 2015, p. 5). Perhaps this rings a bell for you? They are not necessarily talking about producing art and craft, but rather propose that observing craft, design, and architecture can be a tool, a therapeutic medium to help us become better versions of ourselves, learning to look at art in new ways and asking why it matters. The authors propose that we can learn to use art to guide us to certain truths and ideas. Art and craft can guide, cheer, lend solace, and rebalance our characters. An empirical investigation was conducted: to look at art, craft, design, and architecture and ask where their therapeutic impact seemed to be coming from, and then propose some theories. Findings indicate that the esthetic realm can be rebalancing; it can provide that which we may be lacking. Like other tools, art has the power to extend our capacities beyond those that nature has originally endowed us with (deBottom & Armstrong, 2015, p. 5). Viewing art is a therapeutic medium that can help guide, exhort, and console its viewers, enabling them to become better versions of themselves. Perhaps your clients could benefit from a trip into the community where you can put these ideas to the test.

Other authors have provided us with arguments for why craft and art may be "healing." Lambert (2008) has documented several benefits of hand use in producing/creating something, including decreased depression, anxiety, and stress along with increased concentration and self-esteem. Such a homely, simple craft as knitting can calm and destress. The repetitive motions of knitting activate the parasympathetic nervous system, calming the "fight or flight" response. Murphy (2002) provides the metaphor of "knitting myself back together" as she explores the links between knitting, spirituality, and creativity (p. 1). You can probably think of other crafts and activities where repetitive motions and sequences create something "whole." In fact, the processes of crafting and "making" as metaphors for life experiences, pleasures, and disappointments are perhaps obvious to you.

"Making things," says psychiatrist C. Barron, coauthor of *The Creativity Cure* (2012), promotes psychological well-being. As we have modernized, depression has surged. A century ago, according to the best epidemiological evidence, the lifetime rate of depressive illness in the United States was about 1% (Ilardi, 2009). The rate now stands at 23%. The rate of depression has more than doubled in just the past decade. Occupation-centered programming targeting depression and depression-prompting life events seems timely.

Visual Arts to Facilitate the Grieving Process

Bouteiller-Vidal (2013) describes a Lifestyle Redesign group, Grieving the Loss, that included a module titled "Creation of Narratives through the Use of Visual Arts." Visual arts are described by the author as those art forms that create works that are primarily visual in nature (i.e., ceramics, drawing, painting, sculpture, printmaking, design, crafts, photography, video, filmmaking, and architecture).

She utilizes various forms of visual arts to connect clients to the grieving process. Personal narratives that aid individual "remembering" with less pain and more joy are developed with the aid of visual arts. As a closing group cooperative activity, a finger/hand painting is composed of colors that are chosen by the group to represent their pain and suffering (background) and their healing process (foreground).

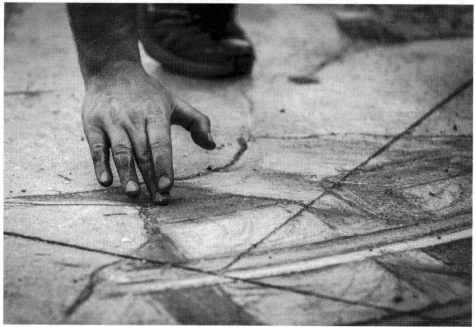

Finger painting to access the grieving process.

Clowning and Drama to Enhance Development and Well-Being

Two other forms of creative art employed by occupational therapy practitioners and others are **clowning** and **creative drama.** Keland Scher, 2013 graduate of the occupational therapy program at Washington University in St. Louis, MO, also has another diploma, this one from the Ringling Brothers and Barnum and Bailey Clown College in Florida. He worked for 5 years with the Big Apple Circus Clown Care unit in hospitals, nursing homes, and camps for children with life-threatening illnesses. Keland also holds advanced degrees in theater and movement for actors. He has expressed the wish to "find a therapeutic container for all of the work he was doing," and found it in occupational therapy (Finch, 2013, p. 25). In his research at Washington University, he has developed a 10-week course to determine how using circus arts as an intervention could help children who are deaf or hard of hearing improve their social skills. In his words, "I enjoy empowering others through physical and vocal expression, helping them to grow, change and transform... occupational therapy in tandem with circus arts has the potential to be a powerful combination" (Finch, 2013, p. 25).

In 2009, occupational therapists Ciukaj, Suarez-Balcazar, and Field (2009) described a community-based program incorporating creative drama in programming for children with disabilities. Often children with disabilities are deprived of the opportunity to engage in creative drama and expressive arts. They may not be able to find accessible accommodations that facilitate participation, they may have limited access to school environments where these programs may be housed, and, generally, just the time they must spend in activities directly related to their disability, such as therapy and tutoring, may limit other engagement. Creative drama and expressive arts can

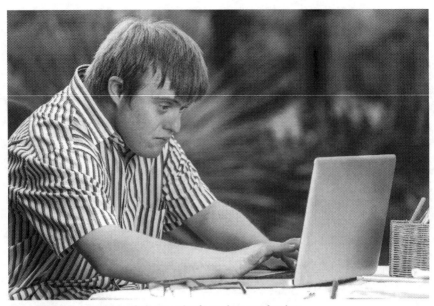

An aspiring playwright works on a script for a class production.

promote self-confidence, literacy skills, and verbal skills, and encourage appropriate interactions with peers (Furman, 2000; Kelin, 2007; Peter, 2003). In 2000, Field created a community program called Special Gifts Theater (SGT). This is a nonprofit organization that invites children with disabilities to participate in creative drama experiences for 25 weeks, concluding in a yearly musical theater production (Ciukaj et al., 2009). SGT is an educationally and therapeutically based program in which students between the ages of 8 and 21 years are matched with typically developing peer mentors or "buddies" of similar age to help them prepare for the final performance, which more than 1000 community members attend.

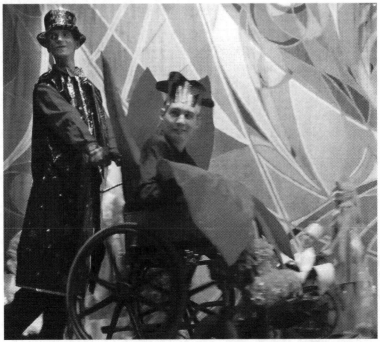

Participants in a creative drama class are ready for opening night.

Restorative Justice Programming in Correctional Centers

At the Jefferson City Correctional Center, a maximum-security state prison just a short distance east of the Missouri State Capitol, a group of male inmates are quilting for charity, attempting to repair a fraction of the damage they have caused. This quilt and others are part of a program called **restorative justice**, an ancient practice that has become a curriculum that equates a crime committed with a debt to be repaid. The world at large was introduced to elements of it by South Africa's Truth and Reconciliation Commission, which sought to heal the wounds of apartheid through conversation and confrontation between the victims of human rights violations and the perpetrators (Knight, 2010).

In the last decade, restorative justice programs, which promote similar dialogues between victims of crime and their offenders and reparative activities like quilting and gardening, have emerged in prisons and communities across America. Prisoners "give back" through a veiled interaction with society. Recipients of quilts are charities such as Backpacks of Love, Boys and Girls Town, and Honor Flight (a nonprofit that flies WWII veterans to their Washington, DC memorial). The quilts are constructed of donated fabric and recycled denim. Typically, the quilts average 4 by 5 feet; however, larger specialty quilts are often made for charity auctions and other causes. One quilt constructed from old army uniforms donated by prison staff formed a lasting partnership between staff and inmates. Restorative justice programs appear to have shown substantial reductions in repeat offending for violent criminals. They are also becoming a popular tool for dealing with juveniles and—amid overcrowding—offenders of lesser crimes in lieu of prison time. For those who are not leaving the prison system, restorative justice has had a significant impact on morale and safety.

According to the Missouri Department of Corrections (2016), offenders volunteered to do reparative activities, which included sewing, gardening, crocheting, and refurbishing wheelchairs and bicycles. The results were donated to shelters, day care centers, nursing homes, hospitals, and schools across the state. As you drive into the prison, the "mission" is displayed along the road on placards with words such as *effective, community, committed,* and *accountable.* In these times, when there appears to be so much violence and anger in the world—violence and anger that is often directed toward innocent and unsuspecting people—perhaps the seeds of ideas such as restorative justice can be used to create innovative programs to heal communities and give people a voice in their own destinies.

ARTS AND CRAFTS FOR LEARNING AND INCLUSION

Museum Collaboration

In the early 1970s, the author was an anthropology graduate student and intern at the Milwaukee Public Museum in Wisconsin. As a part of that experience, a program was designed for the children of museum patrons to learn some of the subsistence techniques employed by early cultures. Arts and crafts traditions were a part of these subsistence technologies and rituals. In the course of planning and talking to families, it was learned that there were children of widely varying abilities, and some with physical and cognitive limitations. I began to analyze the activities that we would do and, through the process, noted where an adaptation might be needed in order for all of the children to be equally engaged and successful. My undergraduate education and work was in occupational therapy and art; however, it was an "ah-hah" moment for me when my supervisor asked how I knew how to do that. I thought like an "occupational therapist." Occupational therapy would provide the foundational thinking for many of the varied practices I would continue to engage in, as it may for you.

Quite similar to my earlier work is a museum-based program at the Betty Brinn Children's Museum in Milwaukee, WI, in more recent years. This museum is a hands-on museum designed for children 10 years of age and under. The museum's education department designs and administers the programs, and at the time this chapter was written, programs included "wind and weather," "cultural traditions from around the world," and a program focusing on "our five senses," among others. Visiting school groups include classes with special needs for which occupational therapist R. Visser has designed an adaptive arts program that has as its primary goal the enhancement of fine and gross motor skills through play with clay (Visser, 2006). She also provides resource materials to parents and teachers. Museum education is a great venue for occupational therapy practitioners who enjoy working with children as well as community-based learning through arts and activities. Museum administrators may not know what you can do, so a measure of self-promotion may be necessary.

Other museum-based, occupation-centered programs have been conducted since. One, designed by student programmers for the Getty Museum in Los Angeles, helps low-vision attendees appreciate the sculpture gallery. Others were designed by G. Orsmond and E. Cohn (2015a), faculty members in the Department of Occupational Therapy at Boston University, Sargent College. These faculty have been working with museums and performing arts institutions to improve accessibility for individuals with autism spectrum disorders and related conditions. Orsmond and Cohn, along with their student A. Boris, produced a story book for families to use when planning a visit to the Boston Children's Museum. This book can be found on the museum's accessibility web page under "Printed Materials" (Orsmond, Cohn, & Boris, 2015). Orsmond and Cohn (2015b) were also invited by the John F. Kennedy Center for the Performing Arts to lend their expertise in the development of a guidebook to help arts administrators provide programs that are inclusive and accessible for individuals with social and cognitive disabilities.

Therapies and Arts and Crafts

What About Art Therapy?

Before we go further, we should address art therapy. The question sometimes comes up in the community-based art venues concerning roles for art therapy and occupational therapy. In fact, art therapy and "art as therapy" may be two sides of the same coin. One focuses on the producer, the other on the spectator; one is coming to art with intention either way (deBotton & Armstrong, 2015, p. 7). However, it may be useful here to point out the distinction between art therapy and occupational therapy, since this chapter is proposing that occupational therapists revitalize their legacy interests in art (as well as craft). **Art therapy,** as described by Moon (2010), is "art as the agent of change" (Foreword). Therapy takes place among clients, media, process, and product. The essence of art therapy group work is beyond the expressive capacity of spoken words; all emphasis is placed on the art experience and product. Occupational therapists may use art and craft as media to bring about change in their clients, but the process of therapy is enhanced by this engagement; the engagement in the art/craft to produce a product is not the goal.

Community Programming That Utilizes Arts and Crafts

Many of the programs described in this text utilize arts, crafts, and creative activities to facilitate participant progress. Some are individualized and some represent a group outcome; many house elements of advocacy and sustainability. They are all occupation-centered programs—art and craft to bring about change.

EMPLOYING THE CREATIVE ARTS IN THERAPIES FOR CLIENTS WITH MENTAL ILLNESS AND COGNITIVE DEFICITS

Minogue and Trussler (2007) describe the Inspire Project, a creativity and mental health project in a Community Health Trust. Artists in residence successfully set up and ran a range of workshops in visual arts, photography, and music, engaging with over 200 service users across a wide range of mental health and learning disability services. The level of user satisfaction was high; there was also evidence that the workshop groups led to increased self-esteem and confidence. Exhibitions of the artwork that was produced were particularly highly valued and were critical in terms of linking with community arts facilities and bringing the art to a wider audience. Some of the intended and achieved outcomes were as follows:

- Social exclusion would be reduced.
- Participants would be linked with mainstream/community arts facilities.
- The program would challenge the stigma and discrimination associated with mental health problems and learning disabilities through exhibitions of the projects work and links with community facilities.

Griffiths (2008) explored the clinical utility of creative activities used as a treatment medium by occupational therapists with people experiencing mental health problems. This was an in-depth grounded theory study of four creative activity groups using observations and semistructured interviews with 5 occupational therapists and 8 of their clients. The study concluded that creative activities can be used to facilitate engagement at different levels. They provide opportunity for experiences of flow, which can be relaxing, refreshing, and peaceful. Strategies to facilitate engagement include discerning and maintaining a balance between perceived skill and perceived challenge, clear expectations, consistent positive feedback, and providing a conducive environment. Such an environment is perceived to be "safe," providing adequate time, space, and privacy.

Potential health gains from using creative activities as a treatment medium include a sense of achievement, growth in self-confidence, the development of skills (both physical and cognitive), and some control of negative thoughts and feelings of stress. In addition, creative activity can become an occupation to an individual, providing purpose and meaning, structuring time, and contributing to self-concept and personal identity. It can also bridge to accessing other groups within the community.

The Creative Works Studio (CWS) is an arts-based occupational therapy and community initiative of the Inner City Health Program of St. Michael's Hospital and operates in partnership with Good Shepherd Non-Profit Homes, Inc. (Fryszberg, 2015). The studio is operated by Isabel Fryszberg, an occupational therapist and practicing artist. Located in Toronto, Ontario, Canada, this community-based arts studio serves people living with severe and persistent mental illness and/or addictions. All of the members are encouraged to reach their highest potential. They are treated as artists first, not as patients. The healing process is based on an integration of principles of occupational therapy, mental health care, visual arts, and vocational counseling. Members are encouraged to develop self-expression through engagement in art as well as greater self-esteem, and improved confidence and efficacy—and, over time, increased participation within the larger community.

A variety of art workshops are offered, including painting, pottery, clay sculpture, songwriting, screen printing, and digital photography. All supplies are provided, and members attend on a drop-in basis. CWS is also actively involved in mental health research, education, and outreach as a means of disseminating information and reducing the stigma of mental illness.

Community-Based Arts Programs for Young Adults Learning to Live With Mental Illness

The Painted Brain

The Painted Brain began as a germinating idea of Dave Leon in 2004. At that time, Leon was a case manager at a large outpatient community mental health agency in Culver City, CA. Leon, a social worker, was most interested in young adults and was struck by how most had known almost nothing about mental illness prior to experiencing one; most had either lost their friends owing to their symptoms and/or the stigma of the diagnoses among their friend groups (Leon, 2014). Most particularly, he saw enormous creativity in both people's actions and thought patterns. These first groups started with some basic drawing and writing activities. Activities were chosen simply to encourage the groups to gain comfort in talking and sharing. Young adults were invited to the group after Leon had developed relationships with them and as they were ready.

Shortly after, Leon replicated the group with college and graduate students who had symptoms associated with schizoid personality, autistic spectrum disorder, depression, and psychosis. Many members first joined as their "social outlet" on campus and, over time, many were able to move on to other campus activities and friendships over a period of some 6 to 12 months in the group. Again, he was struck with the creativity, sensitivity, and compassion for each other and the world that was felt by these young adults, sometimes expressed, sometimes not. The following summer was the first effort to bring together some of the poems and drawings into a published format. The first issue of *The Painted Brain* magazine came out on the night of April 20, 2006, and a celebration party was held in Santa Monica at the Unurban Café. Artists, family members, therapists, case managers, and psychiatrists socialized and performed music and comedy for each other. The magazine was published several times over the next 2 years and celebration parties were hosted.

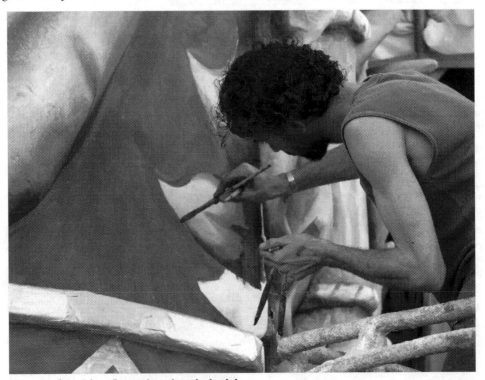

Preparing for a "show," an artist paints the backdrops.

In time, *The Painted Brain* became a separate organization under the fiscal sponsorship of Community Partners. Interns from social work, occupational therapy, and art therapy were added for the 2009–2010 academic year; they provided the additional support for a large-scale downtown Los Angeles gallery event. Also, about this time, artists from the project began holding speakers' panels with occupational therapy and social work students, where they talked about their lived experiences with symptoms and with various care providers.

For a short time, *The Painted Brain* rented a small space in a warehouse in the Downtown Los Angeles toy district. This space made it possible to hold art events and shows. There were ups and downs, and through no fault of the sponsors, the space was lost; however, people had noticed *The Painted Brain*, among them the Los Angeles County Department of Mental Health. They invited the group to explore conducting a large workshop to help instruct mental health professionals in the public system how to run and conduct art groups of their own; the first of these was held in the fall of 2012 and, alongside this, 6 new weekly art or activity groups were started in the South Los Angeles and Hollywood areas.

A new fiscal sponsorship was forged with Special Services for Groups, which proved a better fit and offered more support, including office space. Workshops for providers now included dance, drama, arts, poetry, drumming, and open-studio formats. *The Painted Brain* is alive and well today. Although Leon is never absolutely sure of its future, he is optimistic. Today, the sponsors contract with agencies to conduct group programming, which has helped them to be fiscally sound without reliance on donations. These kinds of partnerships between nonprofit and for profit organizations benefit both entities. At this writing, representatives of the group will soon be coming to the author's class to talk about their lives, their lived experience with mental illness, and their work. You may wish to visit their website for the magazine, which is now online, and other information about current activities (see website at the end of this chapter).

COMMUNITY-BASED ARTS PROGRAMS WITH SOCIAL CHANGE AGENDAS

Nonprofit and For-Profit Companions

The Downtown Women's Center, Los Angeles

Art studios and workshop settings for persons who may be disadvantaged are not uncommon, although the structure and function may vary. Some are sponsored by artists and some by entrepreneurs from the caring professions and the nonprofit world and/or a combination of these. Some of the studios/workshops may be product-oriented, producing articles for sale or exhibition, and some may focus more on process. A coupling of nonprofit and for-profit ventures permits both agendas. An example is the Downtown Women's Center Shop (DWC) on Skid Row in Los Angeles. The shop, called Made by DWC, sells crafts and also food through its gourmet café. All of its products are created by residents and clients of the DWC. The shop contains journals, jewelry, candles, and other crafts created by women who live in or access services at Project Home, the DWC headquarters, which opened in late 2010. A strong theme of the crafts produced is environmental sustainability, particularly sustaining women and the community. The revenue from the store contributes to this sustainability in terms of support for the programs and the work. The shop also raises visibility and encourages people to get involved (Vaillancourt, 2012).

Social Change Artists

The world of community-based arts introduces us to a new term, the **social change artist**. This is an artist or an organization that works alongside students, teachers, workers, villagers, the unemployed, professionals, police officers, prisoners, government leaders, scholars, children, and elders to tangibly transform their communities through art (Knight & Schwarzman, 2015, preface).

Community-based arts live at the crossroads of three things we might normally think of separately: art, learning, and social change. Community-based art requires a determined belief in the power of human beings to overcome problems creatively and collaboratively. Building consensus among people with different perspectives, gifts, talents, and skills is what community-based art does best (Knight & Schwarzman, 2015, introduction). The *Beginners Guide to Community-Based Arts* provides curriculum, program designs, and a general map/guide for how to conceptualize and develop community-based arts programs (Knight & Schwarzman, 2015). **Community-based arts** is "any form or work of art that emerges from a community and consciously seeks to increase the social, economic and political power of that community" (Knight & Schwarzman, 2015, introduction/glossary). Communities housing arts program examples included in this guide include the Zuni Pueblo in New Mexico and other programs in San Francisco, Minneapolis, Charleston, San Antonio, Philadelphia, Seattle, Denver, New York City, and New Orleans. The following are brief descriptions of some of these projects; you may wish to replicate one of them yourself (Knight & Schwarzman, 2015, pp. 29-146):

- Healthy Lifestyles Program (Zuni Pueblo, New Mexico), which uses Zuni stories, signs, symbols, and rituals to motivate changes in living habits that improve the health of all 10,000 residents of the pueblo
- Aerobics, dance, and drama providing venues for successful story making for female inmates in the San Francisco County Jail, California
- Telling stories and healing communities of labor unionists and labor activists in Minneapolis, Minnesota
- Documentary art and storytelling for coal-hauling truckers in Appalachia, West Virginia
- Telling stories from the community through ceramics, The Women of Mujer Arrtes pottery collective in San Antonio, Texas
- Building parks, gardens, and mosaic murals at the Village of Arts and Humanities (a community-based arts, education, and neighborhood organization in inner-city North Philadelphia, Pennsylvania)
- Creating events that celebrate and activate their community through spoken word, dance, music, and visual art: Isangmahal Arts Kollective in Seattle, Washington
- Creating theme-based storytelling "chairs" to provide educational experiences and opportunities that empower artistically talented inner-city youth to be self-sufficient through creative self-expression: Young Aspirations/Young Artists Visual Design Guild (YA/YA), in New Orleans, Louisiana

Art and Craft After School

Teachers, social workers, occupational therapists, artists, and sometimes parents and neighbors will offer art programs after school that respond to varying social and educational agendas. One of the programs previously mentioned in this text, the *Roots and Shoots/4-H Club*, is one such after-school program (see Chapter 19).

After-school programming is often offered to children and youth in high-crime neighborhoods to provide meaningful activity during hours when working parents may not be at home and opportunities for engagement in criminal/gang activity are available. In these times of diminished school budgets, there may be very little opportunity, if any, for children to engage in arts and crafts in school, so these programs can be offered in any neighborhood as enhancement programming. Brite and Jaglinski (2001), authors of *Art After School: A successful Way to Reach Youth in Your*

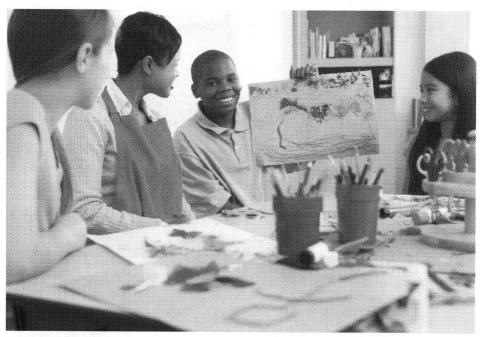

"Art" after school.

Neighborhood, have found that after-school art-based programming can offer a new dimension to intervention and prevention for at-risk youth in particular. They have also found these programs to be useful in building partnerships with schools, public and private agencies, and businesses to form a network of support and growth that can strengthen the entire community. These "stake-holders" also include artists and crafters who contribute to the programs. Many cities have after-school and weekend programs that produce community-shared murals, public art, art in the parks, and various other outlets for the talented graffiti/tagging artists found in many urban areas.

A Glass Artist "Gives Back" to the Community

Therman Statom is a major figure in the studio glass field, with work in the Smithsonian and museums all over the world. Statom says that for him, "art is about much more than the physical objects. I'm interested in how beauty functions as an advocate for change" (Lovelace, 2015). Today, he takes his creative process to hospitals, schools, and communities to empower people and help them heal. His work also encompasses change making in communities, which he describes as activism/advocacy. He suggests that, in all of his projects, there is a discovery process and product. For example, for the lobby of the Children's Hospital of the King's Daughters in Norfolk, VA, he oversaw the making of a suspended sea of colorful glass fish, designed and in some cases even blown by young patients. Giving children a voice in how to make a hospital "fun" is advocacy for well-being, even in the face of pain and discomfort. Other projects have included a series of workshops in collaboration with the U.S. Embassy in Maputo, Mozambique, exploring the ideas of "home," as well as similar work with refugees from Iraq, Afghanistan, and Somalia. *Note*: You may wish to view Statom's permanent installations at the Los Angeles, CA Central Library (fiberglass and aluminum, chandeliers) and the Children's Hospital of the King's Daughters in Norfolk, VA (lobby ceiling display).

"Crafting" Social Statements/Advocacy With Fiber

Yarn Bombing

Perhaps best known in this category is "knit bombing or yarn bombing." It is difficult to know exactly when it began; likely some time after 2000. Some would call it *textile graffiti* (Tapper, 2011). Generally, fiber arts of various kinds are attached to a tree, telephone pole, and street signs. These are orchestrated efforts of community fiber artists but can easily involve others in a neighborhood or community. Often, people randomly add to the display for several weeks or months; it is best to know your area, though, as reactions may be positive or negative. Yarn bombing has been prompted by various concerns including protests of particular events or in support of others. The "bench warmer" project decorated a public bench that included a memorial plaque for a warmly remembered local citizen; "flower power" decorated a telephone pole in support of peace (see website at the end of this chapter).

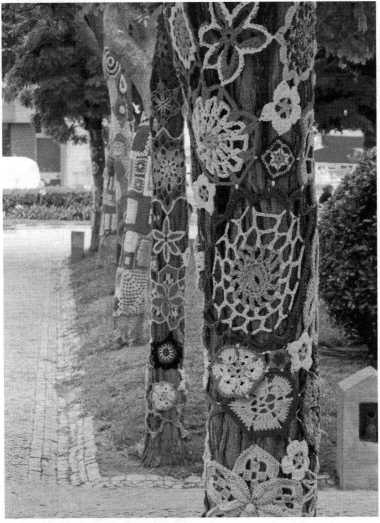

Crafting social statements: "yarn bombing."

Quilts With a Message

The Women of Color Quilters' Network has been crafting stories in quilts as a group since the mid-1980s. According to Carolyn Mazloomi, who brought this group together and continues to advocate for them and to help them sell and show their work, "craft is a social form; and quilting has been a way for women to get together to discuss events, disseminate information, and commune with each other…when you get a gathering of women, it's like a homecoming, a reunion. It's powerful" (Mazloomi, 2011).

Knitting, Crocheting, Quilting, and Sewing for a Cause

This is not a new phenomenon. Volunteers have been knitting for soldiers and sailors for more than a century. Occupational therapists have organized and are organizing groups of patients and volunteers to knit and sew for soldiers, the homeless, and refugees; mobilizing self-concern and personal pain into work for others can be powerful therapy. Today, the Internet is a strong voice when it comes to organizing our communities to take action in response to social concerns and people in need. As an example, S. Pearl-McPhee (Yarn Harlot blog) founded Tricoteuses Sans Frontieres/Knitters Without Borders as a response to the Southeast Asian tsunami of December 26, 2004, and began soliciting donations for Doctors Without Borders (Tapper, 2011, p. 81).

The Red Scarf Project

Every year in February, some 2,500 college students around the United States receive one of their three-per-year care packages from the "Orphan Foundation of America"—a red scarf hand-knitted or crocheted. All of these young adults have aged out of the foster care system and are now on scholarships for their postsecondary education; the scarf is a reminder that someone, somewhere cares about them (Tapper, 2011, p. 83).

Afghans for Afghans

Other similar groups that you may wish to become involved with or encourage your community to participate in are "afghans for Afghans," a humanitarian and educational people-to-people project in the San Francisco Bay Area of California. This group works with experienced relief agencies, transporting thousands of hand-knit and crocheted blankets, sweaters, vests, hats, mittens, and socks to the people of Afghanistan as a gesture of respect and friendship (Tapper, 2011, p. 84).

Friends of Pine Ridge and Mother Bear Project

The Friends of the Pine Ridge Reservation serve the 40,000 members of the Oglala Sioux Tribe on the Pine Ridge Reservation in South Dakota with individual and group contributions of knitted, crocheted, and sewn items. Children with HIV/AIDs in emerging nations are the focus of the Mother Bear Project, which has sent upward of 50,000 hand-knit bears around the world (Tapper, 2011, p. 85).

COLLABORATIVE ART MAKING TO STRENGTHEN COMMUNITIES

Cooper and Sjostrom (2006) describe a project in **collaborative art making**. A First Night sculpture was created by artist Mark Cooper; it represented figures for past and future. It was placed in the city common of Boston. Art markers were handed out and people were encouraged to write New Year's resolutions. The sculpture was completely covered in 3 hours; 1.5 million people had contributed. It seems "human beings yearn to make marks and embellish the world" (Cooper & Sjostrom, 2006, p. 4). Think of the possibilities for building strengths in a community, for bringing people together, and for advocating change—the power of collaborative ritual and art.

Mark Cooper is particularly interested in making collaborative art in schools, with children, and shares five basic organizing principles that we, as occupation-centered practitioners, can also benefit from (Cooper & Sjostrom, 2006):

1. One person/adult (teacher/therapist) serves as master artist.

2. Use a framework/plan to maximize the likelihood of success.

3. Work collaboratively throughout the process.

4. Draw on the perspectives and techniques of contemporary art.

5. Tie the work to the larger world (shared interests and agendas of stakeholders and others in the community).

Collaborative art making with groups of children has included the Whitney Museum Project in New York City. Children initiated the project with a tour of the museum and viewed selected art work relating to significant invention, thought, and historical moments. The children were encouraged to "say something" with their art. After discussions, deliberation, and debate, four billboards and two exhibitions were created with an overall theme of "Getting Along" (Cooper & Sjostrom, 2006, pp. 97-98). A 2001 collaborative art-making project constructed after the 9/11 incident is pertinent today. East Hartford High School in Connecticut engaged in creating a sculpture titled "A Piece for Peace." It became a plea for harmony and a statement for diversity. Five giant puzzle pieces were created out of wood and canvas and relevant messages and images were painted on panels of paper that were glued to the piece (Cooper & Sjostrom, 2006, p. 110).

Potential stakeholders for these kinds of projects include museums, billboard companies, the media, local businesses, parents/families, school administrators and faculty, politicians, and community leaders. Often, artists do this, but you may decide that you would like the children or adults in your particular program to construct the base piece themselves. With some preplanning, this should be easily accomplished.

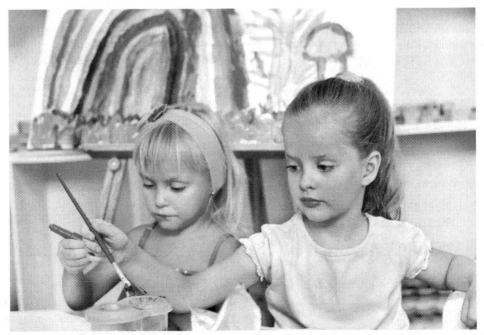

Contributing to a collaborative art project.

PARTICIPATORY, COMMUNITY-BASED, AND COLLABORATIVE ARTS PRACTICES AND RESEARCH

In some of the recent literature describing creative arts practices in the community, the phrase **participatory**, community-based, and collaborative arts practices is used (Conrad & Sinner, 2015). These venues are also often coupled with participatory action research (PAR). The inquiry tradition known as PAR grew alongside the popular education movement of the 1960s and 1970s led by Paulo Freire (1988, 1993). In the early work, PAR aimed at producing practical knowing for the benefit of the community, for education, for community dialogue, and for raising consciousness.

Participatory work in communities in the developing world frequently used popular art forms as ways of engaging community members in inquiry processes, as spaces for cultural exchange, incorporating storytelling, song, dance, photography, puppetry, and theater. Augusto Boal's **Theater of the Oppressed** (1979) is one example of a participatory arts approach known for directly engaging audiences in critical creative processes. In participatory arts by the people and for the people, interactions and relations are key.

Following this tradition, theater games and other activities have been used to create a space for indigenous youths to critically examine the choices they make that affect their health (Linds et al., 2015). In this example, Canadian Indigenous communities (youth in particular) are seen in the context of colonization. One of the effects of this colonization was physical confinement (on reserves and in residential schools) and restricted decision making enacted through the absolute authority of the Indian agent and Indian Affairs. By providing a venue of theater, games, and activities, a space for decolonization and self-determined learning was created. The workshop processes provide a performance-based, theatrical structure for dialogue on significant social, cultural, and health issues (such as peer pressure, drug and alcohol abuse), and create imaginative "blueprints" for possible future choices. These same theater processes also develop leadership skills: youths begin to question habitual thinking as they become aware that, through knowledge, they are better equipped to take appropriate independent action (Linds & Goulet, 2010). The workshops are tailored to the participants; for example, in many indigenous communities, the talking circle is an important ritual that is used to create a space for self-determined sharing (Linds et al., 2015). Participants sit in a circle while an object such as a stone is passed from one to the other, clockwise or counterclockwise, depending on the culture of the community. Each person holds the rock before deciding whether he or she will speak. In the circle, participants connect themselves to their own life experiences and to the workshop community, acknowledging both personal histories and the present moment. This sharing, even if it is only one word, develops an atmosphere of ritual and community. What is said in the circle remains in the circle.

Other examples of participatory arts practices/participatory research include the cocreation of a mural depicting experiences of psychosis (Boydell et al., 2015); designing digital stories together with new immigrant/refugee communities for health and well-being (Mumtaz, 2015); staged photography in community-based participatory research with homeless women (Sakamoto, Chin, Wood, & Ricciardi, 2015); and using drama to build community in Canadian schools (Belliveau, 2012).

THINKING ABOUT CRAFT, ART, AND CREATIVITY: A BROADER PERSPECTIVE

The Occupational Therapy Process/ The Metaphor of Art and Craft

Williams and Paterson (2009) provide a broader view of art and craft as it applies to occupational therapy, and it is worthy of mention as we complete our discussions of engagement in craft and the arts as therapy. They suggest that, if research evidence is to guide practice, then the literature must reflect the "art" as well as the science of occupational therapy. In their phenomenological study of three occupational therapists' views of professional artistry, they examined the "lived experience" of professional artistry.

Higgs, Titchen, and Neville (2001) call this artistry the practice of professional craft knowledge. Three types of knowledge are deemed necessary for professional practice—propositional (theoretical or scientific) knowledge, "knowing that" (Parry, 2001, p. 199); personal knowledge of oneself; and professional craft knowledge, or "knowing how to do something" (Higgs et al., 2001, p. 5). Professional craft knowledge, or "crafting," is a **metaphor** that implies work that can be improved through experience (Titchen & Ersser, 2001). Kielhofner (1983) emphasized the "art of practice." Artistry is inherent in the ability to individualize treatment. The characteristics of professional artistry inherent in occupational therapy practice and identified within the occupational therapy literature reflect the types of knowing described within the concept of professional craft knowledge as well as personal experience and personality traits (Depoy, 1990; Peloquin, 1989, 1995; Titchen & Ersser, 2001). These characteristics included key judgments used in intervention, such as where to start, creation of activities to inspire the client and promote self-direction, choosing the level of challenge, flow between activities, the client/therapist relationship, and decisions about discontinuing therapy. It also included personal traits such as genuineness, creativity, flexibility, warmth, and humor. Clinical reasoning, intuition, caring, empathy, respect, ethics, and esthetics were all identified in the literature as components of professional artistry. This "artistry" is essential to establishing the therapeutic relationship and enabling strong professional judgment.

In occupational therapy, the term *art* is often associated with the skills and activities used in the therapeutic process as well as the historical context of the profession arising from the arts and crafts movement at the turn of the 20th century (Barker-Schwartz, 2003; Fish, 1998). The question, then, would seem to be: How does "professional artistry," the "craft of meaningful therapy," develop in the practitioner? I would propose that it can begin with an introduction to actual art and craft in the occupational therapy educational curriculum where creativity is encouraged and the relationship to skillful "therapy" is emphasized. The metaphor is a powerful one and offers an excellent learning platform to help students understand the complexity of this sometimes vague process that we term *therapeutic use of self, clinical reasoning,* and *intuitive practice.*

SUMMARY

This chapter has offered many ideas and examples using the arts to promote health and well-being for individuals and communities. Occupational therapy practitioners are strongly encouraged to use creative arts options to enrich and extend their practices. The contemporary world of the "makers" is explored to include new perspectives on sustainable living, which offers our clients and members new ways to positively self-identify in this changing environment. Craft and art is explored as a venue for restorative justice, social change, and advocacy. Community, collaboration, and participation are coupled with arts and crafts to provide a gateway to new perspectives for the artist and the therapist.

REFERENCES

Barker-Schwartz, B. (2003). The history of occupational therapy. In E. Crepeau, E. Cohn, & B. Schell (Eds.), *Willard and Spackman's occupational therapy* (pp 5-13). Philadelphia, PA: Lippincott Williams and Wilkins.

Barron, C., & Barron, A. (2012). *The creativity cure.* New York, NY: Scribner.

Belliveau, G. (2012). Shakespeare and literacy: A case study in a primary classroom. *Journal of Social Sciences, 8*(2), 170-177.

Boal, A. (1979). *Theatre of the oppressed* (C. McBride & M. McBride, Trans.). London, UK: Pluto Press.

Bouteiller-Vidal, C. (May 2013). Lifestyle redesign (trademark) group: "Grieving the loss." Unpublished project. Chan Division of Occupational Science and Occupational Therapy, Los Angeles, CA: University of Southern California.

Boydell, K., Gladstone, B., Stasiulis, E., Volpe, T., Dhayanandhan, B., & Cole, A. (2015). The co-creation of a mural depicting experiences of psychosis. In: D. Conrad & A. Sinner (Eds.), *Creating Together* (pp. 39-50). Waterloo, Ontario, Canada: Wilfrid Laurier University Press.

Brite, J., & Jaglinski, M. (2001). *Art after school.* Ann Arbor, MI: Malloy Lithographing, Inc.

Ciukaj, M., Suarez-Balcazar, Y., & Field, S. (2009). Incorporating creative drama into the lives of children with disabilities. *OT Practice, 14*(22), 19-23.

Conrad, D., & Sinner, A. (Eds). (2015). Introduction. *Creating Together.* Waterloo, Ontario, Canada: Wilfrid Laurier University Press.

Cooper, M., & Sjostrom, L. (2006). *Making art together.* Boston, MA: Beacon Press.

Craft and Hobby Association. (2015). Retrieved from https://www.craftandhobby.org/

Cummings, E., & Kaplan, W. (1993). *The arts and crafts movement.* London, UK: Thames and Hudson.

deBotton, A., & Armstrong, J. (2015). *Art as therapy.* New York, NY: Phaedon Press.

Depoy, E. (1990). Mastery in clinical occupational therapy. *American Journal of Occupational Therapy, 44,* 415-422.

Finch, J. M. (2013) Class clown. *Outlook.* St. Louis, MO: Washington University in St. Louis. Retrieved from https://outlook.wustl.edu/

Fish, D. (1998). *Appreciating practice in the caring professions.* Oxford, UK: Butterworth-Heinemann.

Freire, P. (1988). Creating alternative research methods: Learning to do it by doing it. In S. Kemmis & R. McTaggart (Eds.), *The action research reader* (pp. 291-313). Geelong, AU: Deakin University Press.

Freire, P. (1993). *Pedagogy of the oppressed* (M. B. Ramos, Trans.). New York, NY: Continuum.

Fryszberg, I. (2015). About us. *Creative Works Studio.* Retrieved from http://creativeworks-studio.ca/site/about/

Furman, L. (2000). In support of drama in early childhood education, again. *Early Childhood Education Journal, 27*(3), 173-178.

Griffiths, S. (2008). The experience of creative activity as a treatment medium. *Journal of Mental Health, 17*(1), 49-63.

Higgs, J., Titchen, A., & Neville, V. (2001). Professional practice and knowledge. In J. Higgs & A. Titchen (Eds.), *Practice knowledge and expertise in the health professions* (pp. 3-9). Oxford, UK: Butterworth-Heinemann.

Ilardi, S. (2009). *The depression cure: The 6-step program to beat depression without drugs.* Cambridge, MA: DeCapo/Lifelong Press.

Jones, R. (Ed.). (2015). *Handmade Business.* Retrieved from http://handmade-business.com/

Kelin, D.A. (2007). The perspective from within: Drama and children's literature. *Early Childhood Education Journal, 35*(3), 277-284.

Kielhofner, G. (1983). The art of occupational therapy. In G. Kielhofner (Ed.), *Health through occupation: Theory and practice in occupational therapy* (pp. 295-309). Philadelphia, PA: F. A. Davis.

Knight, M. (2010). Breaking patterns. *American Craft.* New York, NY: American Craft Council.

Knight, K., & Schwarzman, M. (2015). *Beginner's guide to community-based arts.* Oakland, CA: New Village Press.

Lambert, K. (2008). *Lifting depression: A neuroscientist's hands-on approach to activating your brain's healing power.* New York, NY: Perseus.

Leon, D. (2014). *Brief history of the painted brain* [unpublished]. Los Angeles, CA: Author.

Linds, W., & Goulet, L. (2010). Intentional spaces: Co-determined leadership through drama/theatre. In W. Linds, L. Goulet, & A. Sammel (Eds.), *Emancipatory practices: Adult/youth engagement for social and environmental justice* (pp. 87-95). Rotterdam, The Netherlands: Sense Publishers.

Linds, W., Goulet, L., Episkenew, J., Schmidt, K., Ritenburg, H., & Whiteman, A. (2015). Sharing the talking stones. In D. Conrad & A. Sinner (Eds.), *Creating together* (pp. 3-19) Waterloo, Ontario, Canada: Wilfrid Laurier University Press.

Lovelace, J. (2015). Art restoration. *American Craft.* New York, NY: American Craft Council.

Mazloomi, C. (2011). *Women of Color Quilt Network.* Retrieved from http://www.wcqn.org/

Minogue, V., & Trussler, T. (2002). *The inspire project: An evaluation of a pilot project* [unpublished]. Yorkshire, UK: Leeds Mental Health Teaching NHS Trust and Southwest Yorkshire Mental Health HITS Trust.

Missouri Department of Corrections. (2016). Restorative justice. Retrieved from http://doc.mo.gov/OD/DD/RJ.php

Moon, B. (2010). *Art-based group therapy.* Springfield, IL: Charles C Thomas.

Mumtaz, N. (2015). Participatory action-based design research: Designing digital stories together with new immigrant/refugee communities for health and well-being. In D. Conrad & A. Sinner (Eds.), *Creating together* (pp. 51-68). Waterloo, Ontario, Canada: Wilfrid Laurier University Press.

Murphy, B. (2002). *Zen and the art of knitting.* Avon, MA: Adams Media Corporation.

Needleman, C. (1979). *The world of craft,* New York, NY: Knopf.

Orsmond, G., & Cohn, E. (2015a). Autism connections. Retrieved from http://www.bu.edu/autismconnections/

Orsmond, G., & Cohn, E. (2015b). *Sensory friendly programming for people with social & cognitive disabilities.* Retrieved from http://education.kennedy-center.org/education/accessibility/lead/sensoryguidebook.pdf

Orsmond, G., Cohn, E., & Boris, A. (2015). Accessibility & special needs. *Boston Children's Museum.* Retrieved from http://www.bostonchildrensmuseum.org/visit/accessibility-special-needs

Parry, A. (2001). Research and professional craft knowledge. In J. Higg & A. Titchen (Eds.), *Practice knowledge and expertise in the health professions* (pp. 199-206). Oxford, UK: Butterworth-Heinemann.

Peloquin, S. M. (1989). Sustaining the art of practice in occupational therapy. *American Journal of Occupational Therapy, 43,* 219-226.

Peloquin, S. M. (1995). The fullness of empathy: Reflections and illustrations. *American Journal of Occupational Therapy, 49,* 24-31.

Peter, M. (2003). Drama, narrative and early learning. *British Journal of Special Education, 30*(1), 21-27.

Ponder, S. (March 2013). Crafty members. *The Costco Connection, 28*(3), 30-35.

Quiroga, V. (1995). *Occupational therapy: The first 30 years.* Bethesda, MD: American Occupational Therapy Association.

Sakamoto, I., Chin, M. Wood, N., & Ricciardi, J. (2015). The use of staged photography in community-based participatory research with homeless women: Methodological learnings. In D. Conrad & A. Sinner (Eds.), *Creating together* (pp. 69-92). Waterloo, Ontario, Canada: Wilfrid Laurier University Press.

Sunset Magazine. (2015). Making it so: Best of the West. Oakland, CA: Sunset Publishing.

Tapper, J. (2011). *Craft activism.* New York, NY: Potter Craft.

Titchen, A., & Ersser, S. J. (2001). Explicating, creating and validating professional craft knowledge. In J. Higgs & A. Titchen (Eds.), *Practice knowledge and expertise in the health professions* (pp. 48-56). Oxford, UK: Butterworth-Heinemann.

Vaillancourt, R. (2012). What's in store: made by DWC. Los Angeles, CA: Downtown News.com

Visser, R. (2006). Museum-based occupational therapy. *OT Practice, 11*(2), 19-20.

Williams, S., & Paterson, M. (2009). A phenomenological study of the art of occupational therapy. *The qualitative report, 14*(3), 689-718. Retrieved from http://nsuworks.nova.edu/tqr/vol14/iss4/5/

Additional Websites Supporting Arts and Crafts

Afghans for Afghans (http://www.afghansforafghans.org/)

American Craft Council (www.craftcouncil.org): nonprofit organization dedicated to promoting contemporary craft.

Arts Business Institute (www.artsbusinessinstitute.org): nonprofit providing education about product design, booth display, event marketing, etc., for art- and craft-making communities.

Craft and Hobby Association (www.craftandhobby.org): International nonprofit trade organization for member companies engaged in the design, manufacture, distribution, and retail sales of products in the craft and hobby industry.

Craft in America (www.craftinamerica.org): nonprofit dedicated to the exploration, preservation and celebration of craft and its impact on the nation's cultural heritage. Located in Los Angeles, California it hosts exhibitions and events and has a research library.

Handmade Business (http://handmade-business.com/): monthly magazine for crafts professionals. Articles and regular columns from how to photograph work to industry trends.

Mother Bear Project (http://www.motherbearproject.org/)

Painted Brain (http://www.thepaintedbrain.com/): magazine and current activities

Red Scarf Project (http://www.redscarfoshawa.com/)

Yarn Bombing/Knit Bombing (https://en.wikipedia.org/wiki/Yarn_bombing)

Arts and Crafts Workshops

Art Camps for Women (www.artcampforwomen.com): held in Colorado includes a variety of workshops and techniques.

Art Is You (http://www.eatcakecreate.com/): mixed media retreats designed to replenish personal creative resources as well as spirit.

Art Unraveled (http://artunraveled.com): week of workshops covering mixed media, jewelry, art books, and more.

Traveling Together, Inc. (www.travelingtogether.net): tours for quilters, miniature-dollhouse collectors, and more. They also arrange tours for Vogue Knitting.

Index

Printed in the United States
by Baker & Taylor Publisher Services